Polymers Enhancing Bioavailability in Drug Delivery

Polymers Enhancing Bioavailability in Drug Delivery

Editors

Ana Isabel Fernandes
Angela Faustino Jozala

MDPI • Basel • Beijing • Wuhan • Barcelona • Belgrade • Manchester • Tokyo • Cluj • Tianjin

Editors

Ana Isabel Fernandes
CiiEM—Interdisciplinary
Research Center Egas Moniz
Instituto Universitário
Egas Moniz
Monte de Caparica
Portugal

Angela Faustino Jozala
LaMInFE—Laboratory of
Industrial Microbiology and
Fermentation Process
University of Sorocaba
Sorocaba
Brazil

Editorial Office
MDPI
St. Alban-Anlage 66
4052 Basel, Switzerland

This is a reprint of articles from the Special Issue published online in the open access journal *Pharmaceutics* (ISSN 1999-4923) (available at: www.mdpi.com/journal/pharmaceutics/special_issues/Polymers_Bioavailability_Drug_Delivery).

For citation purposes, cite each article independently as indicated on the article page online and as indicated below:

LastName, A.A.; LastName, B.B.; LastName, C.C. Article Title. *Journal Name* **Year**, *Volume Number*, Page Range.

ISBN 978-3-0365-5684-0 (Hbk)
ISBN 978-3-0365-5683-3 (PDF)

Contents

About the Editors vii

Ana I. Fernandes and Angela F. Jozala
Polymers Enhancing Bioavailability in Drug Delivery
Reprinted from: *Pharmaceutics* **2022**, *14*, 2199, doi:10.3390/pharmaceutics14102199 1

Desislava Budurova, Denitsa Momekova, Georgi Momekov, Pavletta Shestakova, Hristo Penchev and Stanislav Rangelov
PEG-Modified *tert*-Octylcalix[8]arenes as Drug Delivery Nanocarriers of Silibinin
Reprinted from: *Pharmaceutics* **2021**, *13*, 2025, doi:10.3390/pharmaceutics13122025 9

Mónica G. Simões, Ayelen Hugo, Andrea Gómez-Zavaglia, Pedro N. Simões and Patrícia Alves
Formulation and Characterization of Stimuli-Responsive Lecithin-Based Liposome Complexes with Poly(acrylic acid)/Poly(*N*,*N*-dimethylaminoethyl methacrylate) and Pluronic® Copolymers for Controlled Drug Delivery
Reprinted from: *Pharmaceutics* **2022**, *14*, 735, doi:10.3390/pharmaceutics14040735 27

Yifeng Cao, Xinyan Dong and Xuepeng Chen
Polymer-Modified Liposomes for Drug Delivery: From Fundamentals to Applications
Reprinted from: *Pharmaceutics* **2022**, *14*, 778, doi:10.3390/pharmaceutics14040778 41

Yue Yu, Zhou Wang, Qian Ding, Xiangbin Yu, Qinyan Yang and Ran Wang et al.
The Preparation of a Novel Poly(Lactic Acid)-Based Sustained H_2S Releasing Microsphere for Rheumatoid Arthritis Alleviation
Reprinted from: *Pharmaceutics* **2021**, *13*, 742, doi:10.3390/pharmaceutics13050742 69

Athika Darumas Putri, Pai-Shan Chen, Yu-Lin Su, Jia-Pei Lin, Jing-Ping Liou and Chien-Ming Hsieh
Optimization and Development of Selective Histone Deacetylase Inhibitor (MPT0B291)-Loaded Albumin Nanoparticles for Anticancer Therapy
Reprinted from: *Pharmaceutics* **2021**, *13*, 1728, doi:10.3390/pharmaceutics13101728 81

Alan B. Dogan, Katherine E. Dabkowski and Horst A. von Recum
Leveraging Affinity Interactions to Prolong Drug Delivery of Protein Therapeutics
Reprinted from: *Pharmaceutics* **2022**, *14*, 1088, doi:10.3390/pharmaceutics14051088 97

Ahmad Malkawi, Nasr Alrabadi and Ross Allan Kennedy
Dual-Acting Zeta-Potential-Changing Micelles for Optimal Mucus Diffusion and Enhanced Cellular Uptake after Oral Delivery
Reprinted from: *Pharmaceutics* **2021**, *13*, 974, doi:10.3390/pharmaceutics13070974 113

Muhammad Zaman, Sadaf Saeed, Rabia Imtiaz Bajwa, Muhammad Shafeeq Ur Rahman, Saeed Ur Rahman and Muhammad Jamshaid et al.
Synthesis and Evaluation of Thiol-Conjugated Poloxamer and Its Pharmaceutical Applications
Reprinted from: *Pharmaceutics* **2021**, *13*, 693, doi:10.3390/pharmaceutics13050693 131

Hao Wang, Runwei Li, Yuan Rao, Saixing Liu, Chunhui Hu and Yong Zhang et al.
Enhancement of the Bioavailability and Anti-Inflammatory Activity of Glycyrrhetinic Acid via Novel Soluplus®—A Glycyrrhetinic Acid Solid Dispersion
Reprinted from: *Pharmaceutics* **2022**, *14*, 1797, doi:10.3390/pharmaceutics14091797 151

Nutthapoom Pathomthongtaweechai and Chatchai Muanprasat
Potential Applications of Chitosan-Based Nanomaterials to Surpass the Gastrointestinal Physiological Obstacles and Enhance the Intestinal Drug Absorption
Reprinted from: *Pharmaceutics* **2021**, *13*, 887, doi:10.3390/pharmaceutics13060887 . . . . **173**

Daniela A. Rodrigues, Sónia P. Miguel, Jorge Loureiro, Maximiano Ribeiro, Fátima Roque and Paula Coutinho
Oromucosal Alginate Films with Zein Nanoparticles as a Novel Delivery System for Digoxin
Reprinted from: *Pharmaceutics* **2021**, *13*, 2030, doi:10.3390/pharmaceutics13122030 . . . . **195**

Douweh Leyla Gbian and Abdelwahab Omri
The Impact of an Efflux Pump Inhibitor on the Activity of Free and Liposomal Antibiotics against *Pseudomonas aeruginosa*
Reprinted from: *Pharmaceutics* **2021**, *13*, 577, doi:10.3390/pharmaceutics13040577 . . . . **211**

Gina Tavares, Patrícia Alves and Pedro Simões
Recent Advances in Hydrogel-Mediated Nitric Oxide Delivery Systems Targeted for Wound Healing Applications
Reprinted from: *Pharmaceutics* **2022**, *14*, 1377, doi:10.3390/pharmaceutics14071377 . . . . **229**

About the Editors

Ana Isabel Fernandes

Ana I. Fernandes is an Associate Professor of Pharmaceutics and Head of the PharmSci Lab at Instituto Universitário Egas Moniz, Portugal. She holds a degree in Pharmaceutical Sciences (University of Lisbon) and a Ph.D. in Drug Delivery (University of London). She has been involved in the study of polymers and polymeric systems with biomedical applications, namely, in the delivery of therapeutic proteins and conventional drugs. Her current research is related to formulations in pediatrics, drug solubility enhancement by co-amorphization, and the 3D printing of pharmaceuticals, as well as nutraceuticals and the usage of lifestyle drugs. Over the years, she has been the principal investigator, or collaborator, in several externally financed projects; a scientific consultant; and the author of a number of papers in international journals with referees and oral and poster communications, some of which have been delivered by invitation.

Angela Faustino Jozala

Angela F. Jozala is an Associate Professor in Environmental Technological Processes and Pharmaceutical Sciences Program at Universidade de Sorocaba, São Paulo, Brazil. She holds a degree in Health Technician (University of São Paulo State) and a Ph.D. in Fermentation Process (University of São Paulo). Since 2017, she has been a coordinator of the Laboratory of Industrial Microbiology and Fermentation Processes. Professor Angela is the principal investigator and collaborator in different financed projects, and she has been working on the production, purification, and applications of different biomolecules and biopolymers, especially bacterial cellulose, in the area of pharmaceuticals.

pharmaceutics

MDPI

Editorial

Polymers Enhancing Bioavailability in Drug Delivery

Ana I. Fernandes [1,*] and Angela F. Jozala [2]

1 CiiEM—Interdisciplinary Research Center Egas Moniz, Instituto Universitário Egas Moniz, Monte de Caparica, 2829-511 Caparica, Portugal
2 LaMInFE—Laboratory of Industrial Microbiology and Fermentation Process, University of Sorocaba, Sorocaba 18023-000, SP, Brazil
* Correspondence: aifernandes@egasmoniz.edu.pt; Tel.: +351-212946823

A drug's bioavailability, i.e., the extent to and rate at which it enters the systemic circulation, thus accessing the site of action, is largely determined by the properties of the drug. Many of the drugs currently entering the clinic are highly hydrophobic and/or present high molecular weights; others are highly sensitive and easily degrade upon administration. Pharmaceutical interventions to circumvent poor water solubility and permeability issues, as well as the physicochemical instability or degradation in the body, often rely on the use of polymers, either natural or synthetic, which confer unique properties to the dosage forms and contribute to better clinical outcomes. Therefore, polymeric excipients have been widely introduced in pharmaceutical manufacturing, for the delivery and targeting of many drugs, improving their pharmacokinetics and pharmacodynamics.

This Special Issue aims to provide an update on the state of the art and current trends in polymeric drug-delivery systems specifically designed for improving drug bioavailability. A total of 32 papers were submitted for publication, and those accepted (40.6% acceptance rate) may be found online; this Special Issue comprises 10 original research papers and 3 literature reviews from across the globe.

The majority of the papers (8) report the use of polymeric carriers (e.g., liposomes, microspheres, micelles, nanoparticles, inclusion complexes and supramolecular aggregates) for targeted or controlled delivery. Strategies such as the development and evaluation of novel polymers (some of which with stimuli-responsive attributes), solid-state modifications to enhance drugs' solubility, the promotion of permeation across biological barriers, and polymer–protein drug conjugation are addressed.

Figure 1 summarizes the routes of administration of the systems described in this Special Issue. The parenteral and oral routes are the most prevalent (10 papers), followed by the oromucosal (buccal), topical and pulmonary routes, with 1 publication each. Unsurprisingly, drugs presenting anticancer activity or those effective against inflammation and autoimmune diseases predominate.

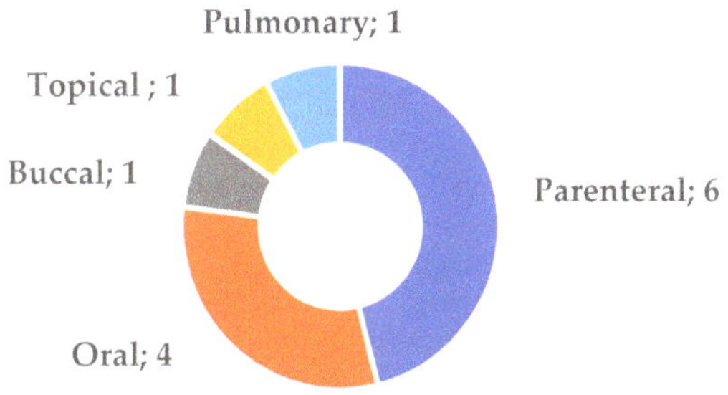

Figure 1. Numbers of papers published by administration route used (or intended).

Citation: Fernandes, A.I.; Jozala, A.F. Polymers Enhancing Bioavailability in Drug Delivery. *Pharmaceutics* **2022**, *14*, 2199. https://doi.org/10.3390/pharmaceutics14102199

Received: 11 October 2022
Accepted: 14 October 2022
Published: 16 October 2022

A concise summary of the polymer-based drug-delivery systems and strategies presented in each paper is provided below.

Silibinin, a hepatoprotective, anticancer and chemopreventive agent with low aqueous solubility, and chemical instability, has been incorporated in PEG-modified tert-octylcalix[8]arenes, as a drug-delivery platform [1]. In the first phase, the novel PEGylated polymers were synthesized by the anionic polymerization of ethylene oxide and characterized using diffusion-ordered NMR spectroscopy. The resulting amphiphilic macromolecules consisted of a hydrophobic calixarene core and eight hydrophilic PEG chains. Inclusion complexes and supramolecular aggregates containing silibinin were then produced by a solvent-evaporation method. The nanosized self-assembled structures, which were formed above the critical micellar concentration, dramatically enhanced the solubility (>1700%) of the drug candidate due to the establishment of hydrophobic non-covalent host–guest interactions, thus promoting the drug's solubilization. In vitro release studies, conducted by membrane dialysis under physiologically relevant conditions, showed a biphasic release of the drug: initial fast release from the aggregates, followed by a delayed drug release from the inclusion complexes, for up to 24 h. The cytotoxicity of drug-loaded and drug-free constructs against human tumor cell lines was evaluated; the constructs were biocompatible and did not compromise the antineoplastic potential of silibinin.

Simões and co-workers developed lecithin-based liposomes complexed with copolymers of Pluronic® and poly(acrylic acid)/poly(N,N-dimethylaminoethyl methacrylate), for controlled drug release [2]. The copolymers, previously synthesized by atom transfer radical polymerization, stabilized the structure of the liposomes, as measured by the leakage of calcein, a fluorescent dye encapsulated in their aqueous compartment. The polymer–liposome complexes presented a homogeneous particle size in the nanometer range, low polydispersity and significantly negative surface charge, preventing agglomeration and promoting stability over time. The absence of cellular toxicity was demonstrated by the maintenance of the viability of human epithelial cells. Moreover, the polymer–liposome complexes showed pH- and temperature-responsive behavior, with higher and faster release of the marker dye. This may be of particular interest for the targeted diagnosis and treatment of diseases whose pathophysiology is characterized by changes in pH/temperature (e.g., tumors, inflammation and infection). Additionally, noteworthy is the possibility of the particles incorporating both hydrophobic and hydrophilic payloads and of presenting long plasma circulating half-lives due to the hydrophilic nature of the polymers used.

Polymer-modified liposomes, as drug-delivery systems, have been thoroughly reviewed by Cao, Dong and Chen [3]. The paper guides the reader from the early days when the first PEGylated liposomal formulation was approved by the FDA (Doxil®, 1995) to the most recent approaches to liposomes' modification and marketed products. While preserving the properties of conventional liposomes (e.g., the incorporation of both hydrophobic and hydrophilic drugs, biocompatibility, tunable physicochemical and biophysical properties, the controlled release of drugs, passive targeting to tumors, and reduced drug toxicity), the surface modification of the carrier modulates its physiological properties. Polymers are mainly grafted or physically adsorbed onto the surfaces of liposomes, to increase the colloidal stability and prevent rapid uptake by the mononuclear phagocytic system and blood clearance. Specific functionalities lent by the surface polymers—e.g., poly(ethylene glycol), hyaluronic acid, chitosan and alginate—include long blood circulation times and targeting and/or stimulus-responsive features, resulting in improved drug pharmacokinetics and pharmacodynamics. The advantages and disadvantages provided by each polymer, and future research and regulatory perspectives are also addressed in this review.

S-propargyl-cysteine has recently been shown to be an outstanding endogenous hydrogen sulfide (H_2S) donor, thus capable of alleviating the symptoms of rheumatoid arthritis, an inflammatory autoimmune disease, which is incapacitating if left untreated. However, to be clinically relevant, H_2S must not be released instantly but rather over a period of time. The sustained release of the molecule was achieved in the work of Yu et al. [4] through the production of poly(lactic) acid microspheres. The microparticulate system was produced using a double emulsion evaporation method. The formulation that produced spherical microparticles of adequate size (≈30 μm; it induced no inflammation at the injection site) and encapsulation efficiency was chosen for further studies. The system was demonstrated to deliver H_2S for up to 4 days in vitro and 3 days in vivo, following a single subcutaneous injection in Sprague Dawley rats. In a rat model for studying anti-inflammatory effects, the therapeutic efficacy against rheumatoid arthritis was also improved and the administration time interval was increased, compared to those of the free molecule.

Histone deacetylase inhibitors, such as MPT0B291, an azaindolysulfonamide, are a new class of antitumor agents currently under investigation; however, MPT0B291′s very low water solubility limits its clinical use and hinders its formulation for the parenteral route. To circumvent this problem, the encapsulation of MPT0B291 into human serum albumin nanoparticles was attempted [5]. Nanoparticles (≈136 nm; polydispersity index < 0.3; high encapsulation efficiency and drug loading) produced by a two-stage emulsification method remained stable for up to 4 weeks in storage, and exhibited in vitro sustained release of the drug. The cytotoxic effect on human pancreatic carcinoma cells was equivalent to that of the free drug. However, the nanoparticulate drug-delivery system provided a higher maximum tolerated intravenous single dose, with reduced side-effects on the normal cells of Balb/c mice. Additionally, in vivo pharmacokinetic studies, in the Sprague Dawley rat model, showed a 5–8-fold increase in bioavailability and a longer blood half-life (2.5 times higher than that of the free drug), which led to a significant improvement of the anticancer efficacy. The authors claim that the controlled-release, nanoscale, biocompatible, biodegradable, targeted, safe and effective injectable preparation developed may be of significant help in bringing other hydrophobic drugs to the clinic.

The effective delivery of peptide and protein therapeutics remains rather challenging and requires frequent administration by the parenteral route. The task becomes more difficult if a local, sustained, controlled delivery of the protein drug is needed. To address these problems, a novel polymer–protein conjugate with poly(ethylene glycol), capped with a high-affinity adamantane, was synthesized; the conjugate was then complexed with a cyclodextrin-based polymer by hydrophobic-driven thermodynamic interactions between the polymeric cyclodextrin cavity and the protein payload cap. Bovine serum albumin and anti-interleukin-10 monoclonal antibodies were used, respectively, as a model protein and as proof of the functionality of the system [6]. The affinity-based construct was capable of maintaining sustained drug release for up to 65 days, largely preserving both structure and protein function. The possibility of leveraging the affinity-driven loading of cyclodextrins with hydrophilic, high-molecular-mass compounds—in turn, prolonging drug release while maintaining antigen specificity (≈70%)—was demonstrated for the first time. Although in vivo experiments are warranted, significant clinical applications of the strategy, for antibody-based treatments in cancer or autoimmune diseases, are expected.

The intestinal mucosal barrier poses a challenge in oral drug delivery, and the development of dual-acting zeta-potential-amphoteric micelles has been proposed to overcome it, by allowing optimal mucopermeation and enhancing cellular uptake [7]. The rationale of the work is that, since the zeta potential of nanoemulsions is known to influence both parameters in opposite directions (cellular uptake is promoted by positively charged and permeation by negatively charged nanodroplets), a system capable of zeta-potential shifting would be beneficial. With this in mind, the study utilized mixed micelles formed by non-ionic surfactants—including Kolliphor, Labrasol (EL and RH 40) and dimethylsulfoxide as a co-solvent—as a drug-delivery method. The anchorage of excess stearic acid (SA) with a hydrophilic carboxylic acid moiety oriented in the hydrophilic shell provided micellar droplets with a high anionic density. A cationic surface was attained by using excess SA, forming hydrophobic ionic complexes with two lipophilic cationic polymers (Eudragit RS 100 and Eudragit RL 100) incorporated within the micellar hydrophobic core, and the exposure of the ammonium groups of polymers. The two types of zeta-potential-changing micellar droplets were loaded with fluorescein diacetate, a hydrophobic model drug, and the diffusion and cellular uptake through porcine intestinal mucus were investigated. The complex-loaded micellar droplets provided a significantly higher cellular uptake of the model drug than blank micelles, and showed no toxicity towards Caco-2 cells. Due to undergoing slow and time-dependent shifts in zeta potential, the modified micelles significantly enhanced the cellular uptake while preserving the mucus-permeating properties, offering dual benefits in drug delivery.

Polymeric drug-delivery systems, which have also emerged as a robust approach to enhancing oral drug bioavailability and intestinal drug absorption, are the focus of the next set of papers. In this respect, the thiolation of polymers, as a means for enhancing their mucoadhesive properties, is one of the most promising approaches to improving the therapeutic indices of drugs, by prolonging the mucosal residence time due to adhesion to mucins at the site of action; additionally, enhanced permeation across mucosa and enzymatic protection from degradation are also provided. Zaman et al. [8] describe the successful thiolation of poloxamer, an amphipathic excipient widely used in pharmacy. The thiomer obtained was evaluated regarding its physicochemical properties, biocompatibility in albino rats and adequacy as an excipient for producing compressed tablets. Tacrolimus, a poorly bioavailable BCS class II immunosuppressant drug, was used as a model. Tacrolimus-containing tablets, produced with the thiomer, showed a satisfactory drug-loading capacity, superior mucoadhesion and an improved in vitro dissolution profile (faster initial release with kinetics independent of the initial drug concentration and a diffusion-type release pattern), indicating that they were suitable for the controlled oral delivery of drugs.

A different strategy, with the same purpose of increasing drug oral bioavailability, is described in the next paper. A stable solid dispersion of the poorly water-soluble glycyrrhetinic acid (GA, a potent anti-inflammatory triterpene saponin) was produced by co-solvent evaporation. L-arginine, used as a low-molecular-weight co-former, produced co-amorphous salts of the drug, which were, in turn, added with Soluplus®, a matrix-forming amphiphilic polymer, to obtain the solid dispersion via hydrogen bonding or complexation reactions [9]. Above the critical micellar concentration, Soluplus® produced micelles encapsulating the hydrophobic drug in the core, promoting solubility and preventing drug crystallization. The solid dispersion was characterized by different microscopic and spectroscopic methods (e.g., FTIR and XRD), and the anti-inflammatory activity was evaluated in a cellular inflammation model and in ear edema and gastric ulcer models in mice. The new oral formulation showed adequate drug loading in the polymer, with dramatically improved solubility, due to the molecular interactions established. The particle size was below 100 nm, allowing the particles to evade rapid clearance by the mononuclear phagocytic system and increasing their cytomembrane penetrability. Furthermore, the immunomodulatory effect of the drug was superior, which translated into improved anti-inflammatory activity both in vitro and in vivo. The authors conclude that this is a safe and effective method for improving the solubility and bioavailability of GA, also providing guidance for other drug candidates showing poor oral bioavailability.

The next work in the Special Issue reviews the gastrointestinal physiological challenges (e.g., poor absorption, metabolic instability, the epithelial mucus layer, intestinal motility, efflux pumps and disease) impacting the bioavailability of drugs and how chitosan-based drug-delivery systems may overcome such barriers, while changing the target sites of absorption [10]. Chitosan is a cationic, biodegradable/biocompatible, atoxic and versatile molecule that has been shown to improve the intestinal assimilation of drugs. Recent advances in the development and application of chitosan-based systems that improve intestinal drug absorption, its mechanisms, and pharmacological applications are extensively discussed. In short, chitosan (or its derivatives) nanoparticles/nanocapsules may be obtained by ionic gelation, chemical modification, and polyelectrolyte complexation methods; the oral drug absorption is improved due to protection from enzymatic degradation, mucoadhesion, efflux inhibition, antimicrobial activity, and enhanced permeation effects of the polymer, which is also capable of controlling the release of the drug. Clinical use in diabetes, cancer, infections and inflammation is envisaged as a new paradigm for nanotechnology-based treatments.

Developing new delivery systems to reduce the risk of intoxication with drugs with narrow therapeutic indices is of the utmost importance. Digoxin is one such drug that is used to treat heart failure and atrial fibrillation, and raises safety concerns, especially in the elderly. However, mucosal drug administration has recently received attention from researchers, as it avoids the hepatic first-pass effect and degradation by gastrointestinal enzymes, providing rapid drug absorption and increasing bioavailability. Additionally, polymeric nanoparticles have wide-ranging potential as carrier systems for bioactive compounds, controlling the drug release profiles and reducing degradation and toxicity. With these premises in mind, the study aimed to demonstrate the potential of sodium alginate films containing digoxin-loaded zein nanoparticles, as a buccal drug-delivery system, to reduce the number of doses and facilitate administration and a rapid onset of action [11]. Sodium alginate was selected for the film matrix, since it is a hydrophilic, biocompatible polysaccharide, with mucoadhesive properties, which may lead to an increased residence time at the site of action. The films were obtained by solvent casting, and the nanoparticles were produced by the nanoprecipitation method. Zein is not only mucoadhesive and biocompatible, but also amphiphilic and thus capable of encapsulating hydrophobic drugs, such as digoxin. In fact, digoxin was efficiently encapsulated (91%) and the particles ($\approx$ 87 nm) were stable and monodisperse and exhibited positive charges, making them capable of interacting with the negatively charged sialic acid residues in mucin and prolonging the buccal residence time. Films were produced with and without a plasticizer (glycerol) and varying concentrations of ethanol; the system containing 10% ethanol presented a swelling profile and mechanical properties compatible with application as a buccal drug-delivery system. The medicated films also showed controlled drug release, with potential for improved therapeutic effects and compliance, with reduced side effects. Though complementary assays are necessary, the system developed seems to be a good alternative to the conventional digoxin solid dosage forms currently available on the market.

Another important strategy addressed in this Special Issue was the use of liposomal formulations to overcome resistance to antibiotics, which results in increasing difficulty in treatment. Gbian and Omri evaluated the efficacy of free and liposome-encapsulated antibiotics—gentamycin (GEN) and erythromycin (ERY)—in combination with a broad-spectrum efflux-pump inhibitor (phenylalanine-arginine β-naphthylamide—PABN)—against *Pseudomonas aeruginosa* strains [12]. Chronic and persistent infections with this opportunistic pathogen are the leading cause of death in cystic fibrosis patients. Antibiotic multiresistance may be due to the poor penetration or active removal of antibiotics from the cells by efflux pumps, justifying the use of inhibitors in this work. Liposomes were prepared by the dehydration–rehydration vesicle method and characterized with respect to size, size distribution and encapsulation efficiency; the antimicrobial activity was determined by the microbroth dilution method. The activity on *P. aeruginosa* biofilms, and the effects of sub-inhibitory concentrations on the virulence factor, quorum-sensing signals and bacterial motility were also studied. The authors showed that the liposomal encapsulation of antibiotics increased the drug penetration and therapeutic effectiveness. PABN combinations potentiated the antibiotics by reducing the minimal inhibitory and bactericidal concentrations by 4 to 32 times in total, for both GEN and ERY. In fact, liposomal antibiotics combined with PABN proved efficacious in inhibiting bacterial growth, eradicating biofilms and reducing virulence factors and motility. Further in vitro and in vivo tests are needed to fully understand the potential impact and utility of the strategy proposed for the clinical management of *P. aeruginosa* infections in cystic fibrosis.

The last paper addresses the relevance of treating chronic wounds in view of the significant burden they represent to healthcare systems and their negative impact on patients' quality of life [13]. The wound-healing cascade and wound-care strategies, such as debridement and especially wound dressing, are reviewed in detail. The properties of the ideal wound dressing are discussed, as well as the use of nitric oxide (NO) for wound healing due to its effects, such as promoting vasodilation, cell proliferation, and angiogenesis, and antimicrobial activity. Polymers may be engineered with an array of materials, fulfilling the required properties of a wound dressing. In this respect, hydrogels, which may be used as storage and delivery matrices for NO, are extensively covered. Such NO-releasing hydrogel-based systems (presenting either physically adsorbed or chemically attached NO donors) have been proven to exhibit bactericidal properties, enhance wound healing, and promote the controlled and sustained release of NO when required. The advantages and disadvantages of NO-donor incorporation in hydrogels and the mechanisms of NO release are also presented. The need for dressings customized according to each type of wound is deemed possible to meet by adjusting the hydrogel. However, extensive characterization of the physicochemical properties, NO-release kinetics and toxicity profile upon chronic exposure will be essential in the future.

Overall, these contributions further strengthen the role of polymers in modern drug delivery and targeting, illustrating the multiple approaches possible and unveiling what the future may bring.

Author Contributions: A.I.F. and A.F.J. contributed equally in summarizing the papers and writing the original draft of the manuscript; A.I.F. made the scientific review and edited the final version of the manuscript. All authors have read and agreed to the published version of the manuscript.

Funding: A.I.F.'s research was supported by Fundação para a Ciência e a Tecnologia, Lisbon, Portugal (Grants PTDC/CTM-BIO/3946/2014 and PTDC/CTM-CTM/30949/2017—Lisboa-010145-Feder-030949); A.F.J. was funded by Fundação de Amparo a Pesquisa do Estado de São Paulo, Process 16/05930-4, 19/22626-5.

Acknowledgments: We would like to thank all the authors of this Special Issue for contributing with their high-quality research.

Conflicts of Interest: Authors declare no competing interest.

References

1. Budurova, D.; Momekova, D.; Momekov, G.; Shestakova, P.; Penchev, H.; Rangelov, S. PEG-Modified tert-Octylcalix[8]arenes as Drug Delivery Nanocarriers of Silibinin. *Pharmaceutics* **2021**, *13*, 2025. [CrossRef] [PubMed]
2. Simões, M.G.; Hugo, A.; Gómez-Zavaglia, A.; Simões, P.N.; Alves, P. Formulation and Characterization of Stimuli-Responsive Lecithin-Based Liposome Complexes with Poly(acrylic acid)/Poly(N,N-dimethylaminoethyl methacrylate) and Pluronic® Copolymers for Controlled Drug Delivery. *Pharmaceutics* **2022**, *14*, 735. [CrossRef] [PubMed]
3. Cao, Y.; Dong, X.; Chen, X. Polymer-Modified Liposomes for Drug Delivery: From Fundamentals to Applications. *Pharmaceutics* **2022**, *14*, 778. [CrossRef] [PubMed]
4. Yu, Y.; Wang, Z.; Ding, Q.; Yu, X.; Yang, Q.; Wang, R.; Fang, Y.; Qi, W.; Liao, J.; Hu, W.; et al. The Preparation of a Novel Poly(Lactic Acid)-Based Sustained H2S Releasing Microsphere for Rheumatoid Arthritis Alleviation. *Pharmaceutics* **2021**, *13*, 742. [CrossRef] [PubMed]
5. Putri, A.D.; Chen, P.-S.; Su, Y.-L.; Lin, J.-P.; Liou, J.-P.; Hsieh, C.-M. Optimization and Development of Selective Histone Deacetylase Inhibitor (MPT0B291)-Loaded Albumin Nanoparticles for Anticancer Therapy. *Pharmaceutics* **2021**, *13*, 1728. [CrossRef] [PubMed]
6. Dogan, A.B.; Dabkowski, K.E.; von Recum, H.A. Leveraging Affinity Interactions to Prolong Drug Delivery of Protein Therapeutics. *Pharmaceutics* **2022**, *14*, 1088. [CrossRef] [PubMed]
7. Malkawi, A.; Alrabadi, N.; Kennedy, R.A. Dual-Acting Zeta-Potential-Changing Micelles for Optimal Mucus Diffusion and Enhanced Cellular Uptake after Oral Delivery. *Pharmaceutics* **2021**, *13*, 974. [CrossRef] [PubMed]
8. Zaman, M.; Saeed, S.; Imtiaz Bajwa, R.; Shafeeq Ur Rahman, M.; Rahman, S.U.; Jamshaid, M.; Rasool, M.F.; Majeed, A.; Imran, I.; Alqahtani, F.; et al. Synthesis and Evaluation of Thiol-Conjugated Poloxamer and Its Pharmaceutical Applications. *Pharmaceutics* **2021**, *13*, 693. [CrossRef] [PubMed]
9. Wang, H.; Li, R.; Rao, Y.; Liu, S.; Hu, C.; Zhang, Y.; Meng, L.; Wu, Q.; Ouyang, Q.; Liang, H.; et al. Enhancement of the Bioavailability and Anti-Inflammatory Activity of Glycyrrhetinic Acid via Novel Soluplus®—A Glycyrrhetinic Acid Solid Dispersion. *Pharmaceutics* **2022**, *14*, 1797. [CrossRef] [PubMed]
10. Pathomthongtaweechai, N.; Muanprasat, C. Potential Applications of Chitosan-Based Nanomaterials to Surpass the Gastrointestinal Physiological Obstacles and Enhance the Intestinal Drug Absorption. *Pharmaceutics* **2021**, *13*, 887. [CrossRef] [PubMed]
11. Rodrigues, D.A.; Miguel, S.P.; Loureiro, J.; Ribeiro, M.; Roque, F.; Coutinho, P. Oromucosal Alginate Films with Zein Nanoparticles as a Novel Delivery System for Digoxin. *Pharmaceutics* **2021**, *13*, 2030. [CrossRef] [PubMed]

12. Gbian, D.L.; Omri, A. The Impact of an Efflux Pump Inhibitor on the Activity of Free and Liposomal Antibiotics against Pseudomonas aeruginosa. *Pharmaceutics* **2021**, *13*, 577. [CrossRef] [PubMed]
13. Tavares, G.; Alves, P.; Simões, P. Recent Advances in Hydrogel-Mediated Nitric Oxide Delivery Systems Targeted for Wound Healing Applications. *Pharmaceutics* **2022**, *14*, 1377. [CrossRef] [PubMed]

pharmaceutics

Article

PEG-Modified *tert*-Octylcalix[8]arenes as Drug Delivery Nanocarriers of Silibinin

Desislava Budurova [1,*], Denitsa Momekova [2], Georgi Momekov [3], Pavletta Shestakova [4], Hristo Penchev [1] and Stanislav Rangelov [1,*]

1 Institute of Polymers, Bulgarian Academy of Sciences, 103 Acad. Georgi Bonchev St., 1113 Sofia, Bulgaria; h_penchev@polymer.bas.bg
2 Department of Pharmaceutical Technology and Biopharmaceutics, Faculty of Pharmacy, Medical University—Sofia, 2 Dunav St., 1000 Sofia, Bulgaria; dmomekova@yahoo.com
3 Department of Pharmacology, Pharmacotherapy and Toxicology, Faculty of Pharmacy, Medical University—Sofia, 2 Dunav St., 1000 Sofia, Bulgaria; gmomekov@gmail.com
4 Institute of Organic Chemistry with Centre of Phytochemistry, Bulgarian Academy of Sciences, Acad. Georgi Bonchev St. Bldg 9, 1113 Sofia, Bulgaria; Pavletta.Shestakova@orgchm.bas.bg
* Correspondence: dbudurova@polymer.bas.bg (D.B.); rangelov@polymer.bas.bg (S.R.)

Abstract: The hepatoprotective properties of silibinin, as well its therapeutic potential as an anticancer and chemo-preventive agent, have failed to progress towards clinical development and commercialization due to this material's unfavorable pharmacokinetics and physicochemical properties, low aqueous solubility, and chemical instability. The present contribution is focused on the feasibility of using PEGylated calixarene, in particular polyoxyethylene-derivatized *tert*-octylcalix[8]arene, to prepare various platforms for the delivery of silibinin, such as inclusion complexes and supramolecular aggregates thereof. The inclusion complex is characterized by various instrumental methods. At concentrations exceeding the critical micellization concentration of PEGylated calixarene, the tremendous solubility increment of silibinin is attributed to the additional solubilization and hydrophobic non-covalent interactions of the drug with supramolecular aggregates. PEG-modified *tert*-octylcalix[8]arenes, used as drug delivery carriers for silibinin, were additionally investigated for cytotoxicity against human tumor cell lines.

Keywords: calix[8]arenes; silibinin; inclusion complexes; PEGylation; cytotoxicity

Citation: Budurova, D.; Momekova, D.; Momekov, G.; Shestakova, P.; Penchev, H.; Rangelov, S. PEG-Modified *tert*-Octylcalix[8]arenes as Drug Delivery Nanocarriers of Silibinin. *Pharmaceutics* **2021**, *13*, 2025. https://doi.org/10.3390/pharmaceutics13122025

Academic Editors: Ana Isabel Fernandes and Angela Faustino Jozala

Received: 19 October 2021
Accepted: 24 November 2021
Published: 27 November 2021

1. Introduction

The plant milk thistle (*Silybum marianum*) has been used since ancient times as a key element for various medical treatments. It has been effectively applied for curing gallbladder disorders and liver dysfunctions. Researchers' findings have repeatedly claimed its effective hepatoprotective action [1]. The World Health Organization has in fact verified silymarin (a milk thistle derivative) as an established medicine [2]. As such, silymarin is present in silimonin, silychristin, silibinin, isosilychristin, isosilybin, and silydianin [3–5]. Silibinin (SBN), the main bioactive component, has proven its antioxidant properties and anticancer activity. It has been established that it possesses therapeutic effects by treating various malignancies, such as skin cancer [6], prostate cancer [7,8], breast cancer cells [9] and gastric tumor cells [10]. SBN is characterized by low bioavailability due to its high hydrophobicity and nonionizable chemical structure [11,12]. It is insoluble in apolar solvents and poorly soluble in water and polar solvents [13]. Its large structure, presented in Figure 1, further reduces its bioavailability and diffusion. Influencing molecules, such as phenol derivatives, amino acids and flavonoids, can improve SBN's bioavailability [14]. To overcome these limitations and to mitigate the unfavorable pharmacokinetic profile, different nanoparticle-based drug delivery approaches are being developed to improve SBN bioavailability [15,16]. Systems based on polymeric nanoparticles demonstrate long-term stability, improved effectiveness, non-toxicity, and targeted drug release in comparison with traditional carriers [17–20]. In addition, when the particle size is under 200 nm, an increased drug accumulation in tumor cells is observed due to enhanced permeability [21].

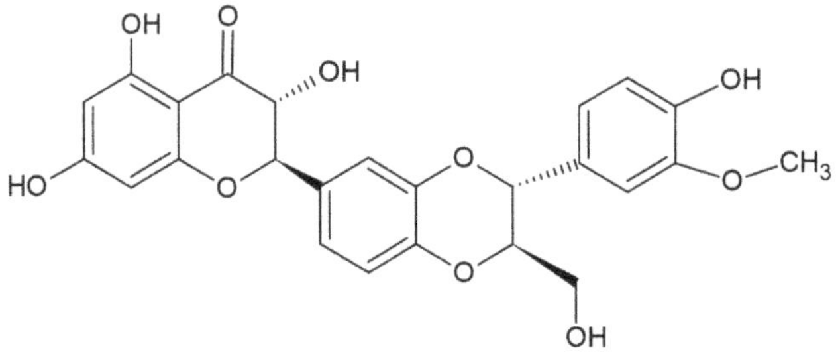

Figure 1. Chemical structure of silibinin.

Recently, extensive research efforts have been focused on supramolecules, such as crown ethers, cyclodextrins, and calix[n]arenes, due to their ability to encapsulate hydrophobic drugs through host–guest interactions [22–25]. The use of such macrocyclic platforms for the solubilization of purely water-insoluble, physiologically active substances is a synthetic approach to forming various types of amphiphilic molecules in a biomimetic way.

Since their discovery, a wide range of applications of calixarenes has been found due to their ability to entrap small molecules. This valuable feature has opened up many opportunities for the design and development of drug delivery. Calix[n]arenes, formed from phenolic units linked by methylene bridges at the 2,6-positions, can self-assemble into different ordered molecular aggregates. These supramolecular compounds have defined lower and upper rims and a large central cavity. They can form guest–host inclusion complexes through the encapsulation of small molecules and ions [26,27]. Calix[n]arenes' most significant disadvantage is their low aqueous solubility. This issue has already been addressed via functionalization with polar substituents, such as sulfonates [28,29], phosphonates [30], amines, amino acids, peptides and saccharides [26,31–33], or poly(ethylene glycol) (PEG) [34,35].

In the present contribution, we are focused on the design of original PEG-modified *tert*-octylcalix[8]arenes and their evaluation as carriers for silibinin. In contrast to the more commonly used calix[4]arenes- and calix[6]arenes-based carriers, the products synthesized by us are characterized by functionalization with long substituents of both the lower and upper rims. The structure of calix[8]arene is identified by its considerably bigger cavity, which allows a higher load with larger molecules and aggregates. The attachment of tert-octyl groups in the upper rim forms a "crown" above the calixarene's cavity through its side methyl-branched groups. This architecture additionally enlarges the actual molecule, and it is highly likely to enlarge the cavity volume of the calixarene basket, which in turn could lead to the inclusion of bigger molecules. The modification of the lower rim through PEG chains leads to the construction of a unique architecture of amphiphilic macromolecules, consisting of a hydrophobic *tert*-octylcalix[8]arene core and eight long arms of hydrophilic PEG chains. Although silibinin has been proven to be a very promising drug candidate, and it is classified as belonging to class II of the Biopharmaceutics Classification System (BCS) (drugs with high permeability and poor solubility), its bioavailability is limited by its poor dissolution and solubility. In this regard, the original PEG-modified *tert*-octylcalix[8]arenes were investigated in detail as a tool for improving the unfavorable aqueous solubility of silibinin. Additionally, both non-loaded and SBN-loaded complexes were investigated for cytotoxicity and against human tumour cell lines.

2. Materials and Methods

2.1. Materials

The PEGylated *tert*-octylcalix[8]arenes were synthesized as described in Section 2.2. Ethylene oxide was supplied by (Clariant, Muttenz, Switzerland). Silibinin, 1,6-diphenyl-1,3,5-hexatriene (DPH), xylene, potassium hydroxide, RPMI-1640 medium, L-glutamine and fetal calf serum (FCS) were purchased from Sigma-Aldrich (St. Louis, MO, USA). The cell lines HL-60 (chronic myeloid leukemia) and CAL-29 (transitional cell urinary bladder cancer) were purchased from the Leibniz Institute-DSMZ German Collection of Microorganisms and Cell Cultures (Braunschweig, Germany).

2.2. Synthesis of Amphiphilic PEGylated tert-Octylcalix[8]arenes

The synthesis of a series of products with different degrees of polymerization of the PEG chains is based on the process of the anionic polymerization of ethylene oxide (EO). *Tert*-octylcalix[8]arene was used as an initiator. The synthetic route, modified to suit the study purposes, was first described by Mustafina et al. [36]. Briefly, a mixture of p-*tert*-octylcalix[8]arene, KOH and xylene was placed into a three-necked flask and was heated to 140 °C under stirring in order to initiate azeotropic water evaporation. After water evacuation, the mixture was cooled to 110 °C. The synthetic route continued with the bubbling of ethylene oxide under a nitrogen atmosphere. The process was maintained for a set period of time in order to achieve PEG chains with the desired total degree of polymerization. The pH of the mixture was adjusted to pH 7 with 5% HCl. After filtration the solvent was evaporated. The product was taken up in dichloromethane and washed several times using deionized water. The solvent was removed under vacuum.

2.2.1. ^{1}H NMR and DOSY Characterization

The NMR spectra were acquired on a Bruker Avance II+ 600 NMR spectrometer equipped with a 5 mm direct detection dual broadband probe, and a gradient coil with maximum gradient strength of 53 G/cm. All spectra were measured at a temperature of 293 K. The DOSY (diffusion-ordered NMR spectroscopy) spectra were acquired with a convection-compensating double-stimulated echo-based pulse sequence, using monopolar gradient pulses (square shaped). The following experimental parameters were used: 32K time domain data points in the direct dimension (t2); 48 gradient strength increments; linear gradient ramp from 4 to 95% of the maximum gradient output (from 1.92 to 45.7 G/cm); 128 scans for each gradient step; relaxation delay of 2 s. To achieve optimal signal attenuation, experiments with different combinations of gradient pulse length, δ, (from 2 to 10 ms) and diffusion delay, Δ, (from 100 to 500 ms) were performed. The following parameters were used for DOSY spectra processing: 64 K data points in F2; exponential window function (line broadening factor 5); 258 data points in the diffusion dimension. The diffusion coefficients were calculated by fitting the diffusion profiles (the normalized intensity of selected signals as a function of the gradient strength G) with an exponential function using a variant of the Stejskal–Tanner equation adapted to the particular pulse sequence used. Assuming a spherical shape, the apparent hydrodynamic diameter, d_h, of the particles was estimated using the Stokes–Einstein equation (Equation (1)) and the obtained value of the diffusion coefficient, D:

$$d_h = \frac{kT}{3\pi\eta D} \tag{1}$$

where k is the Boltzmann constant, T is the temperature (K) and η is the solvent viscosity. In the present experiment, $\eta(D_2O) = 1.2518 \times 10^{-3}$ Pa s at 293 K (NIST, Gaithersburg, MA, USA).

2.2.2. Determination of the Critical Micellization Concentration (CMC)

A series of aqueous solutions of selected PEGylated *tert*-octylcalix[8]arenes with increasing concentrations from 0.008 to 4 wt. % were prepared. In total, 20 μL of a 0.4 mM solution of 1,6-diphenyl-1,3,5-hexatriene (DPH) in methanol was added to 2.0 mL of each of the polymer solutions. Afterwards, the solutions were vortexed briefly and left in the dark overnight. The spectra were recorded at 25 °C on a Beckman Coulter DU® 800 spectrophotometer (Brea, CA, USA) in the wavelength interval 300–500 nm. The main absorption peak, characteristic for DPH solubilized in a hydrophobic environment, was at 356 nm.

2.3. *Preparation of Inclusion Complexes of Silibinin and PEGylated tert-Octylcalix[8]arenes*

Solvent Evaporation Method

For the preparation of inclusion complexes of silibinin and PEGylated *tert*-octylcalix[8] arenes and nanosized aggregates prepared thereof, a solvent evaporation method was chosen as previously described [23]. In brief, a series of samples containing a fixed concentration of SBN (1 mg/mL) and increasing concentrations of PEGylated *tert*-octylcalix[8]arenes (2–12 mg/mL) were prepared in absolute ethanol and evaporated to dryness using a Buchi rotation-type vacuum evaporator. The concentration range was chosen on the basis of the CMCs of the polymers to enable evaluation of their solubilizing capacity, both as a molecular solution (as inclusion complexes) and as a dispersion of supramolecular aggregates. Thereafter, the dried SBN:PEGylated *tert*-octylcalix[8]arenes-containing films were hydrated for 2 h with deionized water at 50 °C and then stirred for a further 24 h at ambient temperature in the absence of light. Afterwards, the undissolved silibinin was separated from the samples by centrifugation for 10 min at 5000 rpm. The clear colorless supernatants containing aggregates of SBN:PEGylated *tert*-octylcalix[8]arene complexes were quantified for SBN by UV–Vis spectroscopy at 286 nm. Phase-solubility graphs were obtained by the correlation of the amount of dissolved silibinin vs. the concentration of calixarenes.

2.4. *Characterization of SBN:PEGylated tert-Octylcalix[8]arenes Inclusion Complexes and Supramolecular Aggregates*

2.4.1. Fourier Transform Infrared (FT-IR) Spectroscopy

The Fourier-transform infrared spectra (FTIR) of pure silibinin, pure PEGylated *tert*-octylcalix[8]arenes, their physical mixtures, and lyophilized inclusion complexes were measured in the range of 400–4000 cm^{-1} on an IRAffinity-1 FTIR spectrophotometer with a MIRacle Attenuated Total Reflectance Attachment (Shimadzu, Kyoto, Japan). The samples were analyzed in attenuated total internal reflection absorbance mode, with an aperture diameter of 3 mm and a spectral resolution of 1 cm^{-1}. For an optimal signal-to-noise ratio, 50 scans were averaged per sample spectrum. All the spectra were normalized thereafter.

2.4.2. Dynamic Light Scattering (DLS)

The size and size distribution patterns of silibinin-loaded supramolecular PEGylated *tert*-octylcalix[8]arenes aggregates were evaluated using a ZetaSizer NanoZS (Malvern Instruments, Malvern, United Kingdom), equipped with a 633 nm laser. The above-mentioned parameters were evaluated at the scattering angle of 175° at 25 °C. The hydrodynamic diameters (d_h) were calculated using the Stokes–Einstein equation (Equation (1)) with $\eta(H_2O) = 0.890 \times 10^{-3}$ Pa s at 293 K.

2.4.3. Electrophoretic Light Scattering

The zeta potentials of silibinin-loaded supramolecular PEGylated *tert*-octylcalix[8] arenes aggregates were determined using a ZetaSizer NanoZS (Malvern Instruments, Malvern, United Kingdom), equipped with a 633 nm laser. The zeta potentials were evaluated at the scattering angle of 175° and 25 °C from the electrophoretic mobility using the Smoluchowski equation (Equation (2))

$$\zeta = 4\pi\eta\nu/\varepsilon, \tag{2}$$

where η is the solvent viscosity, ν is the electrophoretic mobility, and ε is the dielectric constant of the solvent.

2.5. *In Vitro Release Study*

The cumulative release of silibinin from supramolecular OEC-IV and OEC-V aggregates was studied by membrane dialysis under physiologically relevant conditions, namely, 37 °C in acceptor media phosphate-buffered saline (PBS) at pH 7.4, since the possible route of administration of the tested formulations is parenteral. Briefly, 1 mL of each of the tested formulations was placed in a cellophane dialysis membrane tube (MWCO 10,000). The dialysis sacks were then placed in a temperature-controlled vessel in 100 mL PBS. The amount of acceptor phase was selected based on the solubility of silibinin, and thus, the chosen amount of dissolution media was able to dissolve more than 10 times the amount of SBN in the tested formulation. At predetermined time intervals, 2 mL aliquots were taken from the released medium and silibinin content was evaluated by UV–vis spectroscopy at λ = 286 nm from a liner curve (R^2 = 0.9992) (liner eq. A = a + bx).

2.6. *Cytotoxicity Evaluation*

2.6.1. Cell lines and Cultured Conditions

Human promyelocytic (HL-60) and urinary bladder cancer (Cal-29) cells were cultivated in RPMI-1640 culture medium, with the addition of 2 mM L-glutamine and 10% fetal calf serum, and were kept in an incubator (BB 16-FunctionLine' Heraeus (Kendro, Hanau, Germany)) at 37 °C in a 5% CO_2 humidified atmosphere.

2.6.2. MTT Dye Reduction Assay

The cell growth inhibition potentials of free silibinin and its formulations were assessed using the MTT dye reduction assay. The method is based on the biotransformation of the yellow tetrazolium dye (MTT) to a violet formazan product via the mitochondrial succinate dehydrogenase in viable cells. The procedure was performed as described elsewhere [37] with small modifications [38]. Exponentially growing cells were plated in 96-well flat-bottomed microplates (100 µL/well) at a density of 3 × 10^5 cells/mL (HL-60) or 1.5 × 10^5 cells/mL (Cal-29), and after 24 h incubation at 37 °C they were treated with increasing concentrations of a silibinin-free drug (as ethanol solution) or loaded into supramolecular aggregates of PEGylated *tert*-octylcalix[8]arenes for 72 h. For each of the tested formulations a series of 8 wells was used. After the treatment time, samples of 10 µL of MTT solution (10 mg/mL in PBS) were added to each well. Afterwards, the microplates were incubated for an additional 4 h at the same temperature. Then, a 100 µL solution of 5% formic acid in 2-propanol was added to each well to dissolve the formed MTT–formazan crystals. The MTT–formazan absorption was evaluated at 580 nm with a Beckman-Coulter DTX800 multimode microplate reader (Brea, CA, USA). Thereafter, the fractions of surviving cells were calculated as a percentage of the untreated control. The half-inhibitory concentrations (IC50) were calculated from the concentration–response curves.

3. Results and Discussion

3.1. *Synthesis of Amphiphilic tert-Octylcalix[8]arenes*

A series of PEGylated *tert*-octylcalix[8]arenes were synthesized via the "grafting from" approach. By varying the time of polymerization of ethylene oxide (EO), and hence the amount of EO, PEG chains of varying degrees of polymerization were grafted from the lower rim of the *tert*-octylcalix[8]arene macrocycle. The synthetic approach is schematically presented in Figure 2. It yielded polymers of molecular weight distribution (M_w/M_n), as assessed by gel permeation chromatography (GPC) in the 1.40–1.70 range. A small fraction of molecular weight of about 1100 was typically present in the GPC eluograms, which was eliminated after washing with water, to yield M_w/M_n in the range 1.10–1.15 (see ESI, Figure S1). The resulting products were amphiphilic macromolecules, consisting of a hydrophobic *tert*-octylcalix[8]arene core and eight arms of hydrophilic PEG chains.

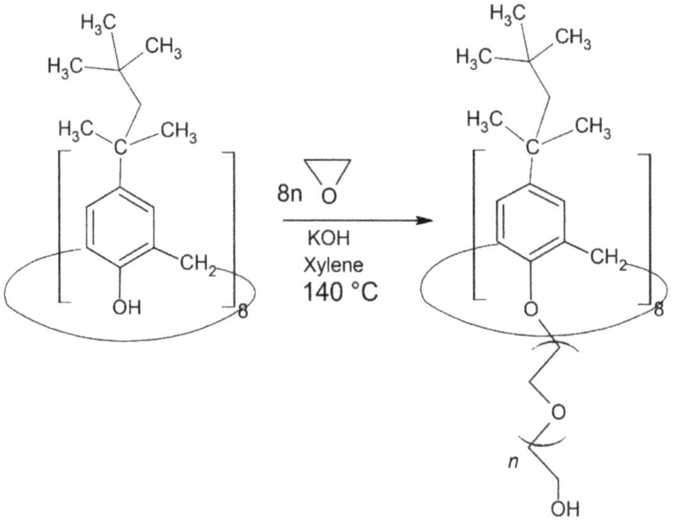

Figure 2. Schematic representation of the synthesis of PEGylated *tert*-octylcalix[8]arenes.

The polymerization degrees of the PEG fragments and the corresponding average molar masses of the obtained PEGylated *tert*-octylcalix[8]arenes were determined from the relative areas of the signals of the CH_2 groups of the PEG fragments at 3.5–3.7 ppm, and the CH_3 protons of the tert-octyl groups at 1.0 ppm. A representative ^1H NMR spectrum is shown in the ESI (Figure S2). The abbreviations of the newly synthesized PEGylated *tert*-octylcalix[8]arenes, as well as theoretical and experimental degrees of polymerization (DP) of the PEG chains and the number average molar masses (M_n) of the investigated products, are given in Table 1. Static light scattering (SLS) measurements of selected samples showed a very good correlation between the molar masses of the products determined by ^1H NMR spectroscopy and SLS (see below and the ESI, Table S1, Figure S3).

Table 1. Abbreviations, theoretical and experimental degrees of polymerization (DP) of the PEG chains and number average molar mass (M_n) of the PEGylated *tert*-octylcalix[8]arenes.

Abbreviation	DP of PEG Chains		Mna
	Theoretical	Experimental [a]	
OEC- I	5	4	3200
OEC-II	7	6	3900
OEC- III	19	14	6700
OEC-IV	22	17	7800
OEC- V	42	41	16,200
OEC- VI	57	52	20,000
OEC- VII	100	96	36,000

[a] Derived from ^1H NMR data in $CDCl_3$.

The successful PEGylation of *tert*-octylcalix[8]arene was evidenced by measuring the DOSY spectra of the new materials in $CDCl_3$. Figure S2 shows as an example the DOSY spectrum of sample OEC-IV, where the PEG units (around 3.7 ppm) and the *tert*-octylcalix[8]arene fragments (0.4–1.7 ppm, 6.9 ppm) show identical diffusion coefficients, indicating that they originate from the same molecules.

3.2. Aqueous Solution Properties

The lowest members of the series of PEGylated *tert*-octylcalix[8]arenes (OEC-I and OEC-II) were not soluble in water. OEC-III exhibited limited solubility at low concentrations, whereas the higher members (OEC-IV–OEC-VII) spontaneously dissolved in water in wide concentration intervals. Considering their non-linear chain topology, the possible steric hindrance caused by the densely functionalized PEG lower rim, and the screening of the hydrophobic moieties, one may anticipate more complicated and complex self-associating behavior compared to that of linear amphiphilic copolymers. The association behavior of the PEGylated *tert*-octylcalix[8]arenes in aqueous solution was investigated by a variety of methods, including dye solubilization, diffusion-ordered NMR spectroscopy, and light scattering. For determination of the CMCs, the sensitivity to changes in the microenvironment of the non-polar dye 1,6-diphenyl-1,3,5-hexatriene(DPH) was exploited [39–43]. Typically, an increase in the absorbance at 356 nm is associated with the formation of hydrophobic domains in which the dye is solubilized. Figure 3a shows a representative absorbance vs. concentration dependence for OEC-IV at 25 °C, from the break of which the CMC was determined. Similarly, the CMC values of all investigated species were determined. They fell in the range 4.4–7.2 mg/mL and showed a gradual increase with increasing M_n (Figure 3b). The lower CMC indicated easier and more favored self-association.

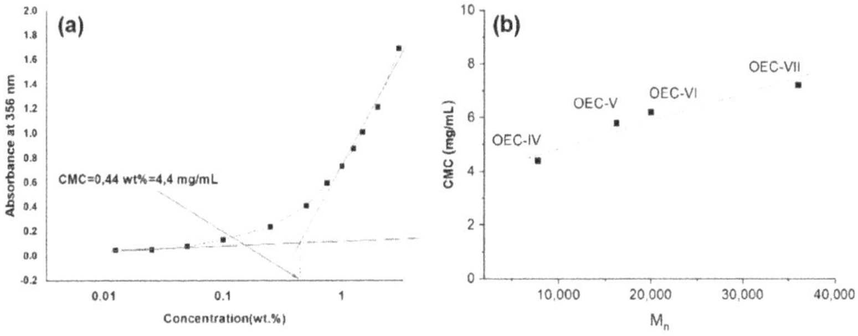

Figure 3. Absorption intensity at 356 nm and CMC determination of OEC-IV (**a**) and CMC versus molar mass of the investigated PEGylated *tert*-octylcalix[8]arenes in aqueous solution (**b**).

Below the CMC, only unimers, that is, unassociated PEGylated *tert*-octylcalix[8]arenes, exist, whereas above the CMC multimolecular aggregates are formed. The transition from unimers to multimolecular aggregates, however, is not sharp, as evidenced by Figure 3a, which could be associated with the polymer nature of the products, their non-linear chain topology, and the presence of a rigid calixarene moiety, as well as some composition dispersity. In this relatively broad transition interval, unimers and multimolecular aggregates were found to co-exist, as evidenced by dynamic light scattering (see ESI, Figure S4 and DOSY. DOSY exploits the differences in the translational diffusion coefficients of various species present in a mixture, thus allowing discrimination between components with different sizes [44]. In the present study, it was used for determination of the diffusion coefficients and sizes of aggregates formed in aqueous solutions of the PEGylated *tert*-octylcalix[8]arenes, containing 14 (OEC-III), 17 (OEC-IV), 41 (OEC-V) and 96 (OEC-VII) oxyethylene units. The DOSY spectra of the systems with 14 and 96 oxyethylene units showed the presence of two components, indicating the formation of two types of aggregates. Figure 4a presents an example of the DOSY spectrum of OEC-III (10 mg in 1 mL D_2O), showing the co-existence of relatively small particles with a diffusion coefficient of 3.38×10^{-11} m^2/s and larger aggregates with a diffusion coefficient of 1.78×10^{-12} m^2/s. The calculated apparent hydrodynamic diameter d_h of the former, of around 10 nm, could be associated with the size of unimers, while the latter, with a d_h of 190 nm, were undoubtedly multimolecular aggregates. Similar results were obtained for the system with

96 (OEC-VII) oxyethylene units (Figure S2 in the ESI). The lack of a diffusion peak for the calixarene fragment in unimers could be explained by the relaxation dynamics of the amphiphilic polymer system in water, which depends in a complex way on the overall and fragmental motion of the unimers and the aggregates. The systems with 17 and 41 oxyethylene units display only one component in their DOSY spectra corresponding to particles with relatively small sizes, and with a d_h of about 10 nm (Figure 4b). The good correlation between the sizes of the co-existing particles determined by DOSY and DLS (see Figure 4 and Figure S4) is noteworthy.

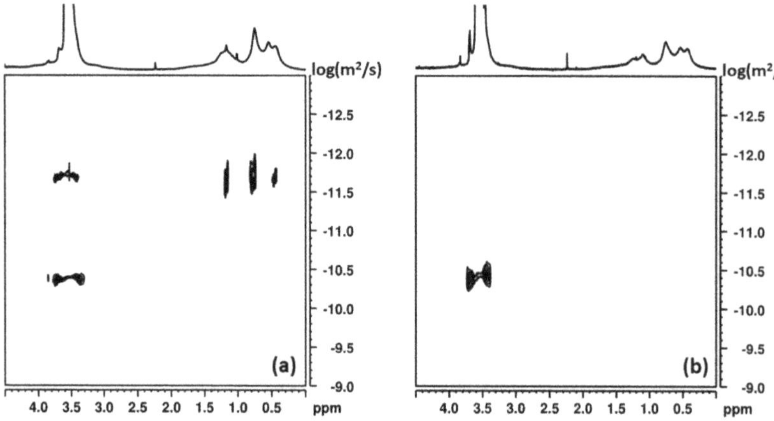

Figure 4. DOSY spectra of (**a**) OEC-III (10 mg/mL in D_2O); (**b**) OEC-V (10 mg/mL in D_2O).

Similar behaviors, i.e., the co-existence of unimers and multimolecular aggregates in relatively wide concentration intervals, were observed for the other three water-soluble PEGylated *tert*-octylcalix[8]arenes.

Static light scattering (SLS) was employed to determine the molar mass and aggregation number of the multimolecular aggregates formed at concentrations well above the CMC. A representative Zimm plot is shown in Figure S3, and the derived parameters are collected in Table S1. The molar mass of the aggregates reached hundreds of kg/mol, corresponding to aggregation numbers (N_{agg}) in the 11–20 range. These are considerably lower figures, corresponding also to the lower density of the materials within the particles, compared to the PEGylated calix[4]arenes studied earlier [45], and can be attributed to the larger size of the calix residue and the enhanced empty volume of the cavity resulting from the functionalization with the tert-octyl side groups at the upper rim.

3.3. Phase Solubility Evaluation

OEC-IV and OEC-V were selected for the preparation of platforms for the delivery of silibinin, and the further investigation and evaluation of their potential, because they are characterized by the lowest CMCs, and thus have enhanced stability upon dilution, larger N_{agg} (that is, larger hydrophobic volume and, hence, possibilities for loading greater drug amounts), and shorter PEG chains, which cause less spatial obstructions upon loading and the formation of inclusion complexes. The phase solubility of SBN in the presence of aqueous solutions of the investigated PEGylated tert-otctylcalix[8]arenes was determined by the method of Higuchi and Connors [46]. Due to their amphiphilic structure, OEC-IV and OEC-V can solubilize silibinin via two mechanisms: by the formation of inclusion complexes at concentrations below their CMC, and additionally by the formation of supramolecular aggregates at concentrations exceeding CMC. Therefore, the concentration range of the PEGylated calixarenes was selected to cover concentrations below and above their critical micellar concentration. The phase solubility profiles are shown in Figure 5.

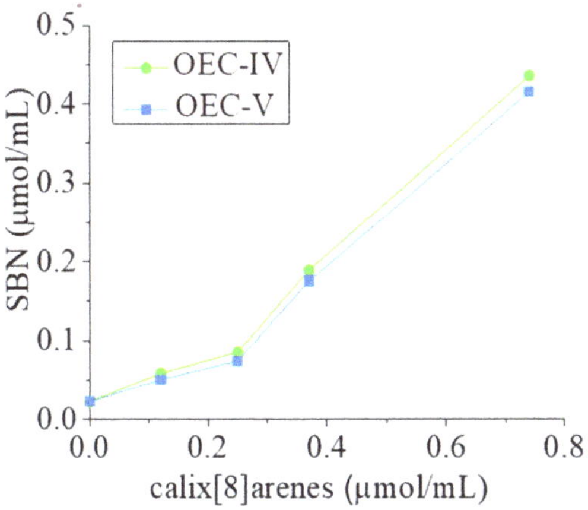

Figure 5. Phase solubility profiles of silibinin (SBN) in aqueous media containing various concentrations of OEC-IV (-•) or OEC-V (-■-) at 25 °C.

As evident from the presented data, the gradual increase in the concentration of the PEGylated *tert*-octylcalix[8]arenes leads to an increase in the solubility of silibinin. Both solubility profiles can be defined as Ap type, as they show a positive deviation from linearity [47]. In the concentration range from 0.0 to 0.25 μmol/mL (concentrations below the CMC), a linear increase in SBN solubility is observed (R^2 above 0.99). From the linear part of the solubility profiles, the slope of the lines can be derived (Table 2). Slopes less than 1 indicates the formation of "host–guest" inclusion complexes, between SBN and PEGylated *tert*-octylcalix[8]arenes, of a stoichiometric ratio of 1:1, following the equation:

$$D + C \overset{Ks}{\Leftrightarrow} [DC], \tag{3}$$

where D is a guest drug molecule, C is the host macrocyclic compound and $[DC]$ is the inclusion complex [46].

Table 2. Stability constants (Ks), thermodynamic parameter (ΔG) and solubility enhancement factor (δ) derived from phase solubility diagrams. *So*—intrinsic solubility of SBN in the absence of complexing agents.

Parameter / Complex	Slope	R^2	Ks (mL/μmol)	ΔG (kJ/mol)	*So* (μmol/mL)	δ (%)
SBN:OEC-IV	0.73556	0.998	126.4	−11.98	0.022	1877
SBN:OEC-V	0.73301	0.996	124.5	−11.84		1786

In addition, the slope values were used to calculate the stability constant (Ks), the main parameter describing the solubility of a drug and the stability of the complex, using the equation:

$$\text{Ks} = \frac{slope}{So(1 - slope)} \tag{4}$$

where *So* is the solubility of silibinin in the absence of a complexing agent.

The Ks values are presented in Table 2. The calculated values for Ks are relatively high, which is an indicator of both the good solubility of silibinin and the sufficient stability of the complexes. In addition, inclusion complexes with Ks values above 100 are considered optimal for biological applications because, in addition to the optimized solubility of the drug, they also provide the ability for controlled release and, respectively, effective drug delivery in the target compartments [48,49]. For more in-depth characterization of the inclusion complexes, the Gibson free energy change of the complexation process was calculated following the equation:

$$\Delta G = -RTlnKs \tag{5}$$

Negative ΔG values (Table 2) indicate the spontaneous complex formation of SBN and the tested PEGylated *tert*-octylcalix[8]arenes in aqueous media.

Although there is no significant difference in the studied parameters between the OEC-IV and OEC-V inclusion complexes, there is a tendency towards the lower solubility of silibinin in the presence of OEC-V. A probable explanation is the spatial obstruction of the longer PEG chains, which may hinder the entry of SBN molecules.

At concentrations above the CMC, a positive deviation in the phase solubility profiles can be clearly seen (Figure 5), evidenced by the formation of supramolecular aggregates, in the hydrophobic domains of which additional amounts of silibinin can be solubilized, leading to a sharp increase in its aqueous solubility. The total solubility improvement of silibinin was studied at OEC-IV and OEC-V concentrations of 1.28 and 0.74 μmol/mL (above CMC), respectively, and was expressed as the solubility enhancement factor (δ), calculated by Equation (6) [47]:

$$\delta = \frac{S - So}{So} \times 100 \tag{6}$$

where *So* and *S* denote silibinin solubility in the absence and presence PEGylated *tert*-octylcalix[8]arenes, respectively.

The solubility enhancement factors are presented in Table 2 and are 100% when the solubility of silibinin exceeds twice its *So* ($S = 2So$). Thus, the addition of the tested PEGylated *tert*-octylcalix[8]arenes at concentrations far exceeding their CMCs leads to a more than 20-fold increase in the aqueous solubility of silibinin via two simultaneously occurring mechanisms: the formation of 1:1 inclusion complexes and the formation of supramolecular aggregates.

3.4. Characterization of OEC:SBN Inclusion Complexes

Fourier Transform Infrared (FT-IR) Spectroscopy

Representative FT-IR spectra of SBN, OEC-IV, the physical mixture of OEC-IV and SBN and the inclusion complex OEC-IV:SBN are shown in Figure 6. The results obtained for other OEC samples are quite similar. The spectrum of free SBN (Figure 6b) shows characteristic peaks at 3452 cm^{-1} (-OH stretching vibration), 1632 cm^{-1} (C=O stretching vibration) and 1506–1468 (skeleton vibration of aromatic C=C ring stretching) [50]. These did not interfere with the bands in the OEC-IV spectrum, and were used as marks for the description of silibinin in the inclusion complex. The characteristic peak at 2873 cm^{-1} in the spectrum of OEC-IV (Figure 6a) is caused by the asymmetric and symmetric stretching vibrations of the CH bonds in calixarene [51]. The FT-IR spectrum of the physical mixture (Figure 6c) is a combination of the spectra of pure SBN and OEC-IV, and shows the characteristic bands of both molecules. In contrast, the spectrum of the inclusion complex (Figure 6d) does not show SBN's characteristic peaks, which is probably due to the restriction of the vibration of the SBN molecule. This observation suggests that the silibinin molecule was entrapped in the hydrophobic calixarene cavity.

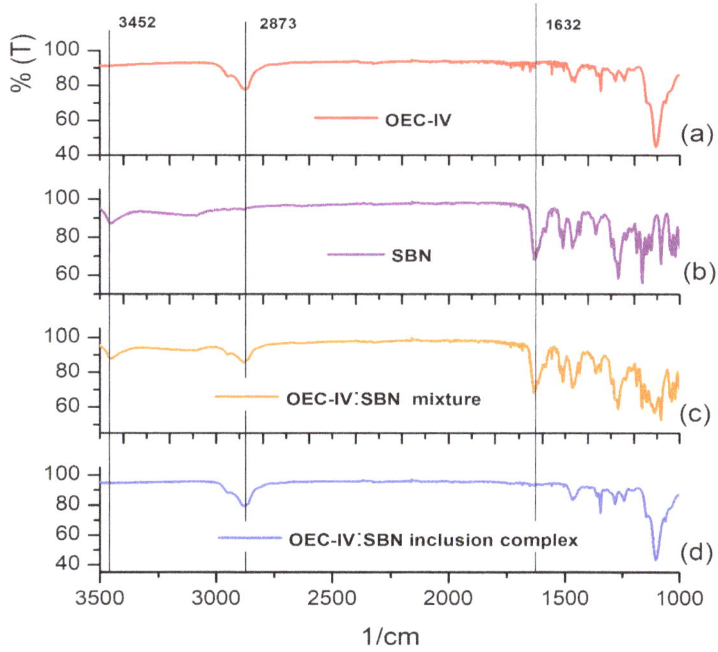

Figure 6. FT-IR spectra in the region 1000–3000 cm^{-1} of (**a**) OEC-IV, (**b**) silibinin, (**c**) the OEC-IV:silibinin physical mixture and (**d**) the OEC-IV:silibinin inclusion complex.

3.5. Characterization of Silibinin-Loaded OEC Supramolecular Aggregates

3.5.1. Size, Size Distribution and Zeta Potential

The size, size distribution patterns and ζ potential of the formed silibinin:OEC aggregates were measured by DLS and electrophoretic light scattering. The results are summarized in Table 3. Representative size distribution curves are depicted in Figure 7.

Table 3. Size, size distribution patterns and ζ potential of empty and silibinin-loaded supramolecular aggregates.

Sample	Diameter (nm)	PDI	ζ Potential (mV)
OEC-IV empty	260.0 ± 5.2	0.54	−32.2 ± 1.55
OEC-IV:SBN	211.0 ± 2.4	0.44	−23.1 ± 0.35
OEC-V empty	295.0 ± 3.8	0,48	−31.5 ± 0.5
OEC-V:SBN	200.0 ± 5.6	0.39	−19.9 ± 1.9

Evident in the presented results are the relatively high PDI values (Table 3) corresponding to the bimodal size distributions (Figure 7): a small fraction (less than 13%) of particles with a size around 10 nm (presumably unimers, see Section 2.2 above) was found to coexist with a dominant fraction (above 87%) of particles with sizes varying from 200 to 295 nm in all of the studied formulations, whether empty or silibinin-loaded. Given the very low percentage distribution of the concomitant fractions of particles and their small sizes, it can be concluded that the presence of these species would not affect the uniform loading of silibinin in the main group of supramolecular aggregates. Another interesting finding from the DLS analysis is that the silibinin loading in the aggregates is accompanied by a decrease in their size (Table 3). A possible explanation for the observed trend is the condensation of the hydrophobic core of the supramolecular aggregates as a result of the binding interactions between the molecules of silibinin and the hydrophobic domains of the calixarene aggregates. These observations are consistent with the findings of other authors who have also shown a reduction in the size of polymer micelles with the inclusion of hydrophobic drugs [52].

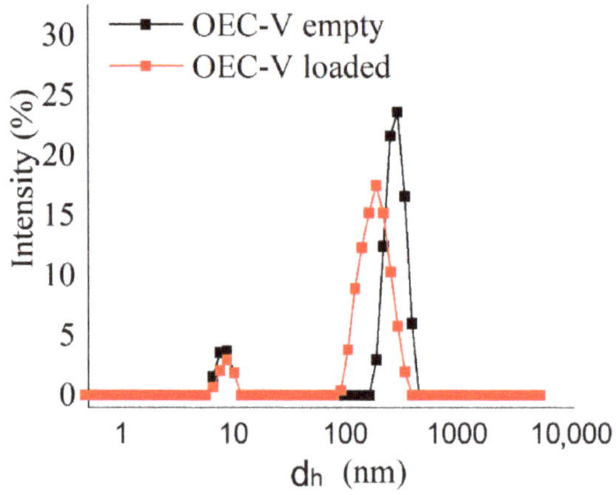

Figure 7. Size distribution curves of non-loaded and silibinin-loaded supramolecular OEC-V aggregates.

Although the PEGylated *tert*-octylcalix[8]arenes under investigation in the present study are nonionic amphiphiles, their supramolecular aggregates, both non-loaded and silibinin-loaded, show a relatively high negative ζ potential (Table 3), which is an indicator of their physical stability. On the other hand, the encapsulation of silibinin was associated with a substantial shift to less negative values. This shift in the ζ potential is probably due not only to the localization of silibinin molecules in the hydrophobic interior of supramolecular aggregates, but also due to their absorption on the surface as a result of the formation of hydrogen bonds between the ether oxygens of the PEG chains of PEGylated *tert*-octylcalix[8]arenes and the OH or keto groups of silibinin molecules. Nevertheless, the absolute value of the ζ potential of the loaded formulations remains relatively high, which is a prerequisite for sufficient physical stability.

3.5.2. Silibinin Release Study

The release behavior of silibinin from supramolecular OEC-IV and OEC-V aggregates was investigated via the dialysis technique against PBS (pH 7.4) at 37 °C for 24 h. The release profiles are shown in Figure 8. The presented results show the two-phase release profiles of silibinin from both types of aggregates. The initial "burst" release, where within 3 h almost 50% of the loaded substance was released, was followed by a delayed silibinin release up to the 24th h. These results are consistent with those of our previous studies of similar nanosized systems of curcumin delivery, which showed the same release behavior [23]. This finding confirms our hypothesis that the initial fast release was due to the release of silibinin from the aggregates, while the slower second phase was due to the release of silibinin from the inclusion complexes, which were characterized with relatively high values of Ks and, as such, mediated a slower drug release (see Section 3.3 and Table 2).

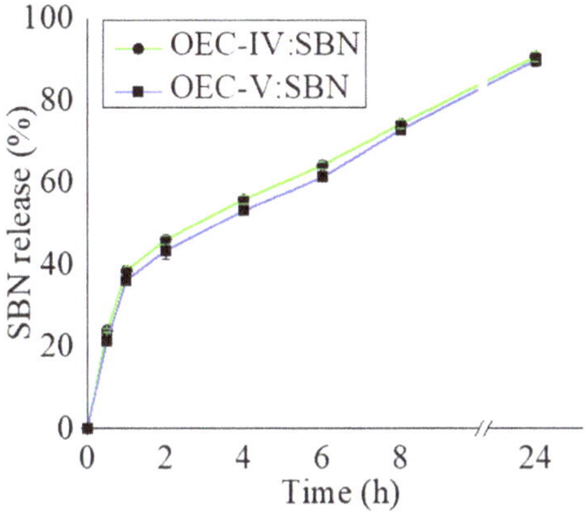

Figure 8. Release profiles of silibinin from supramolecular PEGylated *tert*-octylcalix[8]arenes aggregates.

3.5.3. Cytotoxicity Study

The PEGylated *tert*-octylcalix[8]arenes formulations of silibinin were evaluated in comparison with the free drug for antineoplastic activity against chronic myeloid leukemia (HL-60)- and transitional cell urinary bladder cancer (CAL-29)-derived cell lines after of 72 h continuous exposure, using the MTT dye reduction assay. Both OEC-V and OEC-IV non-loaded systems were tested against these cell lines as well, and as evident from the concentration–response curves depicted in Figure 9a,b, they exerted only marginal intrinsic cytotoxicity. The comparative evaluation of the cell growth inhibition following treatment with the free drug or its formulations (Figure 9c,d, Table 4) showed strong, concentration-dependent cytotoxic effects, with IC_{50} values within the low μg/mL range. Although there was a shift in the dose–response curves towards higher concentrations in the formulated vs. free silibinin, the IC_{50} values thereof were comparable. This suggests that the PEGylated *tert*-octylcalix[8]arenes, although being generally devoid of intrinsic cytotoxicity, did not compromise the antineoplastic potential of the natural compound.

Table 4. IC_{50} values of free and loaded silibinin (μg/mL).

Sample	IC_{50}	
	HL-60	**CAL-29**
SBN	3.01	3.61
OEC-IV:SBN	4.48	4.13
OEC-V:SBN	4.67	4.25

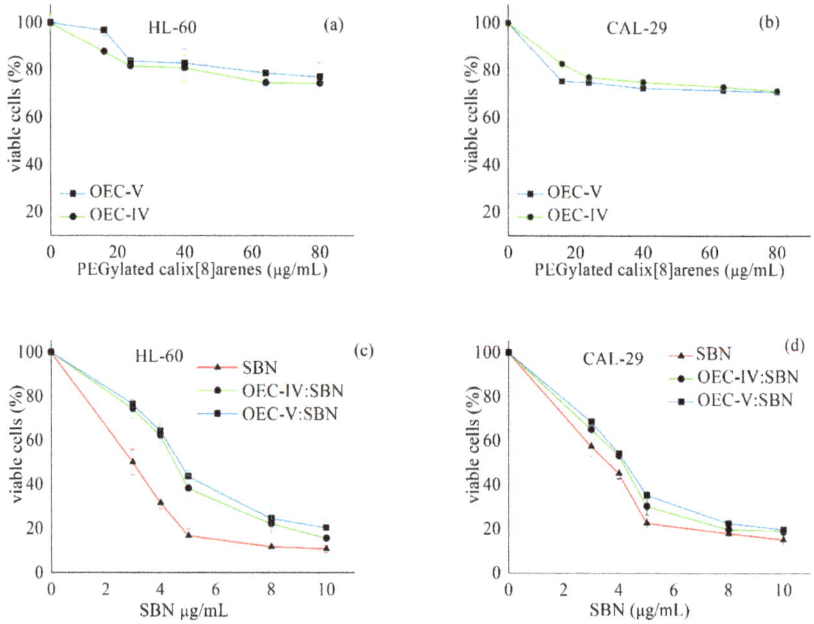

Figure 9. Cytotoxicity of non-loaded supramolecular PEGylated *tert*-octylcalix[8]arenes aggregates (**a**,**b**) and their silibinin-loaded counterparts (**c**,**d**) against human tumor cell lines HL-60 (**a**,**c**) and CAL-29 (**b**,**d**) after 72 h exposure at 37 °C, ±SD from 6 separate experiments.

4. Conclusions

Novel PEGylated *tert*-octylcalix[8]arenes were designed as carriers of silibinin—an anticancer and chemo-protective agent with hepatoprotective properties and high therapeutic potential. The products were obtained by the "grafting from" approach. PEG chains with degrees of polymerization varying from 4 to 96 were grafted from the lower rim of the original *tert*-octylcalix[8]arene macrocycles to produce amphiphilic macromolecules consisting of a hydrophobic *tert*-octylcalix[8]arene core and eight arms of hydrophilic PEG chains. In an aqueous solution, the PEGylated *tert*-octylcalix[8]arenes were found to self-associate above a certain critical concentration into nanosized aggregates. The resulting supramolecular structures were used for the solubilization and delivery of silibinin. Tremendous enhancements in the solubility of silibinin (>1700%) were observed, and were attributed to the simultaneous formation of inclusion complexes and additional solubilization in hydrophobic domains of the supramolecular aggregates. Accordingly, two phases were observed in the release profiles of silibinin: fast release from the aggregates and considerably slower release from the inclusion complexes. The investigated PEGylated *tert*-octylcalix[8]arenes exerted only marginal intrinsic cytotoxicity, and did not compromise the antineoplastic potential of silibinin. Based on a recent review, with a detailed summary of various SBN formulations [53] and focusing on their favorable physico-chemical characteristics, ability to significantly enhance solubility, excellent biocompatibility, and appropriate release profiles, the PEGylated *tert*-octylcalix[8]arenes were found to further expand the experimental knowledge in this field, and can be considered as promising carriers for the delivery of silibinin.

Supplementary Materials: The following are available online: https://www.mdpi.com/article/10.3390/pharmaceutics13122025/s1. Figure S1: GPC eluograms of crude (a) and purified (b) OEC-VI. Figure S2: (a)Representative ^{1}H NMR spectrum of OEC-VII in $CDCl_3$ for determination of the average DP of the PEG chains and number average molar mass (M_n).-; (b) DOSY spectrum of OEC-IV in $CDCl_3$ (10 mg/mL); (c) DOSY spectrum of OEC-VII (10 mg/mL in D_2O) showing the co-existence of two populations of particles—unimers and macromolecular aggregates. Figure S3: (a) Debye plot for OEC-VII in water at 25 °C in the concentration range below the CMC. Measurements were made at an angle of 90°; (b) Zimm plot for OEC-VII in water at 25 °C in the concentration range above the CMC. Figure S4: Particle size distribution from DLS of OEC-VII in water at 25 °C in the transition concentration range. Measurements were made at an angle of 90° and c = 6.2 mg/mL. Table S1: SLS characterization parameters of selected samples in water at 25 °C in the concentration ranges below or above the CMCs.

Author Contributions: Conceptualization, D.B., D.M. and S.R.; formal analysis, D.B., D.M., G.M., P.S. and S.R.; investigation, D.B., D.M., G.M., P.S. and S.R.; writing—original draft preparation, D.B. and S.R.; writing—sections, D.B., D.M., G.M., P.S. and S.R.; writing—review and editing, D.B., D.M., G.M., P.S., H.P. and S.R.; funding acquisition, D.B. and S.R. All authors have read and agreed to the published version of the manuscript.

Funding: This work was supported by the Bulgarian Ministry of Education and Science (Grant D01-217/30.11.2018) under the National Research Programme "Innovative Low-Toxic Bioactive Systems for Precision Medicine (BioActiveMed)" approved by DCM #658/14.09.2018.

Institutional Review Board Statement: Not applicable.

Informed Consent Statement: Not applicable.

Acknowledgments: Research equipment of Distributed Research Infrastructure INFRAMAT, part of the Bulgarian National Roadmap for Research Infrastructures, supported by the Bulgarian Ministry of Education and Science, was used in this investigation.

Conflicts of Interest: The authors declare no conflict of interest. The funders had no role in the design of the study; in the collection, analyses, or interpretation of data; in the writing of the manuscript, or in the decision to publish the results.

References

1. Salmi, H.A.; Sarna, S. Effect of silymarin on chemical, functional, and morphological alterations of the liver. *Scand. J. Gastroenterol.* **1982**, *17*, 517–521. [CrossRef]
2. Weselowska, O.; Łania-Pietrzak, B.; Kuzdzal, M.; Stanczak, K.; Mosiadz, D.; Dobryszycki, P.; Ozyhar, A.; Komorowska, M.; Hendrich, A.B.; Michalak, K. Influence of silybin on biophysical properties of phospholipid bilayers. *Acta Pharmacol. Sin.* **2007**, *28*, 296–306. [CrossRef]
3. Abenavoli, L.; Capasso, R.; Milic, N.; Capasso, F. Milk thistle in liver diseases: Past, present, future. *Phytother. Res.* **2010**, *24*, 1423–1432. [CrossRef] [PubMed]
4. Gazak, R.; Walterova, D.; Kren, V. Silybin and Silymarin—New and emerging applications in medicine. *Curr. Med. Chem.* **2007**, *14*, 315–338. [CrossRef] [PubMed]
5. Hackett, E.S.; Twedt, D.C.; Gustafson, D.L. Milk Thistle and its derivative compounds: A review of opportunities for treatment of liver disease. *J. Vet. Intern. Med.* **2012**, *27*, 10–16. [CrossRef] [PubMed]
6. Liu, W.; Wang, F.; Li, C.; Otkur, W.; Hayashi, T.; Mizuno, K.; Hattori, S.; Fujisaki, H.; Onodera, S.; Ikejima, T. Silibinin treatment protects human skin cells from UVB injury through upregulation of estrogen receptors. *J. Photochem. Photobiol. B Biol.* **2021**, *216*, 112147. [CrossRef] [PubMed]
7. Vue, B.; Zhang, S.; Zhang, X.; Parisis, K.; Zhang, Q.; Zheng, S.; Wang, G.; Chen, Q.-H. Silibinin derivatives as anti-prostate cancer agents: Synthesis and cell-based evaluations. *Eur. J. Med. Chem.* **2016**, *109*, 36–46. [CrossRef] [PubMed]
8. Mahira, S.; Kommineni, N.; Husain, G.M.; Khan, W. Cabazitaxel and Silibinin co-encapsulated cationic liposomes for CD44 targeted delivery: A new insight into nanomedicine based combinational chemotherapy for prostate cancer. *Biomed. Pharmacother.* **2019**, *110*, 803–817. [CrossRef] [PubMed]
9. Binienda, A.; Ziolkowska, S.; Pluciennik, E. The anticancer properties of Silibinin: Its molecular mechanism and therapeutic effect in breast cancer. *Anti-Cancer Agents Med. Chem.* **2020**, *20*, 1787–1796. [CrossRef]
10. Saller, R.; Meier, R.; Brignoli, R. The use of Silymarin in the treatment of liver diseases. *Drugs* **2001**, *61*, 2035–2063. [CrossRef]
11. Bijak, M. Silybin, a major bioactive component of milk thistle (*Silybum marianum* L. Gaernt.)—Chemistry, bioavailability, and metabolism. *Molecules* **2017**, *22*, 1942. [CrossRef]

12. Sahibzada, M.U.; Sadiq, A.; Zahoor, M.; Naz, S.; Shahid, M.; Qureshi, N.A. Enhancement of bioavailability and hepatoprotection by Silibinin through conversion to nanoparticles prepared by Liquid Antisolvent method. *Arab. J. Chem.* **2020**, *13*, 3682–3689. [CrossRef]
13. Biedermann, D.; Vavříková, E.; Cvak, L.; Křen, V. Chemistry of Silybin. *Nat. Prod. Rep.* **2014**, *31*, 1138–1157. [CrossRef] [PubMed]
14. Voinovich, D.; Perissutti, B.; Grassi, M.; Passerini, N.; Bigotto, A. Solid state mechanochemical activation of silybum marianum dry extract with Betacyclodextrins: Characterization and bioavailability of the COGROUND systems. *J. Pharm. Sci.* **2009**, *98*, 4119–4129. [CrossRef] [PubMed]
15. Parveen, R.; Baboota, S.; Ali, J.; Ahuja, A.; Vasudev, S.S.; Ahmad, S. Oil based nanocarrier for improved oral delivery of Silymarin: In vitro and in vivo studies. *Int. J. Pharm.* **2011**, *413*, 245–253. [CrossRef] [PubMed]
16. Nawaz, Q.; Fuentes-Chandía, M.; Tharmalingam, V.; Ur Rehman, M.A.; Leal-Egaña, A.; Boccaccini, A.R. Silibinin releasing mesoporous bioactive glass nanoparticles with potential for breast cancer therapy. *Ceram. Int.* **2020**, *46*, 29111–29119. [CrossRef]
17. Amirsaadat, S.; Jafari-Gharabaghlou, D.; Alijani, S.; Mousazadeh, H.; Dadashpour, M.; Zarghami, N. Metformin and Silibinin co-loaded PLGA-peg nanoparticles for effective combination therapy against human breast cancer cells. *J. Drug Deliv. Sci. Technol.* **2021**, *61*, 102107. [CrossRef]
18. Elshafeey, A.H.; Zayed, R.; Shukr, M.H.; Elsayed, I. Sucrose acetate isobutyrate based nanovesicles: A promising platform for drug delivery and bioavailability enhancement. *J. Drug Deliv. Sci. Technol.* **2020**, *58*, 101806. [CrossRef]
19. Yazdi Rouholamini, S.E.; Moghassemi, S.; Maharat, Z.; Hakamivala, A.; Kashanian, S.; Omidfar, K. Effect of silibinin-loaded nano-NIOSOMAL coated with trimethyl chitosan on mirnas expression in 2D and 3D models of T47D Breast Cancer Cell Line. *Artif. Cells Nanomed. Biotechnol.* **2017**, *46*, 524–535. [CrossRef] [PubMed]
20. Shafiee, M.; Abolmaali, S.S.; Tamaddon, A.M.; Abedanzadeh, M.; Abedi, M. One-pot synthesis of poly(alkyl methacrylate)-functionalized mesoporous silica hybrid nanocomposites for microencapsulation of poorly soluble phytochemicals. *Colloid Interface Sci. Commun.* **2020**, *37*, 100298. [CrossRef]
21. Gohulkumar, M.; Gurushankar, K.; Rajendra Prasad, N.; Krishnakumar, N. Enhanced cytotoxicity and apoptosis-induced anticancer effect of Silibinin-loaded nanoparticles in oral carcinoma (KB) cells. *Mater. Sci. Eng. C* **2014**, *41*, 274–282. [CrossRef] [PubMed]
22. Fan, X.; Guo, X. Development of calixarene-based drug nanocarriers. *J. Mol. Liq.* **2021**, *325*, 115246. [CrossRef]
23. Drakalska, E.; Momekova, D.; Manolova, Y.; Budurova, D.; Momekov, G.; Genova, M.; Antonov, L.; Lambov, N.; Rangelov, S. Hybrid liposomal pegylated calix[4]arene systems as drug delivery platforms for curcumin. *Int. J. Pharm.* **2014**, *472*, 165–174. [CrossRef] [PubMed]
24. Ostos, F.J.; Lebrón, J.A.; López-Cornejo, P.; López-López, M.; García-Calderón, M.; García-Calderón, C.B.; Rosado, I.V.; Kalchenko, V.I.; Rodik, R.V.; Moyá, M.L. Self-aggregation in aqueous solution of amphiphilic cationic calix[4]arenes. potential use as vectors and nanocarriers. *J. Mol. Liq.* **2020**, *304*, 112724. [CrossRef]
25. Shumatbaeva, A.M.; Morozova, J.E.; Syakaev, V.V.; Shalaeva, Y.V.; Sapunova, A.S.; Voloshina, A.D.; Gubaidullin, A.T.; Bazanova, O.B.; Babaev, V.M.; Nizameev, I.R.; et al. The PH-responsive calix[4]resorcinarene-MPEG conjugates bearing acylhydrazone bonds: Synthesis and study of the potential as supramolecular drug delivery systems. *Colloids Surf. A Physicochem. Eng. Asp.* **2020**, *589*, 124453. [CrossRef]
26. Casnati, A.; Sansone, F.; Ungaro, R. Peptido- and glycocalixarenes: playing with hydrogen bonds around hydrophobic cavities. *Acc. Chem. Res.* **2003**, *36*, 246–254. [CrossRef] [PubMed]
27. Da Silva, E.; Lazar, A.N.; Coleman, A.W. Biopharmaceutical applications of Calixarenes. *J. Drug Deliv. Sci. Technol.* **2004**, *14*, 3–20. [CrossRef]
28. Kunsági-Máté, S.; Szabó, K.; Lemli, B.; Bitter, I.; Nagy, G.; Kollár, L. Host–guest interaction between water-soluble calix[6]arene hexasulfonate and p-nitrophenol. *Thermochim. Acta* **2005**, *425*, 121–126. [CrossRef]
29. Perret, F.; Lazar, A.N.; Coleman, A.W. Biochemistry of the para-sulfonato-calix[n]arenes. *Chem. Commun.* **2006**, *23*, 2425–2438. [CrossRef]
30. Martin, A.D.; Raston, C.L. Multifunctional P-phosphonated calixarenes. *Chem. Commun.* **2011**, *47*, 9764. [CrossRef]
31. Fulton, D.A.; Stoddart, J.F. Neoglycoconjugates based on cyclodextrins and Calixarenes. *Bioconjugate Chem.* **2001**, *12*, 655–672. [CrossRef] [PubMed]
32. Křenek, K.; Kuldová, M.; Hulíková, K.; Stibor, I.; Lhoták, P.; Dudič, M.; Budka, J.; Pelantová, H.; Bezouška, K.; Fišerová, A.; et al. Retracted: N-acetyl-D-glucosamine substituted calix[4]arenes as stimulators of NK cell-mediated antitumor immune response. *Carbohydr. Res.* **2007**, *342*, 1781–1792. [CrossRef] [PubMed]
33. Shahgaldian, P.; Sciotti, M.A.; Pieles, U. Amino-substituted Amphiphilic Calixarenes: Self-assembly and interactions with DNA. *Langmuir* **2008**, *24*, 8522–8526. [CrossRef] [PubMed]
34. Gao, Y.; Li, Z.; Sun, M.; Li, H.; Guo, C.; Cui, J.; Li, A.; Cao, F.; Xi, Y.; Lou, H.; et al. Preparation, characterization, pharmacokinetics, and tissue distribution of curcumin nanosuspension with TPGS as stabilizer. *Drug Dev. Ind. Pharm.* **2010**, *36*, 1225–1234. [CrossRef] [PubMed]
35. Taton, D.; Saule, M.; Logan, J.; Duran, R.; Hou, S.; Chaikof, E.L.; Gnanou, Y. Polymerization of ethylene oxide with a Calixarene-based precursor: Synthesis of eight-arm poly(ethylene oxide) stars by the core-first methodology. *J. Polym. Sci. Part A Polym. Chem.* **2003**, *41*, 1669–1676. [CrossRef]

36. Mustafina, A.; Zakharova, L.; Elistratova, J.; Kudryashova, J.; Soloveva, S.; Garusov, A.; Antipin, I.; Konovalov, A. Solution behavior of mixed systems based on novel amphiphilic cyclophanes and Triton X100: Aggregation, Cloud Point Phenomenon and cloud point extraction of lanthanide ions. *J. Colloid Interface Sci.* **2010**, *346*, 405–413. [CrossRef]
37. Mosmann, T. Rapid colorimetric assay for cellular growth and survival: Application to proliferation and cytotoxicity assays. *J. Immunol. Methods* **1983**, *65*, 55–63. [CrossRef]
38. Konstantinov, S.M.; Eibl, H.; Berger, M.R. BCR-abl influences the antileukaemic efficacy of alkylphosphocholines. *Br. J. Haematol.* **1999**, *107*, 365–374. [CrossRef]
39. Alexandridis, P.; Holzwarth, J.F.; Hatton, T.A. Micellization of poly(ethylene oxide)-poly(propylene oxide)-poly(ethylene oxide) Triblock copolymers in aqueous solutions: Thermodynamics of Copolymer Association. *Macromolecules* **1994**, *27*, 2414–2425. [CrossRef]
40. Chattopadhyay, A.; London, E. Fluorimetric determination of critical micelle concentration avoiding interference from detergent charge. *Anal. Biochem.* **1984**, *139*, 408–412. [CrossRef]
41. Halacheva, S.; Rangelov, S.; Tsvetanov, C. Poly(glycidol)-based analogues to pluronic block copolymers. synthesis and aqueous solution properties. *Macromolecules* **2006**, *39*, 6845–6852. [CrossRef]
42. Scherlund, M.; Brodin, A.; Malmsten, M. Micellization and gelation in block copolymer systems containing local anesthetics. *Int. J. Pharm.* **2000**, *211*, 37–49. [CrossRef]
43. Svensson, M.; Linse, P.; Tjerneld, F. Phase behavior in aqueous two-phase systems containing micelle-forming block copolymers. *Macromolecules* **1995**, *28*, 3597–3603. [CrossRef]
44. Johnson, C.S. Diffusion ordered nuclear magnetic resonance spectroscopy: Principles and applications. *Prog. Nucl. Magn. Reson. Spectrosc.* **1999**, *34*, 203–256. [CrossRef]
45. Momekova, D.; Budurova, D.; Drakalska, E.; Shenkov, S.; Momekov, G.; Trzebicka, B.; Lambov, N.; Tashev, E.; Rangelov, S. Aggregation behavior and in vitro biocompatibility study of octopus-shaped macromolecules based on tert-butylcalix[4]arenes. *Int. J. Pharm.* **2012**, *436*, 410–417. [CrossRef] [PubMed]
46. Connors, K.A. Correlation and prediction of solvent effects on paper chromatographic RF values. *Anal. Chem.* **1965**, *37*, 261–264. [CrossRef]
47. Ukhatskaya, E.V.; Kurkov, S.V.; Matthews, S.E.; El Fagui, A.; Amiel, C.; Dalmas, F.; Loftsson, T. Evaluation of a cationic calix[4]arene: Solubilization and self-aggregation ability. *Int. J. Pharm.* **2010**, *402*, 10–19. [CrossRef]
48. Wang, L.; Yan, J.; Li, Y.; Xu, K.; Li, S.; Tang, P.; Li, H. The influence of hydroxypropyl-β-cyclodextrin on the solubility, dissolution, cytotoxicity, and binding of riluzole with human serum albumin. *J. Pharm. Biomed. Anal.* **2016**, *117*, 453–463. [CrossRef]
49. Suvarna, V.; Kajwe, A.; Murahari, M.; Pujar, G.V.; Inturi, B.K.; Sherje, A.P. Inclusion complexes of Nateglinide with HP–β–CD and L-arginine for solubility and dissolution enhancement: Preparation, characterization, and Molecular Docking Study. *J. Pharm. Innov.* **2017**, *12*, 168–181. [CrossRef]
50. Wu, W.; Zu, Y.; Wang, L.; Wang, L.; Li, Y.; Liu, Y.; Wu, M.; Zhao, X.; Zhang, X. Preparation, characterization and antitumor activity evaluation of Silibinin nanoparticles for oral delivery through Liquid Antisolvent precipitation. *RSC Adv.* **2017**, *7*, 54379–54390. [CrossRef]
51. Furer, V.L.; Vandyukov, A.E.; Zaripov, S.R.; Solovieva, S.E.; Antipin, I.S.; Kovalenko, V.I. FT-IR and FT-raman study of hydrogen bonding in P-alkylcalix[8]arenes. *Vib. Spectrosc.* **2018**, *95*, 38–43. [CrossRef]
52. Ahmad, Z.; Shah, A.; Siddiq, M.; Kraatz, H.-B. Polymeric micelles as drug delivery vehicles. *RSC Adv.* **2014**, *4*, 17028–17038. [CrossRef]
53. Di Costanzo, A.; Angelico, R. Formulation Strategies for Enhancing the Bioavailability of Silymarin: The State of the Art. *Molecules* **2019**, *24*, 2155. [CrossRef] [PubMed]

pharmaceutics

MDPI

Article

Formulation and Characterization of Stimuli-Responsive Lecithin-Based Liposome Complexes with Poly(acrylic acid)/Poly(*N*,*N*-dimethylaminoethyl methacrylate) and Pluronic® Copolymers for Controlled Drug Delivery

Mónica G. Simões [1], Ayelen Hugo [2], Andrea Gómez-Zavaglia [2], Pedro N. Simões [1,*] and Patrícia Alves [1,*]

[1] CIEPQPF, Department of Chemical Engineering, University of Coimbra, Rua Sílvio Lima, Pólo II-Pinhal de Marrocos, 3030-790 Coimbra, Portugal; simoesmonica91@gmail.com

[2] Center for Research and Development in Food Cryotechnology (CIDCA, CCT-CONICET), La Plata 1900, Argentina; ayelen_h@yahoo.com.ar (A.H.); angoza@qui.uc.pt (A.G.-Z.)

* Correspondence: pnsim@eq.uc.pt (P.N.S.); palves@eq.uc.pt (P.A.)

Abstract: Polymer–liposome complexes (PLCs) can be efficiently applied for the treatment and/or diagnosis of several types of diseases, such as cancerous, dermatological, neurological, ophthalmic and orthopedic. In this work, temperature-/pH-sensitive PLC-based systems for controlled release were developed and characterized. The selected hydrophilic polymeric setup consists of copolymers of Pluronic®-poly(acrylic acid) (PLU-PAA) and Pluronic®-poly(*N*,*N*-dimethylaminoethyl methacrylate) (PLU-PD) synthesized by atom transfer radical polymerization (ATRP). The copolymers were incorporated into liposomes formulated from soybean lecithin, with different copolymer/phospholipid ratios (2.5, 5 and 10%). PLCs were characterized by evaluating their particle size, polydispersity, surface charge, capacity of release and encapsulation efficiency. Their cytotoxic potential was assessed by determining the viability of human epithelial cells exposed to them. The results showed that the incorporation of the synthesized copolymers positively contributed to the stabilization of the liposomes. The main accomplishments of this work were the innovative synthesis of PLU-PD and PLU-PAA by ATRP, and the liposome stabilization by their incorporation. The formulated PLCs exhibited relevant characteristics, notably stimuli-responsive attributes upon slight changes in pH and/or temperature, with proven absence of cellular toxicity, which could be of interest for the treatment or diagnosis of all diseases that cause some particular pH/temperature change in the target area.

Keywords: polymer–liposome complexes; Pluronic®-poly(acrylic acid); Pluronic®-poly(*N*,*N*-dimethylaminoethyl methacrylate); stimuli-responsive; intelligent drug delivery systems

Citation: Simões, M.G.; Hugo, A.; Gómez-Zavaglia, A.; Simões, P.N.; Alves, P. Formulation and Characterization of Stimuli-Responsive Lecithin-Based Liposome Complexes with Poly(acrylic acid)/Poly(*N*,*N*-dimethylaminoethyl methacrylate) and Pluronic® Copolymers for Controlled Drug Delivery. *Pharmaceutics* **2022**, *14*, 735. https://doi.org/10.3390/pharmaceutics14040735

Academic Editors: Juan José Torrado and Alyssa Panitch

Received: 11 February 2022
Accepted: 24 March 2022
Published: 29 March 2022

1. Introduction

The so-called smart drug delivery systems aim at targeting effectively a given active agent into a specific location by responding to stimuli such as variations in pH, temperature, light, etc. [1,2]. The role of controlled-release systems in areas such as gene therapy, the treatment and/or diagnosis of cancer, neurological, dermatologic, ophthalmologic and orthopedic diseases, as well as cosmetic products and food engineering, contributes to explaining the hundreds of publications related to this matter [3,4] and also to addressing different challenges of the food and cosmeceutical industries (the targeted release of unstable bioactives, e.g., antioxidants) [5,6]. The importance of these studies came from the continuing need to find more reliable, effective and selective drug release solutions.

Controlled delivery systems can be based on polymeric, inorganic or lipid compounds. Among them, lipids have unique properties that allow the relatively easy formation of nano-sized structures such as liposomes. They are biocompatible, biodegradable, non-immunogenic and non-toxic vesicles, ideal for the encapsulation, transport, storage and release of hydrophilic and/or lipophilic substances [7,8]. In addition, the use of liposomes as carriers enhances the solubility and stability of encapsulated drugs, and reduces their side effects and toxicity [9,10]. However, there are some drawbacks in the in vivo application of these nanocarriers since they are easily attacked and uptaken by phagocytic cells of the immune system. This instability represents a major issue and compromises the efficiency of the drug delivery at the desired target location [2]. To overcome this problem, the anchoring of polymers into the lipid bilayers of liposomes, leading to the so-called polymer–liposome complexes (PLCs), has been a successful strategy [9,11]. The presence of polymers in the liposome surface brings more mechanical resistance and prevents the capture by the phagocyte system, thus increasing the residence time of PLCs in the bloodstream, which is an essential condition for a successful treatment. Poly(ethylene glycol) (PEG)-coated liposomes represent the paradigmatic case of long-circulation liposomes that are commercialized for cancer treatment [12–14]. PEGylation involves the grafting of PEG to the surfaces of nanoparticles/liposomes, wherein ethylene glycol units form tight associations with water molecules, resulting in the formation of a hydrating layer [15].

Over the past few decades, PEG has been considered to be non-immunogenic. However, there is growing evidence that it might be more immunogenic than previously recognized. This is supported by the presence of anti-PEG antibodies in healthy humans who are increasingly exposed to PEG additives. Furthermore, there is evidence that formulations containing anticancer drugs in PEGylated liposomes (Doxil®, DaunoXome® and Ambisome®) could induce CARPA (complement activation-related pseudoallergy), which is classified as a non-IgE-mediated pseudoallergy caused by the activation of the complement system [16]. Therefore, it is very important to find new non-immunogenic, generally recognized as safe (GRAS) polymers capable of extending the half-life of liposomes.

The development of alternative intelligent-release systems based on stimuli-responsive polymers, namely those sensitive to pH and/or temperature, has been rather well accepted in the medicine and pharmaceutical fields [17]. Poly(*N*-substituted acrylamides) are among the most studied thermosensitive polymers [18], and liposomes functionalized with this class of polymers can accurately release the encapsulated drug at temperatures above the lower critical solution temperature [8]. Poly(2-(*N*,*N*-dimethylamino)ethyl methacrylate) (PDMAEMA) has been investigated for gene delivery materials [19], anticancer drug delivery by micelles [20], coating magnetic nanoparticles in cancer treatments [21] and more recently for incorporation into drug delivery liposomes [22]. Poly(acrylic acid) (PAA) is another polymer suitable to deliver and release drugs in tumors and inflammation sites due to its inherent biocompatibility, pH sensitivity and mucoadhesive properties [23–25]. PAA has been studied in the form of hydrogels and nanoparticles, and incorporated into liposomes, the latter case corresponding to pH-sensitive PLCs [24–26]. Pluronic® (PLU), also known as Poloxamer, is a biocompatible and non-toxic triblock copolymer of polypropylene oxide and ethylene oxide, with known applications in delivery systems [27]. PLU can be incorporated into liposomes to form PLCs due to the hydrophobic nature of polypropylene oxide, which promotes the polymer anchoring into the lipid bilayer [28–30]. It has been reported that PLU increases the permeation of a drug through the blood–brain barrier, affects the micro-viscosity of cells and is also capable of sensitizing and accumulating in multidrug-resistant cancer cells [31,32].

In this work, we are proposing a novel step that goes beyond previous attempts (e.g., [33]) towards the conjugation of these polymers. Here, we formulate PLCs that combine all benefits of both polymers and liposomes in just one control release system. Therefore, we are employing PLU, as a nuclear element, conjugated with PAA and PDMAEMA segments, as stimuli-responsive copolymers that can be used to formulate long-circulation pH-/temperature-sensitive PLCs. Moreover, the synthetized PLU-PAA and PLU-PD are hydrophilic polymers that could form three-dimensional networks capable of holding a large amount of water. It is possible that these polymers could also form a hydrating layer in our liposomes, as PEG does, protecting them from protein adsorption and the subsequent opsonization and destabilization.

PLU was used as an initiator in the PDMAEMA/PAA polymerization reaction, after esterification with bromide 2-bromoisobutyryl (2-BiB) [22]. The copolymers were synthesized under mild reaction conditions by control/living radical polymerization (LRP), particularly by atom transfer radical polymerization (ATRP) [34,35]. This technique allows one to obtain low molecular weights and low dispersity (Đ), which are crucial parameters to achieve an efficient polymer-based drug delivery system.

Liposomes were formulated with soybean lecithin (LC), which is a non-toxic, natural phospholipid found in the organism and is also used as a food supplement [36,37]. Given the intended drug delivery applications, release profiles, calcein loading capacity (CLC), stability at different pH/temperatures and cell viability were evaluated to select the most appropriate copolymer and copolymer/lipid ratio for the proposed PLC systems.

2. Materials and Methods

The following materials were used in the different stages of polymeric synthesis and PLC formulation: 1,1,4,7,7-pentamethyldiethylenetriamine (98%, Alfa Aesar, Kandel, Germany), 3-(4,5-dimethylthiazol-2-yl)-2,5-diphenyltetrazolium bromide (MTT, Sigma-Aldrich, St. Louis, MO, USA), 4-(2-hydroxyethyl)-1-piperazineethanesulfonic acid (HEPES, Amresco®, Seattle, WA, USA), 4-(dimethylamino)pyridine (PMDETA, 99%, Merck, Darmstadt, Germany), bromide 2-bromoisobutyryl (2-BiB, 97%, Alfa Aesar, Kandel, Germany), calcein (Acros Organics, Geel, Belgium), chloroform (99.2%, VWR Chemicals, Fontenay-sous-Bois, France), copper (I) bromide (99%, Alfa Aesar, Kandel, Germany), deuterated dimethyl sulfoxide (99.9%, Sigma-Aldrich, St. Louis, MO, USA), dialysis membranes (MWCO 3500 Da, Medicell Membranes Ltd., London, UK), dichloromethane (99.8%, VWR Chemicals, Fontenay-sous-Bois, France), dimethyl sulfoxide (DMSO, 99.6%, VWR Chemicals, Fontenay-sous-Bois, France), Dulbecco's Modified Eagle Medium (GIBCO BRL Life Technologies, Rockville, MD, USA), fetal bovine serum (FBS, PAA Laboratories, GmbH, Pasching, Austria), hydrochloric acid (37%, VWR Chemicals, Fontenay-sous-Bois, France), methanol (99%, VWR Chemicals, Fontenay-sous-Bois, France), *N,N*-dimethylaminoethyl methacrylate (DMAEMA, ≥99%, Merck, Darmstadt, Germany), n-hexane (99.3%, VWR Chemicals, Fontenay-sous-Bois, France), non-essential amino acids (GIBCO BRL Life Technologies, Rockville, MD, USA), penicillin–streptomycin solution (GIBCO BRL Life Technologies, Rockville, MD, USA), Pluronic® F68 (Sigma-Aldrich, St. Louis, MO, USA), sodium chloride (99%, Sigma-Aldrich, St. Louis, MO, USA), soybean lecithin (LC, Acros Organics, Fair Lawn, NJ, USA), tert-butyl acrylate (tBA, 99%, Alfa Aesar, Kandel, Germany), tetrahydrofuran (VWR Chemicals, Fontenay-sous-Bois, France), toluene (99%, VWR Chemicals, Fontenay-sous-Bois, France), triethylamine (99%, Merck, Darmstadt, Germany), trifluoracetic acid (99%, VWR Chemicals, Fontenay-sous-Bois, France) and Triton® X-100 (Sigma-Aldrich, St. Louis, MO, USA).

2.1. Synthesis of Pluronic®-2-Bromoisobutyrate (PLU-Br)

The initiator was obtained by the esterification of Pluronic® F68 (PLU) with bromide 2-bromoisobutyryl (2-BiB) (Figure 1A). This approach is based on the synthesis of cholesterol-2-bromoisobutyrate (CHO-Br) reported by Alves et al. [18]. Briefly, a 1 g sample of 4-(dimethylamino)pyridine (previously recrystallized from toluene) in 10 mL of dry dichloromethane was mixed with 0.7 mL of triethylamine (dried over CaH_2 and vacuum-distilled). The solution was transferred to a 250 mL three-neck round-bottom flask equipped with a condenser, dropping funnel, gas inlet/outlet and a magnetic stirrer. After cooling to 0 °C, 1.5 mL of 2-BiB in 10 mL of dry dichloromethane was added. Then, 21 g of PLU in 50 mL of dry dichloromethane was added dropwise to the formed yellow dispersion, for 1 h under dry nitrogen; subsequently, the temperature was raised to 28 °C. The reaction was kept under stirring for 22 h. Afterwards, the mixture was washed with a saturated aqueous sodium chloride solution and dried over magnesium sulfate, followed by evaporation of half of the solvent. The PLU-Br initiator was precipitated in ethanol and finally filtered and dried in vacuum. The final product was obtained in the form of a white powder and characterized by ^{1}H NMR.

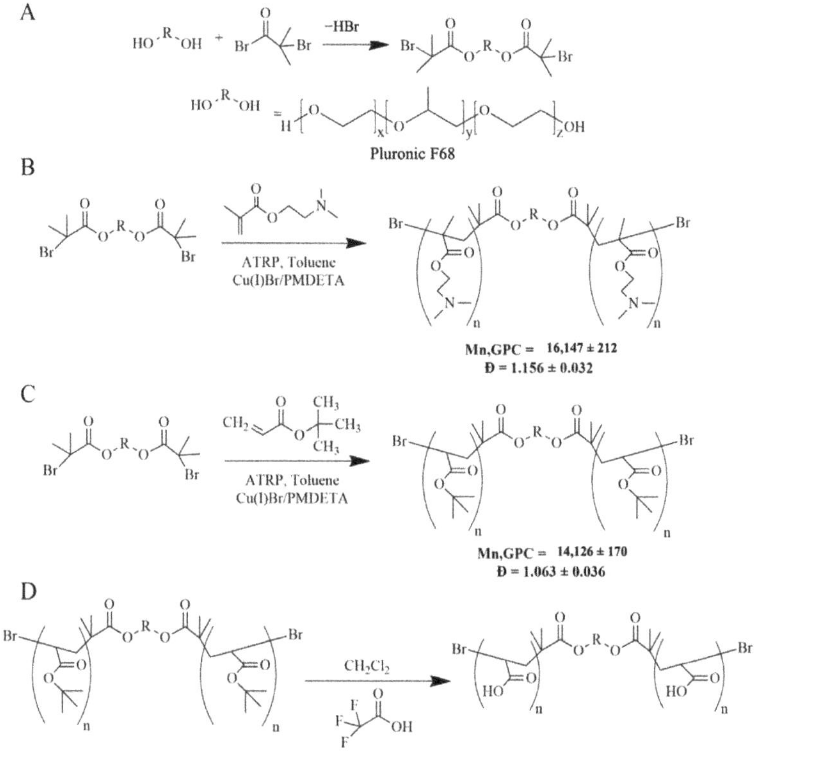

Figure 1. Schematic representation of the (**A**) synthesis of Pluronic®-2-bromoisobutyrate (PLU-Br), (**B**) synthesis of Pluronic®-poly(*N*,*N*-dimethylaminoethyl methacrylate) (PLU-PD), (**C**) synthesis of Pluronic®-poly(tert-butyl acrylate) (PLU-PtBA) and (**D**) synthesis of Pluronic®-poly(acrylic acid) (PLU-PAA). Molecular weight and dispersity obtained by GPC analysis of PLU-PD and PLU-PtBA are also presented.

2.2. Synthesis of Pluronic®-Poly(N,N-dimethylaminoethyl methacrylate) (PLU-PD)

PLU-PD was synthesized by ATRP (Figure 1B) according to Eugene et al. [33]. To obtain the copolymer, the previously prepared PLU-Br was used as an initiator, copper (I) bromide as a catalyst, 1,1,4,7,7-pentamethyldiethylenetriamine (PMDETA) as a ligand and toluene as a solvent. Succinctly, the monomer *N*,*N*-dimethylaminoethyl methacrylate (DMAEMA, 2 mL freshly passed through a Al_2O_3 column) and 600 mg of the initiator PLU-Br were added to a 25 mL Schlenk flask equipped with a magnetic stirrer, and frozen and bubbled with N_2 to eliminate oxygen. Then, 30 mg of copper (I) bromide, 26 mg of PMDETA and 2 mL of toluene (previously bubbled with N_2) were added under N_2 atmosphere to the Schlenk flask, which was then sealed and deoxygenated under reduced pressure and then filled with N_2. The reaction proceeded for 24 h at 80 °C, after which it was quenched by the addition of acetone and exposure to air. Purification was achieved by passing the obtained product through a neutral alumina column using acetone as the eluent, then dialyzed for 48 h, dried by evaporation, dissolved in water, frozen at −20 °C for 24 h and freeze-dried at −50 °C and 0.04 mbar in an Alpha 1–2 LD Plus (CHRIST, Osterode am Harz, Germany) for an additional 48 h. The obtained polymer was analyzed by gel permeation chromatography (GPC) and nuclear magnetic resonance (^{1}H NMR).

2.3. Synthesis of Pluronic®-Poly(tert-butyl acrylate) (PLU-PtBA)

PLU-PtBA was also obtained via ATRP (Figure 1C) from the same procedure used in the synthesis of PLU-PD previously described, except for the monomer used, which was tert-butyl acrylate (tBA) instead of DMAEMA; also different were the reagent quantities (500 mg of PLU-Br, 24 mg of copper (I) bromide and 30 mg of PMDETA) and reaction time, which, in this case, was 30 min. Once purified and isolated, the obtained polymer was analyzed by GPC and ^{1}H NMR.

2.4. Synthesis of Pluronic®-Poly(poly(acrylic acid) (PLU-PAA)—PLU-PtBA Hydrolysis

PLU-PtBA was hydrolyzed in order to obtain PLU-PAA (Figure 1D) [38]. Briefly, PLU-PtBA was added to a round-bottom flask with three necks (equipped with a condenser, an addition funnel and magnetic stirring) with 10 mL of dichloromethane, in a bath at 0 °C under N_2 atmosphere. A 5-fold molar excess of trifluoroacetic acid was added dropwise to the flask, and then the temperature was slowly raised to 30 °C. After 48 h of reaction, the polymer was precipitated in n-hexane, filtered and dried under vacuum at 40 °C until a constant weight. PLU-PAA was characterized by ^{1}H NMR.

2.5. Characterization of the Initiator and Polymers

2.5.1. Nuclear Magnetic Resonance (NMR)

^{1}H NMR spectra were collected in a Bruker Avance III 400 MHz spectrometer (Bruker, Billerica, MA, USA), by using deuterated dimethyl sulfoxide as a solvent and tetramethylsilane (TMS) as an internal standard, in 5-mm-diameter tubes.

2.5.2. Gel Permeation Chromatography (GPC)

The number-average molecular weight (M_n) and dispersity ($Đ = M_w/M_n$) of PLU-PtBA and PLU-PD were determined by GPC, in a Viscotek (Dual detector 270, Viscotek, Houston, TX, USA), with THF as the eluent at 30 °C (1.0 mL/min). Narrow polystyrene standards were used for the calibration. OmniSEC software (Malvern Instruments, Malvern, UK) was used along with the TriSEC calibration to determine the $M_{n,GPC}$ and Đ of the obtained polymers.

2.6. Preparation of Liposomes and Polymer–Liposome Complexes (PLCs)

Liposomes were prepared according to the hydration film method [3,22,24], which consists of dissolving soybean lecithin (LC) in chloroform (2.9 mM) in a round-bottom flask. A N_2 stream was then used to evaporate all the chloroform, thus allowing the formation of a thin lipid film. Bare liposomes (LIP) were obtained by rehydrating the lipidic film in a buffered solution of 50 mM 4-(2-hydroxyethyl)-1-piperazineethanesulfonic acid (HEPES) at pH 7.0, vigorously stirred and incubated for 24 h above the transition temperature (ca. 37 °C). PLCs were obtained by adding the copolymer solution of PLU, PLU-PD or PLU-PAA in HEPES (10 mg/mL) to the LIP in copolymer/LC molar ratios of 2.5, 5 and 10%. The formulations were further vigorously stirred and left for a further 24 h at 37 °C for the incorporation of polymers into the liposome bilayers, leading to PLCs.

2.7. Particle Size and ζ-Potential Measurements

A Malvern Instrument Zetasizer Nano-Z (Malvern Instruments, Malvern, UK) was used to evaluate particle size and ζ-potential measurements, at 37 °C. The average hydrodynamic particle size (Z-average) and polydispersive index (PdI) were determined by dynamic light scattering at backward scattering (173°) with the Zetasizer 6.20 (Malvern Instruments, Malvern, UK). ζ-potential was determined using a combination of measurement techniques: electrophoresis and laser Doppler velocimetry (Laser Doppler Electrophoresis) (Malvern Instrument Zetasizer Nano-Z, Malvern Instruments, Malvern, UK). ζ-potential outcomes were provided directly by the instrument. The results presented are the average and standard deviation of at least 10 replicates per sample.

2.8. Retention Capacity and Leakage Experiments

Calcein was used as a fluorescent dye for the release experiments by means of its encapsulation into the aqueous compartment of the liposomes. Briefly, the lipid films obtained after chloroform evaporation were hydrated with 60 mM calcein in HEPES (50 mM, pH 7.0), vigorously stirred and incubated for 24 h above the transition temperature (ca. 37 °C) to obtain calcein-loaded LIPs. The incorporation of the copolymers into calcein-loaded PLCs followed the procedure previously described. To eliminate the non-entrapped calcein from the external medium, LIPs and PLCs were centrifuged (10,000 rpm for 5 min, three times; Centurion Scientific Ltd., Stoughton, UK). Washed PLCs were resuspended in 200 μL of HEPES (50 mM, pH 7.0) [22,39].

Release profiles and drug retention capacity along time (up to 35 h) of all formulations were determined fluorometrically on a Synergy HT fluorescence microplate reader (Bio-Tek Instruments, Winooski, VT, USA) with excitation and emission wavelengths at 485/20 nm and 528/20 nm, respectively.

Calcein-loaded LIPs and PLCs were used to evaluate the stability of the liposomes after 15 min incubation time under physiological conditions (37 °C, pH 7.0), and at pH 2, 4, 7 and 11 (37 °C), and at 42 °C (pH 7.0). The fluorescence intensity was determined along time. After the last recording, to induce its total lysis (100% release of calcein), 20 μL of a solution of Triton X-100 (10%, *v*/*v*) was added to each sample [22]. Calcein release percentage was obtained according to Equation (1).

$$\%\ Release = \frac{(F - F_i)}{(F_t - F_i)} \times 100 \quad (1)$$

where (F) is the fluorescence intensity of the sample after each incubation time, (F_i) is the initial fluorescence intensity of the sample, and (F_t) is the total fluorescence intensity of the sample after the addition of Triton-X100. The calcein loading capacity, *CLC* (%), of each test was determined as the molar concentration of calcein per molar concentration of lipid (Equation (2)).

$$CLC(\%) = \frac{[Calcein]}{[Lipid]} \times 100 \quad (2)$$

A calibration curve ($[Calcein] = 1 \times 10^{-3}\ (F_t - F_i)$, $R^2 = 0.99$) was used to obtain the molar concentration of the encapsulated calcein. The molar concentrations of lipids in LIPs and PLCs were obtained by using a commercial kit (CHO-POD enzymatic colorimetric from Spinreact, Lisbon, Portugal) following the instructions of the manufacturer, and the concentrations were normalized to the total lipid content [40,41].

2.9. Cytotoxicity Assays

Cell viability was determined by assessing mitochondrial dehydrogenase activity, using 3-(4,5-dimethylthiazol-2-yl)-2,5-diphenyltetrazolium bromide (MTT). For use in the assays, human epithelial HEp-2 cells (ATCC, Manassas, VA, USA) were cultured in DMEM (Gibco, Grand Island, NY, USA) supplemented with 10% (*v*/*v*) heat-inactivated (30 min/60 °C) fetal bovine serum, and 1% (*w*/*v*) non-essential amino acids and 1% (*v*/*v*) penicillin–streptomycin solution (100 U/mL penicillin G, 100 μg/mL streptomycin). HEp-2 cells were seeded in 48-well plates at 1×10^5 cells per well and incubated at 37 °C in a 5% CO_2 95% air atmosphere, to early post-confluence.

LIP and PLCs (75, 375 and 750 μM, in both cases) were added to the cells, in triplicate, and incubated for 24 h. The cells were then washed twice with PBS and the medium replaced with DMEM (without phenol red dye) containing 0.5 mg/mL MTT. After 2 h incubation, 0.2 mL dimethylsulfoxide was added to each well and stirred for 20 min at 25 °C on a plate shaker to solubilize the cells and the formed formazan crystals. The optical density

(OD) values were collected in a Synergy HT fluorescence microplate reader at 490 nm (Bio-Tek Instruments, Winooski, VT, USA). *Cell viability* was calculated by Equation (3).

$$Cell\ Viability\ (\%) = \frac{OD_t}{OD_c} \times 100\% \quad (3)$$

where OD_t is the optical density of the cells treated with liposomes, and OD_c is the optical density of the non-treated control cells.

3. Results

The synthesis success of the two copolymers was confirmed by ^1H NMR (Figure 2). From PLU (Figure 2A) to PLU-Br spectra (Figure 2B), a peak at 2.1 ppm appears (d, CH_3C–Br), indicating the presence of the 2-bromo-2-methylpropionyl groups from the esterification of the PLU with the 2-BiB, confirming the modification/initiator synthesis [22,33]. Figure 2C shows the PLU-PtBA spectrum with a new peak at 1.45 ppm. This chemical shift is ascribed to the methyl protons (e, $-C(CH_3)$) of the tBA segments. PLU-PAA (Figure 2D) was obtained by removing the tert-butyl groups of PLU-PtBA by acidic hydrolysis, as shown in Figure 2C. In Figure 2D, after the hydrolysis, the chemical shift of tert-butyl groups (1.45 ppm) vanishes completely, which confirms its success. In Figure 2E, the signals at 2.2–2.4 ppm are ascribed to methyl (f, N–CH_3) and methylene (g, N–CH_2) protons of DMAEMA segments, and at 4.2 ppm to the methylene protons adjacent to the oxygen moieties of the ester linkages (h, H_2CO–C=O). The number-average molecular weight (M_n) and dispersity (Đ = M_w/M_n) of PLU-PtBA and PLU-PD obtained from GPC analysis are included in Figure 1. The success of the polymerization approach is supported by both Đ close to one and the high conversion level (99% and 84% for PLU-PD and PLU-PAA, respectively), the latter obtained by peak integration of the ^1H NMR spectra.

LIPs' and PLCs' particle size and ζ-potential were assessed at 37 °C and pH 7.0. PLCs were prepared with copolymer/lipid ratios of 2.5, 5 and 10%, and the corresponding Z-average, PdI and ζ-potential are gathered in Table 1. Comparing LIPs with PLCs, an increase in particle size is observed after the functionalization. Generally, PLCs' Z-average increases with the percentage of copolymer added. On the other hand, PdI changes slightly, although it is below 0.5 in every case. Vesicles with a higher percentage of PLU-PD exhibit lower absolute values of ζ-potential. The opposite effect can be noticed in PLU-PAA PLCs, while LIPs are the most negative vesicles studied. The CLC results are also summarized in Table 1. PLCs present higher EE than LIP for all copolymer/lipid ratios, and the PLCs with 5% of PLU-PD/PLU-PAA are those with the highest CLC (ca. 27%).

PLCs' stability was estimated by measuring calcein release at 37 °C and pH 7 (Figure 3). All samples exhibit lower releases when compared to LIPs. PLCs with 10% of PLU-PD/PLU-PAA show a release of ca. 25% after 30 h, which contrasts with LIPs, which release around 60% of their encapsulated calcein after the same time. Moreover, the increase in the PLCs' copolymer/lipid ratio also lowers the release rate, which indicates enhanced efficiency in retaining the content. Among copolymers, PLU-PD was demonstrated to be more effective than PLU-PAA, considering that, for the same incubation time and amount of copolymer, the PLU-PAA PLCs are faster releasers (i.e., 5% PLCs, Figure 3).

Calcein release was also determined at different pHs (from 2 to 11, at 37 °C) and different temperatures (37 and 42 °C, at pH 7), as shown in Figures 4 and 5a, respectively. When slight changes in pH were applied (either higher or lower then 7.0), PLCs became significantly less stable (Figure 4). As expected, the same outcome was not observed in LIPs (Figure 4). Among the copolymers, the pH destabilization is more evident with PLU-PAA PLCs (i.e., 10% PLCs, Figure 4). On the other hand, PLU-PD PLCs exhibit a faster and higher calcein release at 42 °C (ca. 22%) for the same incubation time (Figure 5a).

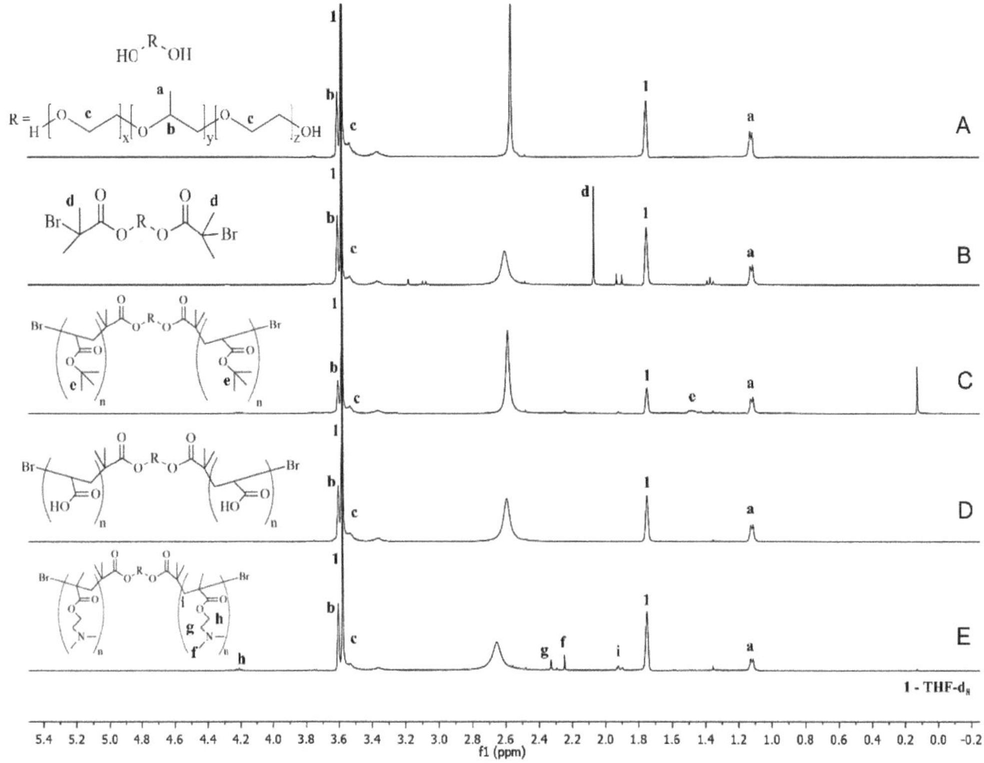

Figure 2. ^{1}H-NMR spectra of (**A**) Pluronic® F68, (**B**) PLU-Br, (**C**) PLU-PtBA, (**D**) PLU-PAA and (**E**) PLU-PD, where (a) –CH_3 is the methyl protons of PPO units; (b) –CH is the methine proton of PPO units; (c) –CH_2 is the methylene proton of PEO units; (d) CH_3C–Br, from 2-bromo-2-methylpropionyl group; (e) –$C(CH_3)$ is the methyl protons of tBA units; (f) N–CH_3 is the methyl protons of DMAEMA units; (g) N–CH_2 is the methylene protons of DMAEMA units; (h) H_2C–O–C=O is the methylene protons of DMAEMA units; (i) −CH_2− from PDMAEMA backbone.

Table 1. Physical characterization of LIPs and PLCs at 37 °C and pH = 7. Molar concentration of encapsulated calcein, molar concentration of lipids and CLC. Data denoted as mean ± standard deviation (SD), n = 5.

Formulation	Z-Average (nm)	PdI	ζ-Potential (mV)	[Calcein] (mM)	[Lipid] (mM)	CLC (%)
LIP	236.1 ± 7.1	0.439 ± 0.06	−28.2 ± 4.6	0.029 ± 0.002	0.259 ± 0.04	11.1 ± 0.4
PLU-PD 2.5%	267.7 ± 8.9	0.377 ± 0.05	−24.5 ± 6.4	0.064 ± 0.004	0.256 ± 0.05	25.1 ± 1.5
PLU-PD 5%	351.0 ± 8.0	0.433 ± 0.03	−21.0 ± 3.2	0.074 ± 0.005	0.269 ± 0.02	27.3 ± 1.7
PLU-PD 10%	362.5 ± 7.7	0.426 ± 0.04	−18.9 ± 8.2	0.054 ± 0.006	0.246 ± 0.07	21.9 ± 2.5
PLU-PAA 2.5%	244.9 ± 8.3	0.484 ± 0.08	−20.3 ± 2.5	0.041 ± 0.002	0.210 ± 0.03	19.6 ± 0.8
PLU-PAA 5%	225.1 ± 2.8	0.436 ± 0.07	−24.8 ± 3.1	0.064 ± 0.006	0.236 ± 0.03	27.0 ± 2.7
PLU-PAA 10%	253.7 ± 7.2	0.397 ± 0.08	−26.2 ± 8.8	0.041 ± 0.002	0.226 ± 0.05	18.1 ± 0.9

Regarding cell viability studies, Figure 5b depicts the percentage survival of HEp-2 cells when exposed to different concentrations of LIPs and 10% PLU-PD/PLU-PAA PLCs, after 24 h. The results demonstrate that, for the tested concentrations, LIPs and/or PLCs are revealed to be non-cytotoxic to HEp-2 cells.

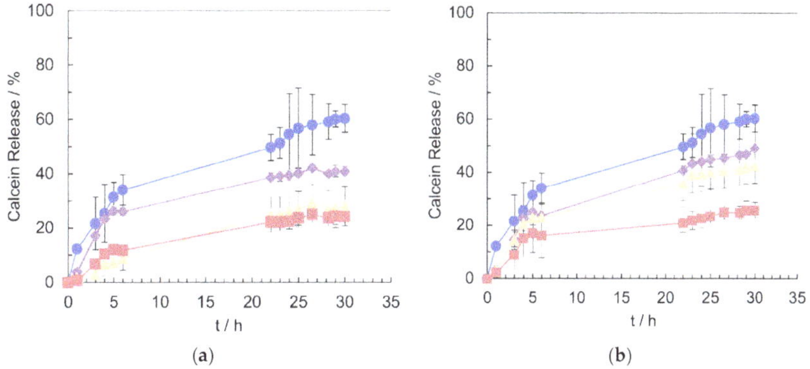

Figure 3. Calcein release profiles at 37 °C and pH = 7. Blue circles: LIP; purple diamonds: 2.5% of copolymer; orange triangles: 5% of copolymer; pink squares: 10% of copolymer. (**a**) PLU-PD PLCs. (**b**) PLU-PAA PLCs. Results are expressed as mean ± standard deviation (SD), n = 3.

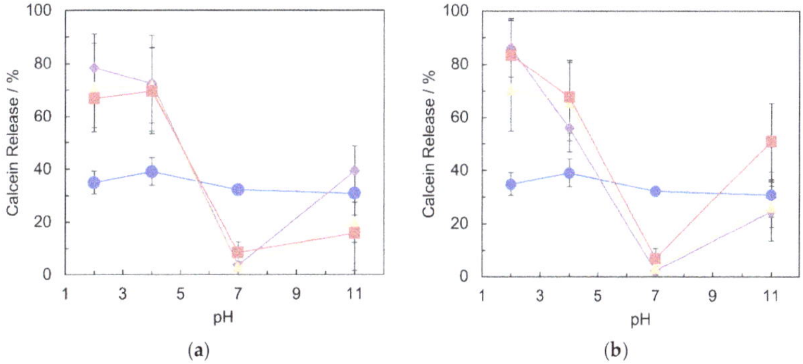

Figure 4. Calcein release profiles after 2 h of incubation at 37 °C and different pHs. Blue circles: LIP; purple diamonds: 2.5% of copolymer; orange triangles: 5% of copolymer; pink squares: 10% of copolymer. (**a**) PLU-PD PLCs. (**b**) PLU-PAA PLCs. Results are expressed as mean ± standard deviation (SD), n = 3.

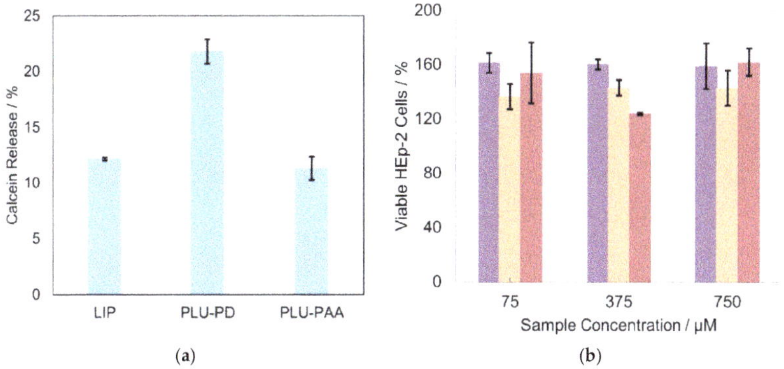

Figure 5. (**a**) Calcein release of LIP, PLCs with 10% PLU-PD and PLCs with 10% PLU-PAA after 2 h of incubation at 42 °C and pH = 7. Results are expressed as mean ± standard deviation (SD), n = 3. (**b**) Viability of HEp-2 cells after 24 h of incubation with LIP (purple bars), PLCs of 10% PLU-PD (orange bars) and PLCs of 10% PLU-PAA (pink bars). Results are expressed as mean ± standard deviation (SD), n = 3.

4. Discussion

As far as we are aware, the synthesis of PAA or PDMAEMA copolymers using the ATRP method with PLU-Br as an initiator has never been reported in the context of PLC formulation. Compared with other LRP methods, e.g., oxyanion-initiated polymerization [35,42] and reversible addition-fragmentation chain transfer (RAFT) polymerization [43], ATRP (Figures 1 and 2) is simpler and avoids severe conditions. Moreover, the LRP approach stands out due to the strict control of the copolymer homogeneity in terms of both structure and molecular weight, allowing low Đ values and high conversion levels to be achieved. The advantage of using PLU-PD and PLU-PAA copolymers for the formulation of PLCs rests on the PLU hydrophobic segment and its high affinity with the lipid membranes, which enables and facilitates their incorporation [44]. Furthermore, thanks to the stimuli-responsive character of PAA and PDMAEMA segments [22,24], pH-/temperature-sensitive PLCs could be developed.

The low Z-average and PdI results (Table 1) reveal acceptable homogeneity and size distributions of the formulated PLCs, which are key parameters for several biomedical applications. For instance, small particles (e.g., liposomes) are able to accumulate in tumors due to their higher permeation capacity [3,4,45]. Nevertheless, further studies are necessary in order to tune these parameters according to the targeted application.

Concerning the ζ-potential, the observed trends can be explained by the positive and negative character of PDMAEMA and PAA, respectively (Table 1). The PDMAEMA and PAA segments of the synthesized copolymers, PLU-PD and PLU-PAA, are located at the external side of the liposomes. Therefore, the surface charge of PLCs is determined by the polymer and tuned according to the copolymer/lipid ratios (Table 1). In addition, the ζ-potential values are significantly negative, which contributes to preventing the agglomeration of the developed PLCs, and thus to keeping them stable over time, as desired. Taking into account both surface charge distribution and copolymer size, the stabilization of electrosteric quality is plausible [46].

The stabilizing effect of PLU-PD and PLU-PAA was confirmed by the PLCs' improved CLC (Table 1) and low release profiles obtained at 37 °C and pH 7.0, when compared with LIPs (Figure 3). The copolymers incorporated on the LIP surface avoid cell uptake and act as an extra barrier to the encapsulated dye, preventing its escape. Even if, during the PLC washing, some calcein is lost [3,9,47], a larger amount of dye is kept in the inner aqueous compartment of the liposomes when conjugated with the copolymers, thus explaining the significant difference between LIPs' and PLCs' CLC (Table 1).

In a simulated physiological medium for release (37 °C and pH 7.0), LIPs and PLCs show again a distinct behavior (Figure 3). LIPs, which present a low CLC (ca. 11%), are also less stable than any PLC formulation, releasing up to 60% of their content after 30 h (Figure 3). On the contrary, PLU-PD and PLU-PAA PLCs show lower release profiles. Moreover, increasing the copolymer/lipid ratio in the complex, the release becomes slower, ca. 25% after 30 h for 10% PLU-PDMAEA/PAA (Figure 3), which indicates that, from both formulations, the PLCs' content release can be controlled and tuned.

Additionally, in acid and alkaline medium, at 37 °C, PLCs show pH stimuli-responsive properties in the form of a sharp and high percentage release profile at certain pH values (Figure 4). A possible explanation for this behavior lies in the conformational changes of PDMAEMA/PAA when exposed to mild to acidic or alkali conditions (Figure 4) [22,24]. The fast release at low pH is especially relevant for cancer treatments, because tumor areas are typically acidic, which can promote the drug release only in that specific zone [48]. The PLCs' destabilization above pH 7 may appear less interesting, although, for other purposes, such as diagnosis or therapeutic monitoring, it might be a relevant attribute.

These results confirm the development of pH stimuli-responsive PLCs both with PLU-PD and PLU-PAA, which are possible candidates for pH-sensitive drug delivery systems [35,42,49].

Contrariwise, for the thermal stimuli experiments at 42 °C and pH 7, the difference between PLU-PD and PLU-PAA PLCs is notorious, as shown in Figure 5a. LIP and PLU-

PAA PLCs released a low percentage of calcein after 2 h of incubation (ca. 10%), comparable to the release profiles observed at 37 °C (Figures 3 and 4), indicating no sensitivity to the temperature change. In contrast, PLU-PD PLCs released ~23% of the total encapsulated calcein in the same 2 h, which is a result substantially different from that observed at 37 °C (ca. 5% after 2 h and ~25% after 30 h of incubation) (Figures 3 and 4), revealing a clear sensitivity to higher temperatures [43]. This characteristic of PLU-PD PLCs is interesting, particularly for cases where the desired release site presents higher temperatures, above 37 °C as, e.g., in tumors and adjacent regions or local infections [22].

Cell viability studies are essential in the development of appropriate PLC formulations. The results presented in Figure 5b demonstrate that all studied PLCs reveal no cytotoxicity towards HEp-2 cells within the range of the tested concentrations. The percentages above 100% indicate that all cells were able not only to survive but also to reproduce in the presence of the LIP and PLCs (Figure 5b). Therefore, all the results of this work consolidate the potential of the developed PLU-PDMAEMA and PLU-PAA PLCs as long-circulation stimuli-responsive drug delivery systems for biomedical applications.

5. Conclusions

PLU-PD and PLU-PAA copolymers were successfully synthesized by ATRP with PLU-Br as the initiator, the latter obtained by esterification of PLU with 2-BiB. Low-molecular-weight and -dispersity copolymers were obtained, which is a crucial feature towards the formulation of PLCs.

The incorporation and anchoring of these copolymers in liposomes resulted in long-term functional PLCs with acceptable average size and polydispersity and without a tendency to aggregate. The achieved low and controlled release, considerable retention (CLC) and pH/temperature sensitivity are distinctive factors given that temperatures above physiologic levels and low pH are common in tumors and inflammation regions. Furthermore, no cytotoxicity towards HEp-2 cells was detected.

Overall, safe and stable PLCs with pH/thermal stimuli-responsive properties were developed, which can be loaded with any type of hydrophilic or hydrophobic active compound for the treatment and/or diagnosis of a large number of diseases.

Author Contributions: Conceptualization, M.G.S., A.H. and P.A.; methodology, M.G.S. and A.H.; validation, A.G.-Z., P.N.S. and P.A.; formal analysis, M.G.S. and A.H.; investigation, M.G.S., A.H. and P.A.; resources, A.G.-Z. and P.N.S.; writing—original draft preparation, M.G.S., A.H. and P.A.; writing—review and editing, M.G.S., A.H., A.G.-Z., P.N.S. and P.A.; visualization, M.G.S. and P.A.; supervision, A.G.-Z., P.N.S. and P.A.; project administration, P.N.S. and P.A.; funding acquisition, A.G.-Z., P.N.S. and P.A. All authors have read and agreed to the published version of the manuscript.

Funding: This research was funded by the Argentinean Agency for the Scientific and Technological Promotion (ANPCyT) [Projects PICT (2017)/1344; PICT start-up (2016)/4808]. A.H. and A.G.-Z. are members of the research career CONICET. The authors from CIEPQPF were supported by FCT—Fundação para a Ciência e a Tecnologia (Portuguese Foundation for Science and Technology) UIDB/00102/2020.

Institutional Review Board Statement: Not applicable.

Informed Consent Statement: Not applicable.

Data Availability Statement: The raw/processed data required to reproduce these findings cannot be shared at this time due to technical or time limitations, but will be sent upon request.

Acknowledgments: NMR data were collected at the UC-NMR facility, which is supported in part by FEDER—European Regional Development Fund—through the COMPETE Programme (Operational Programme for Competitiveness) and by national funds through FCT—Fundação para a Ciência e a Tecnologia (Portuguese Foundation for Science and Technology) through grants RECI/QEQ-QFI/0168/2012 and CENTRO-07-CT62-FEDER-002012, and also through support to Rede Nacional de Ressonância Magnética Nuclear (RNRMN) and to Coimbra Chemistry Centre through grant UID/QUI/00313/2019.

Conflicts of Interest: The authors declare no conflict of interest. The funders had no role in the design of the study; in the collection, analyses, or interpretation of data; in the writing of the manuscript, or in the decision to publish the results.

References

1. Pattni, B.S.; Chupin, V.V.; Torchilin, V.P. New Developments in Liposomal Drug Delivery. *Chem. Rev.* **2015**, *115*, 10938–10966. [CrossRef] [PubMed]
2. Bakker-Woudenberg, I.A.J.M. Long-circulating sterically stabilized liposomes as carriers of agents for treatment of infection or for imaging infectious foci. *Int. J. Antimicrob. Agents* **2002**, *19*, 299–311. [CrossRef]
3. Laouini, A.; Jaafar-Maalej, C.; Limayem-Blouza, I.; Sfar, S.; Charcosset, C.; Fessi, H. Preparation, Characterization and Applications of Liposomes: State of the Art. *J. Colloid Sci. Biotechnol.* **2012**, *1*, 147–168. [CrossRef]
4. Storm, G.; Crommelin, D.J.A. Liposomes: Quo vadis? *Pharm. Sci. Technol. Today* **1998**, *1*, 19–31. [CrossRef]
5. Hougeir, F.G.; Kircik, L. A review of delivery systems in cosmetics. *Dermatol. Ther.* **2012**, *25*, 234–237. [CrossRef]
6. Awulachew, M.T.; Desta, A.B.; Sefefe, M. *Encapsulation and Control Release in Food Engineering*; LAP Lambert Academic Publishing: Chisinau, Moldova, 2021.
7. Torchilin, V. Multifunctional nanocarriers. *Adv. Drug Deliv. Rev.* **2006**, *58*, 1532–1555. [CrossRef] [PubMed]
8. Akbarzadeh, A.; Rezaei-Sadabady, R.; Davaran, S.; Joo, S.W.; Zarghami, N.; Hanifehpour, Y.; Samiei, M.; Kouhi, M.; Nejati-Koshki, K. Liposome: Classification, preparation, and applications. *Nanoscale Res. Lett.* **2013**, *8*, 102. [CrossRef] [PubMed]
9. Kulkarni, P.R.; Yadav, J.D.; Vaidya, K.a. Liposomes: A Novel Drug Delivery System. *Int. J. Curr. Pharm. Res.* **2011**, *3*, 10–18.
10. Vemuri, S.; Rhodes, C. Preparation and characterization of liposomes as therapeutic delivery systems: A review. *Pharm. Acta Helv.* **1995**, *70*, 95–111. [CrossRef]
11. Lee, S.M.; Chen, H.; O'Halloran, T.V.; Nguyen, S.T. "Clickable" polymer-caged nanobins as a modular drug delivery platform. *J. Am. Chem. Soc.* **2009**, *131*, 9311–9320. [CrossRef]
12. Immordino, M.L.; Dosio, F.; Cattel, L. Stealth liposomes: Review of the basic science, rationale, and clinical applications, existing and potential. *Int. J. Nanomed.* **2006**, *1*, 297–315.
13. Torchilin, V.P. Multifunctional, stimuli-sensitive nanoparticulate systems for drug delivery. *Nat. Rev. Drug Discov.* **2014**, *13*, 813–827. [CrossRef] [PubMed]
14. Lee, S.M.; Chen, H.; Dettmer, C.M.; O'Halloran, T.V.; Nguyen, S.T. Polymer-Caged Lipsome: pH-Responsive Delivery System High Stability. *J. Am. Chem. Soc.* **2007**, *129*, 15096–15097. [CrossRef] [PubMed]
15. Blanco, E.; Shen, H.; Ferrari, M. Principles of nanoparticle design for overcoming biological barriers to drug delivery. *Nat. Biotechnol.* **2015**, *33*, 941–951. [CrossRef] [PubMed]
16. Mohamed, M.; Abu Lila, A.S.; Shimizu, T.; Alaaeldin, E.; Hussein, A.; Sarhan, H.A.; Szebeni, J.; Ishida, T. PEGylated liposomes: Immunological responses. *Sci. Technol. Adv. Mater.* **2019**, *20*, 710–724. [CrossRef]
17. Cabane, E.; Zhang, X.; Langowska, K.; Palivan, C.G.; Meier, W. Stimuli-Responsive Polymers and Their Applications in Nanomedicine. *Biointerphases* **2012**, *7*, 9. [CrossRef]
18. Ta, T.; Porter, T.M. Thermosensitive liposomes for localized delivery and triggered release of chemotherapy. *J. Control. Release* **2013**, *169*, 112–125. [CrossRef]
19. Agarwal, S.; Zhang, Y.; Maji, S.; Greiner, A. PDMAEMA based gene delivery materials. *Mater. Today* **2012**, *15*, 388–393. [CrossRef]
20. Car, A.; Baumann, P.; Duskey, J.T.; Chami, M.; Bruns, N.; Meier, W. pH-Responsive PDMS- b -PDMAEMA Micelles for Intracellular Anticancer Drug Delivery. *Biomacromolecules* **2014**, *15*, 3235–3245. [CrossRef]
21. Ioana Lungu, I.; Rădulescu, M.; Dan Mogoşanu, G.; Mihai Grumezescu, A. pH sensitive core-shell magnetic nanoparticles for targeted drug delivery in cancer therapy. *Rom. J. Morphol. Embryol.* **2016**, *57*, 23–32.
22. Alves, P.; Hugo, A.A.; Tymczyszyn, E.E.; Ferreira, A.F.; Fausto, R.; Pérez, P.F.; Coelho, J.F.J.; Simões, P.N.; Gómez-Zavaglia, A. Effect of cholesterol-poly(N,N-dimethylaminoethyl methacrylate) on the properties of stimuli-responsive polymer liposome complexes. *Colloids Surf. B Biointerfaces* **2012**, *104*, 254–261. [CrossRef] [PubMed]
23. Zhu, L.; Torchilin, V.P. Stimulus-responsive nanopreparations for tumor targeting. *Integr. Biol.* **2012**, *5*, 96–107. [CrossRef]
24. Simões, M.G.; Alves, P.; Carvalheiro, M.; Simões, P.N. Stability effect of cholesterol-poly(acrylic acid) in a stimuli-responsive polymer-liposome complex obtained from soybean lecithin for controlled drug delivery. *Colloids Surf. B Biointerfaces* **2017**, *152*, 103–113. [CrossRef] [PubMed]
25. Vasi, A.-M.; Popa, M.I.; Tanase, E.C.; Butnaru, M.; Verestiuc, L. Poly(Acrylic Acid)–Poly(Ethylene Glycol) Nanoparticles Designed for Ophthalmic Drug Delivery. *J. Pharm. Sci.* **2014**, *103*, 676–686. [CrossRef] [PubMed]
26. Lo, Y.-L.; Hsu, C.-Y.; Lin, H.-R. pH-and thermo-sensitive pluronic/poly(acrylic acid) in situ hydrogels for sustained release of an anticancer drug. *J. Drug Target.* **2013**, *21*, 54–66. [CrossRef]
27. Zhirnov, A.E.; Demina, T.V.; Krylova, O.O.; Grozdova, I.; Melik-Nubarov, N.S. Lipid composition determines interaction of liposome membranes with Pluronic L61. *Biochim. Biophys. Acta Biomembr.* **2005**, *1720*, 73–83. [CrossRef]
28. Zhang, Y.; Lam, Y.M.; Tan, W. Poly(ethylene oxide)–poly(propylene oxide)–poly(ethylene oxide)-g-poly(vinylpyrrolidone): Association behavior in aqueous solution and interaction with anionic surfactants. *J. Colloid Interface Sci.* **2005**, *285*, 74–79. [CrossRef]

29. Bonacucina, G.; Cespi, M.; Mencarelli, G.; Giorgioni, G.; Palmieri, G.F. Thermosensitive Self-Assembling Block Copolymers as Drug Delivery Systems. *Polymers* **2011**, *3*, 779–811. [CrossRef]
30. Hosseinzadeh, H.; Atyabi, F.; Dinarvand, R.; Ostad, S.N. Chitosan-Pluronic nanoparticles as oral delivery of anticancer gemcitabine: Preparation and in vitro study. *Int. J. Nanomed.* **2012**, *7*, 1851–1863.
31. Krupka, T.M.; Exner, A.A. Structural parameters governing activity of Pluronic triblock copolymers in hyperthermia cancer therapy. *Int. J. Hyperth.* **2011**, *27*, 663–671. [CrossRef]
32. Batrakova, E.V.; Kabanov, A. Pluronic block copolymers: Evolution of drug delivery concept from inert nanocarriers to biological response modifiers. *J. Control. Release* **2008**, *130*, 98–106. [CrossRef] [PubMed]
33. Choo, E.S.G.; Yu, B.; Xue, J. Synthesis of poly(acrylic acid) (PAA) modified Pluronic P123 copolymers for pH-stimulated release of Doxorubicin. *J. Colloid Interface Sci.* **2011**, *358*, 462–470. [CrossRef] [PubMed]
34. Coessens, V.; Pintauer, T.; Matyjaszewski, K. Functional polymers by atom transfer radical polymerization. *Prog. Polym. Sci.* **2001**, *26*, 337–377. [CrossRef]
35. Siegwart, D.J.; Oh, J.K.; Matyjaszewski, K. ATRP in the design of functional materials for biomedical applications. *Prog. Polym. Sci.* **2012**, *37*, 18–37. [CrossRef] [PubMed]
36. Van Meer, G.; Voelker, D.R.; Feigenson, G.W. Membrane lipids: Where they are and how they behave. *Nat. Rev. Mol. Cell Biol.* **2008**, *9*, 112–124. [CrossRef]
37. Rabasco Álvarez, A.M.; González Rodríguez, M.L. Lipids in pharmaceutical and cosmetic preparations. *Grasas Y Aceites* **2000**, *51*, 74–96. [CrossRef]
38. Bertrand, O.; Schumers, J.-M.; Kuppan, C.; Marchand-Brynaert, J.; Fustin, C.-A.; Gohy, J.-F. Photo-induced micellization of block copolymers bearing 4,5-dimethoxy-2-nitrobenzyl side groups. *Soft Matter* **2011**, *7*, 6891. [CrossRef]
39. Alves, P.; Hugo, A.A.; Szymanowski, F.; Tymczyszyn, E.E.; Pérez, P.F.; Coelho, J.; Simões, P.N.; Gómez-Zavaglia, A. Stabilization of polymer lipid complexes prepared with lipids of lactic acid bacteria upon preservation and internalization into eukaryotic cells. *Colloids Surf. B Biointerfaces* **2014**, *123*, 446–451. [CrossRef]
40. Corvo, M.L.; Mendo, A.S.; Figueiredo, S.; Gaspar, R.; Larguinho, M.; da Silva, M.F.C.G.; Baptista, P.V.; Fernandes, A.R. Liposomes as Delivery System of a Sn(IV) Complex for Cancer Therapy. *Pharm. Res.* **2016**, *33*, 1351–1358. [CrossRef]
41. Vicario-De-La-Torre, M.; Benítez-Del-Castillo, J.M.; Vico, E.; Guzman, M.; De-Las-Heras, B.; Herrero-Vanrell, R.; Molina-Martinez, I.T. Design and Characterization of an Ocular Topical Liposomal Preparation to Replenish the Lipids of the Tear Film. *Investig. Opthalmol. Vis. Sci.* **2014**, *55*, 7839–7847. [CrossRef]
42. Nayak, S.; Lyon, L.A. Soft Nanotechnology with Soft Nanoparticles. *Angew. Chem. Int. Ed.* **2005**, *44*, 7686–7708. [CrossRef] [PubMed]
43. Sepehrifar, R.; Boysen, R.I.; Danylec, B.; Yang, Y.; Saito, K.; Hearn, M.T.W. Application of pH-responsive poly(2-dimethylaminoethylmethacrylate)-block-poly(acrylic acid) coatings for the open-tubular capillary electrochromatographic analysis of acidic and basic compounds. *Anal. Chim. Acta* **2016**, *917*, 117–125. [CrossRef]
44. Chandaroy, P.; Sen, A.; Hui, S.W. Temperature-controlled content release from liposomes encapsulating Pluronic F127. *J. Control. Release* **2001**, *76*, 27–37. [CrossRef]
45. Shrestha, H.; Bala, R.; Arora, S. Lipid-Based Drug Delivery Systems. *J. Pharm.* **2014**, *2014*, 801820. [CrossRef] [PubMed]
46. Elbayoumi, T.A.; Torchilin, V.P. *Liposomes*; Oxford University Press: Oxford, UK; New York, NY, USA, 2003.
47. Maherani, B.; Arab-Tehrany, E.; Mozafari, M.R.; Gaiani, C.; Linder, M. Liposomes: A Review of Manufacturing Techniques and Targeting Strategies. *Curr. Nanosci.* **2011**, *7*, 436–452. [CrossRef]
48. Di Paolo, D.; Pastorino, F.; Brignole, C.; Marimpietri, D.; Loi, M.; Ponzoni, M.; Pagnan, G. Drug Delivery Systems: Application of Liposomal Anti-Tumor Agents to Neuroectodermal Cancer Treatment. *Tumori J.* **2008**, *94*, 246–253. [CrossRef]
49. Allen, T.M.; Cullis, P.R. Liposomal drug delivery systems: From concept to clinical applications. *Adv. Drug Deliv. Rev.* **2013**, *65*, 36–48. [CrossRef]

pharmaceutics

Review

Polymer-Modified Liposomes for Drug Delivery: From Fundamentals to Applications

Yifeng Cao [1,*], Xinyan Dong [2] and Xuepeng Chen [3,*]

[1] Department of Electronic Chemicals, Institute of Zhejiang University-Quzhou, Quzhou 324000, China
[2] School of Biological and Chemical Engineering, NingboTech University, Ningbo 315100, China; dxyan@zju.edu.cn
[3] The Affiliated Hospital of Stomatology, School of Stomatology, Zhejiang University School of Medicine, Clinical Research Center for Oral Diseases of Zhejiang Province, Key Laboratory of Oral Biomedical Research of Zhejiang Province, Cancer Center of Zhejiang University, Hangzhou 310006, China
* Correspondence: caoyf@zju.edu.cn (Y.C.); cxp1979@zju.edu.cn (X.C.)

Abstract: Liposomes are highly advantageous platforms for drug delivery. To improve the colloidal stability and avoid rapid uptake by the mononuclear phagocytic system of conventional liposomes while controlling the release of encapsulated agents, modification of liposomes with well-designed polymers to modulate the physiological, particularly the interfacial properties of the drug carriers, has been intensively investigated. Briefly, polymers are incorporated into liposomes mainly using "grafting" or "coating", defined according to the configuration of polymers at the surface. Polymer-modified liposomes preserve the advantages of liposomes as drug-delivery carriers and possess specific functionality from the polymers, such as long circulation, precise targeting, and stimulus-responsiveness, thereby resulting in improved pharmacokinetics, biodistribution, toxicity, and therapeutic efficacy. In this review, we summarize the progress in polymer-modified liposomes for drug delivery, focusing on the change in physiological properties of liposomes and factors influencing the overall therapeutic efficacy.

Keywords: liposome; polymer; drug delivery; long circulation; polymer–lipid conjugates; targeting; stimulus-responsive

Citation: Cao, Y.; Dong, X.; Chen, X. Polymer-Modified Liposomes for Drug Delivery: From Fundamentals to Applications. *Pharmaceutics* **2022**, *14*, 778. https://doi.org/10.3390/pharmaceutics14040778

Academic Editors: Tomáš Etrych, Ana Isabel Fernandes and Angela Faustino Jozala

Received: 25 February 2022
Accepted: 29 March 2022
Published: 2 April 2022

1. Introduction

Efficient drug delivery systems are highly demanded in treating human diseases by satisfying pharmacological properties and therapeutic efficiencies [1]. Liposomes (Figure 1), first discovered in 1961 and reported in 1965 by Bangham et al. [2], are vesicles of closed lipid bilayer(s) composed mainly of phospholipids (PLs) with or without cholesterol (Chol), the major components of mammalian cell membranes. The hydrophobic interior of the lipid bilayer and the internal aqueous phase of liposomes enable the encapsulation of respective hydrophobic and hydrophilic drugs with relatively high drug encapsulation. Together with their good biocompatibility, tunable physicochemical and biophysical properties, as well as controlled release of drugs, liposomes are among the most feasible and extensively studied drug-delivery systems that are promising for advanced drug delivery in the treatment of cancers and other diseases [3,4]. More significantly, a number of liposomal formulations have been approved for clinical practice by the Food and Drug Administration (FDA) of the United States and the European Medicines Agency (EMA) of Europe since the first nanosized drug delivery system based on poly(ethylene glycol)-modified (PEGylated) liposome, Doxil®, was approved in 1995 [5,6]. More promising formulations are under clinical trials [7]. Meanwhile, more administration routes, such as nasal [8], inner ear [9], skin [10], oral [11], intra-articular [4,12], and gastrointestinal drug delivery [13], have been designed. Combination therapy by co-delivery of multiple therapeutic agents with liposomal formulations has also become an emerging research area [14].

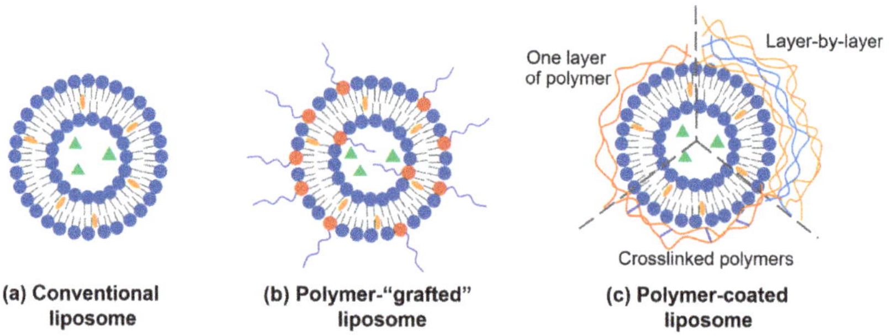

Figure 1. Liposomes for drug delivery: (**a**) conventional liposome, (**b**) polymer-"grafted" liposome, and (**c**) polymer-coated liposome, where liposomes are coated by a layer of adsorbed polymer, by the layer-by-layer (LbL) assembly, or by crosslinked polymers (polymer-"caged"). Liposomes can encapsulate hydrophobic drugs (orange ovals) in the hydrophobic region and hydrophilic ones (green triangles) in the interior aqueous region.

2. Conventional Liposomes as Drug-Delivery Carriers

The concept in designing liposomal formulations (Figure 2) [15] clearly depicts the complexity. The vesicle composition plays a central role in determining the physicochemical properties, surface structure, interactive properties, and in vivo performance, including pharmacokinetics, biodistribution, toxicity, and therapeutic efficacy.

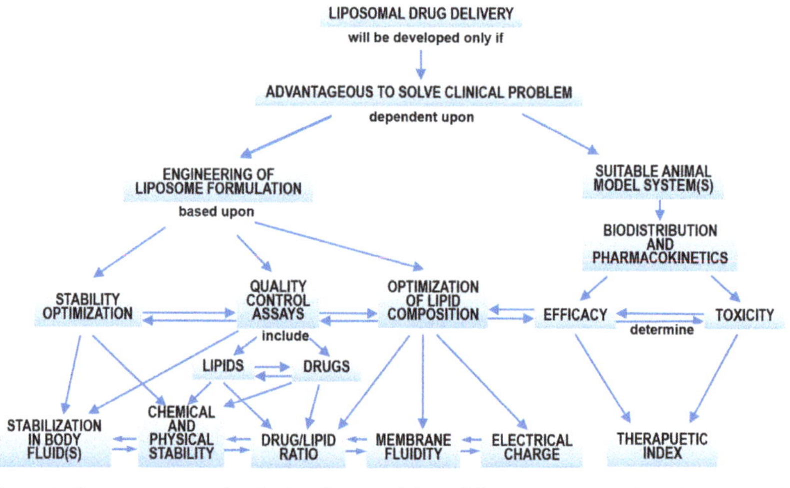

Figure 2. Concept map on developing liposomal drug delivery systems. Adapted from Ref. [15], published by Elsevier, 1993.

The physicochemical properties of liposomes, including phase state of the membranes, surface charge, and rigidity of lipid membranes, are determined by the lipid composition and size distribution of the vesicles and impact the physiological and pharmacokinetics performances of liposomal formulations, and consequently the efficacy of encapsulated drugs and toxicity [3,16]. The bilayer composition of conventional liposomes (Figure 1a)—also called the first-generation liposomes—is purely lipid-based. The major component of conventional liposomes is zwitterionic PL, including phosphatidylcholine (PC), phosphatidylethanolamine (PE), and sphingomyelin (SM), as well as nonionic lipids, such as cholesterol. The phase state of the bilayer, which characterizes the permeability, is determined by the structure of PLs (including headgroup, alkyl chain length, degree of unsaturation, and the ratio of cholesterol inserted in the bilayer [17]). A small amount of charged

PLs, including negatively charged phosphatidylserine (PS) and phosphatidylglycerol (PG), as well as positively charged, double-chain surfactant carrying a trimethylammonium (TAP) headgroup, directly regulates the surface charge characteristics of liposomes [6]. Electrostatic repulsion between the charged liposomes prevents the prepared liposome dispersion from aggregating and governs the interaction between liposomes and the surrounding biological substances, further influencing the toxicity. Briefly, positively charged liposomes are relatively more toxic than negatively charged ones [18]. Additionally, the size distribution of liposomes plays a less significant role in influencing their toxicity, but largely determines the biodistribution and circulation time of liposomes [7]. Liposomes of sizes ranging from 100 to 200 nm can take advantage of the enhanced permeability and retention (EPR) effect of tumor blood vessels and passively accumulate at the tumor sites (Figure 3), thereby resulting in targeted drug delivery and reduced systemic toxicity [19–21].

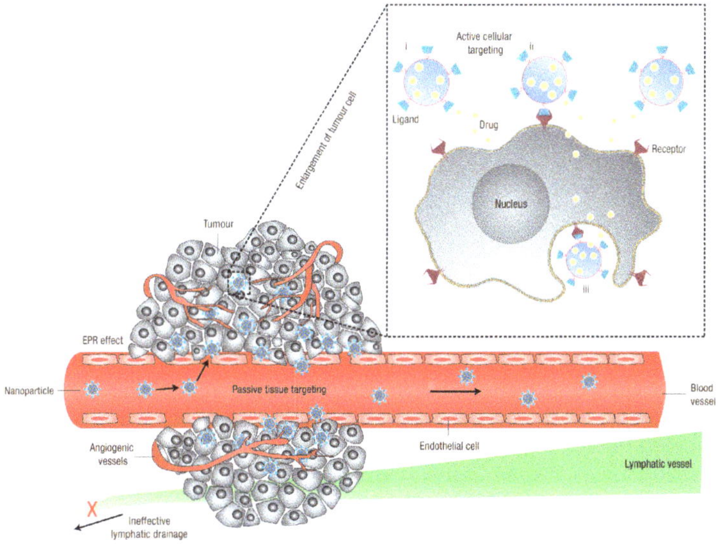

Figure 3. Nanoparticles, including liposomes, passively penetrate the blood vessel through the gaps between endothelial cells by the enhanced permeation and retention (EPR) effect at the tumor site, followed by endocytosis by the tumor cell. Adapted with permission from Ref. [22]. Published by Nature Publishing Group, 2007.

Efficient loading of therapeutic agents (payload), including hydrophobic, ionic, and zwitterionic ones, into liposomes to obtain a reasonable drug-to-lipid ratio is critical for the drug delivery system [3,23]. The encapsulated molecules by liposomes show improved solubility in aqueous media, particularly for the hydrophobic drugs, enhanced stability and bioavailability, as well as reduced side effects. Efficient drug-loading methods, depending on the nature of drugs, have been developed [24–27]. Drug-free liposomes can be prepared using hydration–extrusion, sonication, reverse phase evaporation, microfluidics, and supercritical carbon-dioxide-mediated processes [28–30]. Drug-loading is performed during liposome formation (passive loading) or afterward (such as active loading). Water-insoluble drugs or therapeutic agents, which are incorporated in the center of the hydrophobic region of the lipid bilayer, are generally encapsulated into liposomes passive way, resulting in high encapsulation effectiveness. During this process, interactions between lipid and drug molecules play a key role, whereas hydrophobic lipid molecules, such as PCs with longer and saturated alkyl chains, favor encapsulation [31]. Hydrophilic drugs can be encapsulated by passive or active loading [25]. For water-soluble weak acids and bases, remote loading of these molecules into liposomes takes advantage of the ion gradient across the bilayer, forming a stable (semi-)solid phase (gel-like) precipitate in the interior of the liposome, thereby resulting in high loading efficiency and avoiding burst/fast release [24,32].

The effectiveness of liposomal drug formulation is achieved mainly via the uptake of liposomes by target cells, mediated by liposome adsorption onto the cell surface, followed by cellular uptake via membrane fusion or endocytosis, or other methods [33]. Drugs are released from the liposomal formulation by passive permeation and diffusion, and exert their therapeutic effects [26]. Controlled and prolonged drug release can be achieved by tuning the physicochemical properties of the liposomal carriers, modification with stimulus-responsive and/or targeting moieties, and so on.

Despite the advantages mentioned previously, there are still some problems associated with using conventional liposomes as drug delivery platforms. Their colloidal and in vivo stabilities are vital issues (Figure 2). One problem associated with conventional liposomes, especially the neutral ones, is the colloidal instability of aqueous dispersion over time, giving rise to vesicle fusion and aggregation, causing limited shelf time [34]. After administration, the interactions between liposomes and biomacromolecules or cells in the surrounding biological environment, i.e., plasma proteins and cells, play a key role in the pharmacokinetics of liposomes. Another problem is that liposomes bind to proteins and other biomolecules in the biological fluid (such as serum albumin) via electrostatic, hydrophobic, and other specific interactions, forming a "protein corona" about the surface, which alters the characteristics of the liposomal formulation (size, surface charge, and properties, etc.) [35,36]. The formed complex may disrupt liposomes, promote drug pre-release [37], and determine biodistribution and cellular uptake pathways. The protein corona enables non-specific rapid clearance of administered liposomes from circulation by the mononuclear phagocyte system (MPS) before reaching the target sites other than the MPS tissues (i.e., liver and spleen) [38–40], resulting in low efficacy. Characteristics of liposomes, including lipid composition, size, surface charge, fluidity, and hydrophobicity, influence the circulation time [41,42].

To overcome the problems associated with using conventional liposomes as drug-delivery carriers, the outer surface of conventional liposomes provides sites for functionalization. Tuning the physiochemical properties, most importantly, the interfacial properties of liposomes by varying lipid composition (the second-generation liposomes), by surface modification with gangliosides or sialic acid (the second-generation liposomes), and surface modification of liposomes with polymers, has been intensively investigated to modify liposome-involved interactions (i.e., liposome–liposome, liposome–serum proteins) [43–47]. Versatile polymers, including natural and synthetic ones, have long been used as drug delivery carriers due to their tailorable structures, properties, and functionalities [48]. Depending on the characteristic of the incorporated polymer, the polymer-modified liposomes show superior performances in improved colloidal stability, prolonged circulation, and targeted and triggered release [49]. Briefly, surface modification of liposomes with polymers uses at least one of the following strategies: polymer grafting on the surface of liposomes and liposomes coated with physically adsorbed polymers (Figure 1b,c). Additionally, multi-functional liposomes have also been engineered by incorporating polymers with more than one specific functionality.

3. Polymer-"Grafted" Liposomes

For polymer-grafted liposomes, hydrophilic polymers bear one nonadsorbing end with the other end attached to the liposome surface either by the "grafting to" approach, where the hydrophobic anchors are inserted into the lipid bilayer mainly in forms of amphiphilic polymer-lipid conjugates (Figure 4a) and bola amphiphiles composed of two hydrophilic chains connected by a hydrophobic domain [50,51], or by the "grafting from" approach through directly grafting polymers from the liposomal surface (liposome-surface-initiated atom-transfer radical polymerization) [52]. The hydrophilic polymers form a thicker hydration layer surrounding the liposome surface, which inhibits the interactions between nearby liposomes, and between liposome and proteins and/or cells in the biological environment by steric, hydration, and/or electrostatic repulsion [34].

The interactions between surface-grafted nanocarriers and biomolecules are determined by the grafting density, molecular weight, and configuration of grafted hydrophilic polymers [53,54]. The configuration of polymers bound to a surface, whether forming a mushroom or polymer brush, is mainly dependent on the ratio between the Flory dimension (R_f) and the averaged distance between adjacent chains (D) (Figure 4b) [55].

$$R_f = aN^{3/5} \tag{1}$$

$$D = (A/M)^{1/2} \tag{2}$$

where a is the monomer size or persistence length, N is the degree of polymerization, A is the area per grafted polymer chain in the bilayer, and M is the molar fraction of polymer-lipid conjugates. The R_f/D values below and above 1.0 indicate mushroom and brush configurations, respectively [55]. In general, increasing chain length and grafting density is beneficial for suppressing protein adsorption and/or macrophage uptake, reducing liposome uptake by MPS, and obtaining prolonged circulation time. Such liposomes are also referred to as "stealth liposomes".

Quite a large number of hydrophilic polymers and their derivatives have been investigated to prolong the circulation of liposomes. PEGylated liposome is the most extensively studied and most successfully commercialized one. The PEGylated liposomal formulations approved include Doxil®/Caelyx® for the delivery of doxorubicin (DOX, Figure 4c) and Onivyde® for irinotecan [5]. More are under clinical or preclinical studies.

3.1. *Stealth Liposomes*

Surfaces modified with antifouling polymers can effectively resist the non-specific adsorption of proteins and/or adhesion of cells [56,57], therefore overcoming the problems associated with rapid clearance of conventional liposomes by the RES system. Such polymers include PEG-based materials, zwitterionic polymers, and polyampholytes [56,57]. In general, the antifouling performance of the surface-grafted polymer is positively correlated with the hydration level of the polymeric moieties [57]. The configuration of grafted polymers, whether in brush or mushroom configuration, also greatly influences the physiochemical and biological performance [53,54].

3.1.1. PEGylated Liposomes

PEGylation has been recognized as the "gold standard" for steric protection of liposomes [58]. PEG ((-O-CH_2-CH_2-)$_n$) is hydrophilic, highly flexible, and inexpensive. The antifouling property of PEG is attributed to its hydrophilic nature and hydration ability under aqueous conditions. In contrast, hydrogen bonding dominates the interaction between water molecules and PEG chains [59], and entropic origin, where the high flexibility of PEG chains will be suppressed upon fouling. The thick hydration layer surrounding the polymers, particularly the tightly bound water molecules lying the outmost interfacial layer, inhibits non-specific protein adsorption. In contrast, the mobility of polymers plays a less significant role in the antifouling property [60]. Consequently, PEGylated liposomes show decreased RES uptake and increased blood circulation time, depending on the molecular weight and content of grafted PEG in the vesicles [61].

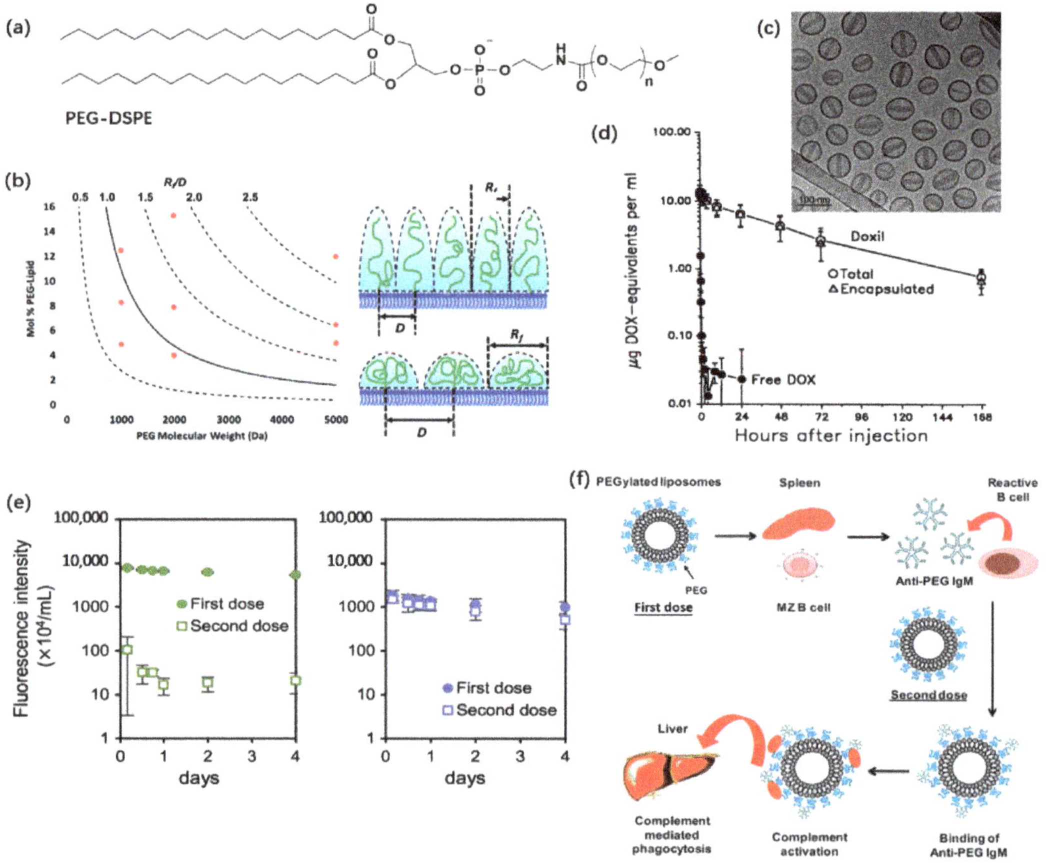

Figure 4. PEGylated liposomal formulation. (**a**) Chemical structure of PEG-DSPE conjugate, where *n* represents the number of repeating units; (**b**) Determination of the configuration of surface-grafted polymer; (**c**) TEM image of PEGylated doxorubicin; (**d**) Pharmacokinetics of PEGylated liposomal doxorubicin (open symbols) and free drug (solid symbols); (**e**) Blood concentration after the first and second doses (solid and open symbols, respectively) for PEGylated liposome induces ABC while poly(sarcosine)-modified liposomes do not cause ABC; (**f**) Mechanism of ABC induced by repeated administration of PEGylated liposomes. The panel (**b**) is adapted with permission from Ref. [54], published by Royal Society of Chemistry, 2018. The panel (**c**) is adapted with permission from Ref. [5]; Copyright © 2012 Elsevier B.V. All rights reserved. The panel (**d**) is adapted from Ref. [62]; Copyright © 1994, American Association for Cancer Research. The panel (**e**) is adapted with permission from Ref. [63]; Copyright © 2020 Elsevier B.V. All rights reserved. The panel (**f**) is adapted from Ref. [64], an Open Access article distributed under the terms of the Creative Commons Attribution License; Copyright © 2019 Mohamed et al.

The configuration of grafted PEG, as illustrated in Figure 4b, is determined by the molecular weight and grafting density. The PEG extension length is given by Equation (1) for the mushroom configuration and by Equation (3) for the polymer brushes:

$$L_{\text{brush}} \approx aN^{3/5}/D^{2/3} \tag{3}$$

where D is the distance between grafted PEG polymers. For the most widely used conjugation of PEG_{2000} and 1,2-distearoyl-*sn*-glycero-3-phosphoethanolamine (DSPE), the configuration of surface-grafted PEG undergoes a transition from mushroom (3.5 nm) to brush (10 nm, fully PEGylated) when the content of PEG_{2000}-DSPE exceeds 4 mol%, and the liposomes transit to micelles when PEG_{2000}-DSPE is more than ca. 8 mol% [65].

Incorporating PEG–lipid conjugates may also change the phase state of the lipid bilayers, which in turn changes the permeability, bending modulus of the bilayer, and other properties of the liposomes [65–67]. Adding DSPE into distearoylphosphatidylcholine (DSPC) bilayer changes the phase state of the bilayer from gel-phase (<ca. 10 mol%) to tilted gel phase ($L\beta'$), interdigitated gel phase ($L\beta I$), untitled gel phase ($L\beta$), or micellar phase, depending on the content and molecular weight of the PEG moieties [68]. A previous study has demonstrated that the fluid-phase PEGylated liposomes interact more weakly with human serum albumin than those in gel-state [67].

Steric interaction plays an essential role in the improved colloidal stability and favorable pharmacokinetic and therapeutic properties of PEGylated formulation [34,69]. Direct measurement of the normal forces between PEG functionalized DMPC (1,2-dimyristoyl-*sn*-glycero-3-phosphocholine) bilayers (DMPC + 7.5 mol% DMPE-PEG_{2000}, either in gel- or in fluid-phase, where DMPE is the abbreviation of 1,2-dimyristoyl-*sn*-glycero-3-phosphoethanolamine) using a surface-force apparatus revealed the presence of roughly exponentially decayed long-range electrostatic (Debye length ca. 20 nm across 0.25 mM $NaNO_3$) originating from the phosphate group of PE molecules (Figure 4a) and short-range steric repulsion [70]. Steric interaction between PEG-grafted liposomes increases as PEG-lipid concentration and the molecular weight of the PEG chain increase [55]. Similarly, PEGylated liposomes also exhibit diminished protein and cellular interactions and favorable pharmacokinetic behaviors and therapeutic effects, including very long circulation/elimination time, low RES-uptake, and specific accumulation at tumor sites. The blood clearance curve of liposomes shows a $T_{1/2}$ up to 15.3 h for PEG-DSPE incorporated ones and a 4-fold increase compared to those without PEGylation. Meanwhile, the inclusion of PEG-DSPE also decreases the amount of liposome in liver but promotes the accumulation in the tumor tissues [71]. Compared with free doxorubicin drug molecules which are rapidly cleared from blood circulation, the elimination half-life of PEGylated liposomal doxorubicin is ca. 45 h in humans (Figure 4d) [62]. These features account for the broad application of PEGylated liposomes as drug delivery carriers.

Despite these advantages, increasing studies on PEG polymer and PEGylated products also reveal some unfavorable effects. The most significant one is that the administration of PEGylated liposomes can cause complement activation, which leads to an accelerated blood clearance (ABC) phenomenon (Figure 4f) and hypersensitivity reactions upon repeated administration, resulting in decreased therapeutic efficacy [72,73]. Different approaches have been investigated to eliminate complement activation by playing with PEGylated formulations and designing alternative polymers as grafting moieties for long-circulating liposomes.

3.1.2. Accelerated Blood Clearance (ABC)

The first injection of PEGylated liposomes induces the production of PEG-specific Immunoglobulin M (IgM) antibodies by the spleen [74]. Upon the second injection, anti-PEG antibodies can bind to PEGylated liposomes, giving rise to complement activation, which in turn enhances the rapid clearance of vesicles from the systemic circulation by complement-mediated phagocytosis [75]. This phenomenon is called accelerated blood clearance (ABC, Figure 4e,f) [64,76]. The plasma concentrations of PEGylated liposome after the second dose drop dramatically than those after the first dose, as shown in Figure 4e [63]. Moreover, possibly due to the prevalent application of PEG in consumer and pharmaceutical products, anti-PEG antibodies, IgG, and/or IgM have been detected in ~72% of the individuals who have never received PEGylated drug treatment [77,78]. These pre-existing antibodies may also induce allergic reactions after individuals receive the first dose [79].

The ABC phenomenon is influenced by many factors, including the backbone of the polymers, PEGylation of the liposomes, molecular weight of PEG, PEG-lipid linkages, animal species, the time interval between administrations, lipid dose, the physicochemical properties (size and charge, for example) of the formulation, as well as the encapsulated drugs [64,69,73,80–83]. Studies have shown that, for empty PEGylated liposomes (HSPC/Chol/mPEG$_{2000}$-DSPE = 1.49:1.00:0.134, molar ratio, where HSPC is the abbreviation for hydrogenated soy phosphatidylcholine), no ABC was observed at high doses of >5 μmol PLs/kg, but was observed for low doses of <1 μmol PLs/kg; a time interval of 4–7 days between the first and second doses induces a much more pronounced ABC phenomenon [84]; encapsulation of cytotoxic or tolerogenic agents, such as doxorubicin and rapamycin, also inhibits the ABC phenomenon, possibly due to the released doxorubicin in spleen impairing the production of anti-PEG IgM; prolonging the administration interval from 7 days to 4 weeks also eliminates ABC [73,85,86]. More recently, researchers also found that using high-molecular-weight free PEG to saturate already-existing anti-PEG antibodies offers a window for up to 2 months for the practical application of PEGylated therapeutics [85,87].

More strategies have been developed to address the ABC phenomenon. Inserting ganglioside into PEGylated liposome prevents the immunogenicity of PEG and induces B cell tolerance to subsequent doses, thereby preserving the therapeutic efficacy upon repeated administration [88].

As the negative charge on PEG–phospholipid, the most commonly used PEG-incorporating amphiphile has proven to play a key role in complement activation [89], PEG–nonphospholipid conjugates, such as PEG$_{2000}$-conjugated hexadecylcarbamoylmethyl hexadecanoate (HDAS-PEG) and cleavable PEG-cholesterol, and can also lessen or eliminate ABC phenomenon [90,91]. On the contrary, introducing a hydroxyl group at the end of the PEG chain can cause enhanced clearance of the subsequent doses [92].

As alternatives to PEG, a number of hydrophilic polymers have been used to fabricate long-circulating liposomes. Poly(carboxybetaine) (PCB), branched PEG, poly(sarcosine) (PSar, Figure 4e, right panel), polyglycerol, poly(hydroxyethyl-l-asparagine) (PHEA), poly(vinylpyrrolidone) (PVP), poly(*N*,*N*-dimethylacrylamide) (PDMA), poly(*N*-acryloyl morpholine) (PAcM), poly[*N*-(2-hydroxypropyl)) methacrylamide] (HPMA), and poly(2-methyl-2-oxazoline) (PMOX) can effectively reduce or eliminate immunogenic response upon repeated injections [63,80,93–96]. However, PMOX was proved to induce a pronounced ABC effect in rats [80].

3.1.3. Zwitterionic Polymer-Lipid Conjugates

Compared with uncharged PEG polymers, which form hydrogen bonds with water molecules and cannot completely prevent protein binding [97], zwitterionic polymers interact with water molecules mainly via charge–dipole interaction. Therefore, they are more hydrated than PEG. Water molecules surrounding the zwitterionic moieties are more ordered, forming a physical and energy barrier resistant to the adsorption of biological proteins, such as bovine serum albumin and lysozyme [98]. In contrast to the ABC phenomenon associated with PEGylated liposomes, the highly hydrophilic zwitterionic polymers are expected to exhibit improved immunological safety meanwhile maintaining the stealth properties [99]. Consequently, zwitterionic polymer-grafted liposomes incorporating PCB- and poly-(2-(methacryloyloxy)ethyl phosphorylcholine) (PMPC)-grafted liposomes have been designed and investigated as alternatives to PEGylated ones [34,100].

Cao et al. [100] synthesized superhydrophilic zwitterionic PCB–DSPE conjugate with a sharp polarity contrast between the PCB and alkyl chains of DSPE. The highly hydrophilic PCB brushes can stabilize liposome structure more so than amphiphilic PEG chains. Similar to PEGylated liposomes, PCB$_{5000/2000}$-stabilized liposomes are stable at 4 °C for over half a year, and have a longer blood circulation half-life (ca. 3–7 h) than that of the small unilamellar vesicles (SUVs) of DSPC (<1 h). Moreover, doxorubicin encapsulated in DSPC/PCB$_{5000}$-DSPE 10% eliminated tumors by a single i.v. injection, and cured mice faster than commercial Doxil® [100]. Unlike PEGylated liposomes, the pH-sensitive PCB-stabilized liposomes were internalized into cells via endocytosis with superior cellular uptake and drug release. Meanwhile, surface-grafted PCB avoided the ABC phenomenon and promoted accumulation of drug-loaded liposomes to tumor sites [101].

Taking into consideration of the 2-(methacryloyloxy)ethyl phosphorylcholine (MPC) moieties that resemble the highly hydrated headgroups of PC lipids, which largely account for the extreme hydration lubrication of synovial joints [102–104], Lin et al. [34] designed and synthesized PMPC–DSPE conjugates, aiming to improve the colloidal stability of conventional liposomes while simultaneously improving the lubrication behavior of the polymer-grafted surface. Compared with bare HSPC-SUVs, which aggregate shortly after preparation, incorporating 2 mol% DSPE-PMPC can significantly inhibit SUV aggregation for more than 90 days [34]. The PMPCylated liposomes exhibit superior in vivo retention time to the commonly used PEGylated ones. The in vivo intra-articular retention time (half-life, $T_{1/2}$) of HSPC/PMPC (2%) is 85 h, much longer than HSPC/PEG (<20 h) and commonly administrated HA (<1 h) [12]; size-dependent retention behavior was also observed for HSPC/PMPC (2%), of which the $T_{1/2}$ is 85 h and 18–22 h for diameters of 170 and 80 nm, respectively, but not for HSPC/PEG (17 $\pm$ 4 h). More interestingly, PMPCylated liposome-coated surfaces are capable of affording extremely low friction coefficients (at 10^{-4} level) under physiologically high pressures, which is one order of magnitude better than those for PEGylated liposomes (friction coefficients 0.006–0.011), attributed to the higher hydration level of MPC moieties [34]. These results together indicate that PMPCylated liposomes are more appropriate as drug carriers for intraarticular drug delivery and as efficient boundary lubricants for treating osteoarthritis (OA), a degenerative joint disease characterized by slowly disrupted synovial cartilage and undermined lubrication performance [4].

As the hydration level of zwitterionic polymer plays a central role in antifouling ability, recently developed antifouling polymers, such as strong-hydration materials (poly trimethylamine *N*-oxide, PTMAO) [105], amino acid-based zwitterionic polymers prepared from L-serine, lysine, ornithine, asparagine, hydroxyethyl-L-asparagine, glutamine, and repeated glutamic acid and lysine motifs [106–108], as well as poly(ectoine) [109], also provide feasible options for polymer-grafted liposome, in the context of developing long-circulating formulations. Moreover, further studies on the immunogenic and toxicological performances of the modified liposomes are highly demanded.

4. Polymer-Coated Liposomes

The outer surface of liposomes allows adsorption of polymers through non-specific (electrostatic, dipole-charge, hydrogen-bonding, van der Waal's) interactions. As a consequence of the adsorbed polymers, the interfacial and physiochemical properties of liposomes are modified, thereby attaining colloidal, biological, and mechanical stability, prolonged circulation half-life, reduced permeability and controlled release of the payload, as well as targeting [45,110–112]. Direct adsorption of single-component hydrophilic polymers on the liposome surface, incorporating polymers modified with multiple hydrophobic anchors ("comb-like" structure) into a lipid bilayer, layer-by-layer (LbL) deposition of complementary polymers, and caged liposomes with cross-linked polymers are among the most commonly used approaches.

4.1. Liposomes Coated with One Layer of Polymer

Coating liposomes with polymer adsorption is performed by adding polymer solution dropwise into already-prepared liposome dispersion, which avoids pre-functionalization of the polymers and is a feasible way of modifying the properties of liposomes. The chemical structure, charge, and molecular weight of polymers predominately determine their interaction with liposomes and the polymer–liposome configuration. As shown in Figure 5a, as the content of low-molecular-weight hyaluronic acid (HA) increases, the configuration of cationic liposome-polymer dispersion changes from aggregation, to phase separation, then dispersion, along with an increase followed by a decrease in the colloidal size (Figure 5a) [113].

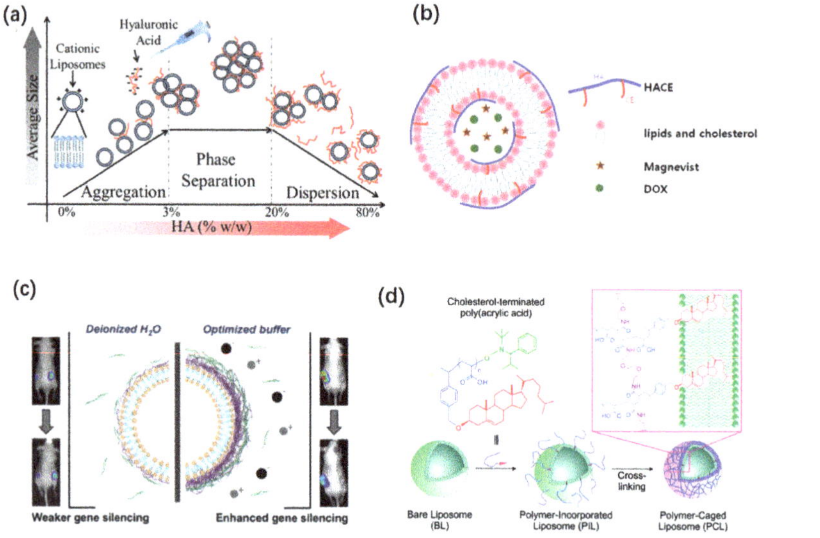

Figure 5. Schematic of liposomes coated with polymers. (**a**) Schematic of the configuration of low-molecular-weight HA/liposome complex. Reprinted with permission from Ref. [113]. Copyright © 2015, American Chemical Society. (**b**) Liposomes modified with hyaluronic acid–ceramide (HA–CE), whereas multiple hydrophobic anchors were introduced to HA. Reprinted with permission from Ref. [114]. Copyright © 2013 Elsevier B.V. All rights reserved. (**c**) Layer-by-layer (LbL) deposition of appositively charged polyelectrolytes. Enhanced therapeutic efficacy was obtained under optimized LbL deposition conditions. Reprinted with permission from Ref. [115]. Copyright © 2019, American Chemical Society. (**d**) Polymer-caged liposomes. Liposomes were modified with poly(acrylic acid)-cholesterol, followed by cross-linking with diamine. Reprinted with permission from Ref. [116]. Copyright © 2007, American Chemical Society.

Polymers can adsorb on the oppositely-charged liposomes by electrostatic, hydrophobic, and hydrogen-bonding interactions, and bind to zwitterionic PC vesicles, introducing charges to the surface [117]. Therefore, liposomes modified with charged polymers are electrostatically repulsive and are supposed to be colloidal-stable. The coating layer also serves as a barrier controlling the release rate of encapsulated drugs. For example, prolonged release of encapsulated *N*-acetylcysteine was observed for chitosan-coated liposomes compared to the uncoated ones (DPPC/Chol/DPPG, whereas DPPC and DPPG refer to 1,2-dipalmitoyl-*sn*-glycero-3-phosphocholine and 1,2-dipalmitoyl-*sn*-glycero-3-phosphoglycerol sodium salts, respectively) [118].

Strong polymer–liposome interaction may cause leakage of the entrapped agents [119], while weak attachment may cause polymer detachment after injection, leading to a shorter circulation time [120]. For a polymer-coated liposome drug-delivery system, sufficient polymer molecules (saturation concentration) are required to cover the liposomal surfaces. Meanwhile, special attention should be paid to avoid the following problems: inhomogeneous distribution of polymers along with the same vesicle and on vesicles from the same batch [121], dehydration, and fusion of vesicles [122], and bridging or depletion flocculation of the liposome–polymer mixture [123].

Charged polysaccharides, including HA, chitosan, and alginate, have attracted much attention for liposome-based drug delivery systems. In addition to biocompatibility, biodegradability, good aqueous solubility, and charge characteristics, certain polysaccharides also exhibit specific properties without functionalization, such as reinforced mucoadhesion for chitosan and CD44 targeting for HA. Surface-functionalized polysaccharide derivatives could enable the coated liposomes with specific properties. Biocompatible synthetic polymers, such as polyvinyl alcohol (PVA), zwitterionic polymers, and dendrimers [124,125] have also been investigated. It was found that coating with zwitterionic polymer can also inhibit nonspecific protein adsorption to liposomes [124], while polyphenylene dendrimer-coated liposomes (DOPE:Egg PC:Chol = 1:1:1, molar ratio, whereby DOPE is the abbreviation of 1,2-dioleoyl-*sn*-glycero-3-phosphoethanolamine) could inhibit the binding of specific opsonins while increasing the adsorption of proteins that control cellular uptake [125].

To reinforce the attachment between polymer and lipid and form a stable coating layer, one solution is to introduce more anchors to polymer–lipid conjugates [114,120,126]. Liposomes modified with PVA-conjugated hydrophobic anchors (PVA-R) are resistant to aggregation or fusion, and prolong the circulation time in lungs after pulmonary administration, possibly through reduced clearance by macrophage, whereas higher molecular-weight PVA is more effective [120]. To stabilize the coated HA layer, amphiphilic hyaluronic acid derivative and hyaluronic acid–ceramide (HA-CE) were involved in the encapsulation of the anti-cancer drug doxorubicin, and a contrast agent for magnetic resonance imaging, Magnevist, was used. which enabled simultaneous targeted drug delivery and cancer imaging (Figure 5b) [114]. To overcome the problems associated with coating by one polymer layer, the layer-by-layer (LbL) technique (Figure 5c) and polymer-caging (Figure 5d) have also been investigated (Figure 1c).

4.2. *Layer-by-Layer (LbL)*

LbL coating is a simple process achieved by subsequent adsorption materials to form a stable layer on the substrate/surface. Electrostatic attraction is the most commonly used driving force fabricating LbL structures. Other assemblies by virtue of hydrophobic, charge–transfer, host–guest, biologically specific, coordination chemistry, and covalent bonding interactions have also been reported [127]. The versatility of LbL assembly, particularly of the outermost layer, provides a wide range of properties and functions to the drug delivery systems, including but not limited to steric stability, stealth properties, active targeting, and environmental responsiveness [115,128,129].

For the self-assembly of alternatively deposited charged polymers on liposomes, an ion-exchange phenomenon whereby the associated counterions about the substrates are replaced by the next layer of charged polyelectrolytes, the main driving force is entropy gain from the released counterions [130]. The internal charge balance of the system is therefore maintained by the intrinsic lipid/polymer and polymer/polymer ion pairs, and extrinsic polymer/counterion pairs. As surface-charge reversal has been commonly observed in such systems [131,132], charge overcompensation is considered to play a significant role in successfully building the multilayers [133]. However, it was reported that charge overcompensation during the growth of multilayers poly(diallyldimethylammonium chloride)/poly(styrene sulfonate) (PDADMAC/PSS) took place only on the adsorption of polycations, due to the differences lying in the reaction-diffusion ranges of charges from positive and negative polyelectrolytes [134].

Competitive interactions between polyelectrolyte–liposome and oppositely charged polyelectrolytes also drive the formed structures and the colloidal stability of the liposomes. Despite charge reversal revealed by measuring zeta-potential values after each coating, sequential adsorption of biopolyelectrolytes with respectively high and low charge densities, dextran sulfate-sodium salt and poly-L-arginine, onto cationic liposomes composed of 1,2-dioleoyl-*sn*-glycero-3-phosphocholine and 1,2-dioleoyl-3-trimethylammonium-propane (DOPC/DOTAP, 1:1, molar ratio) resulted in the formation of heterogeneous polyelectrolyte patches [135]. The number of polymers adsorbed on the surface is determined by the surface–polymer interaction and is self-regulated due to electrostatic repulsion. Charges on the liposome core control the adsorption amount of polymer in the first layer. However, no template effect was observed for the second and following layers, namely, the amount of adsorbed polymers for the subsequent layers is independent of the liposomal membrane composition [133]. Taking together the "soft" nature of lipid bilayer into consideration, rational selection of a polycation/polyanion pair with reasonable charge densities is of crucial importance to the successful fabrication of multilayers. A summary of representative studies on LbL-coated liposomes for drug delivery is listed in Table 1.

Table 1. Presentative studies on LbL-coated liposomal systems designed for drug delivery.

Liposome Composition	Polycations	Polyanions	Encapsulated Agents	Properties	Ref.
Soya lecithin (24.5 mg), Chol (11.5 mg), stearyl amine (SA, 2 mg)	Chitosan	Polyacrylic acid (PAA)	Paclitaxel (PTX)	Good stability in simulated gastrointestinal fluids after lyophilization, sustained release with a 3-h lag time compared with PTX-liposome, enhanced cytotoxicity by PTX due to cell affinity of chitosan	[136]
DPPC/Chol/DDAB	Chitosan	Alginate	Bovine serum albumin (BSA)	Increased colloidal stability, Enhanced drug encapsulation efficacy, sustained linear release of BSA	[137]
DPPC/Chol/DDAB	Chitosan	Alginate	Recombinant human (rh) osteogenic protein-1/rhOP-1	Locally restricted release of rhOP-1 and resulting effect	[138]
DMPC/DLPA	Chitosan	Dextran sulfate (DXS) or deoxyribonucleic acid (DNA)	1-Hydroxy pyrene-3,6,8-trisulfonic acid (HPTS), alendronate, and glucose	Temperature-dependent release achieved by DNA denaturation	[131]
EYPC/Chol (5:1, mass ratio)	Trimethyl chitosan (TMC)	Pectin	Celastrol	Ideal resistibility to GI conditions, rapid drug release as a response to colonic pH, strong mucoadhesive causing better colon localization and prolonged colonic retention, improved cytotoxicity and visceral toxicity	[139]
EYPC/Chol/EYPG	Poly-L-lysine (PLL)	Poly(L-glutamic acid) PGA	-	Biocompatible and biodegradable polyelectrolytes	[140]
DLPA/DMPC	PLL	Poly-L-aspartic acid (PAsp)	A fluorescent probe, 1-hydroxypyrene-3,6,8-trisulfonic acid (HPTS)	Controlled release of HPTS by the coverage of the first layer and the ratio of DLPA	[119]
DOTAP/DOPE/Chol (35:35:30, molar ratio)	PLL	Hyaluronan or DXS	AZD6244 (selumetinib), an allosteric inhibitor of Mek1/2, and PX-866, a covalent inhibitor of PI3K	Combination chemotherapy, CD44 receptor targeting, hypoxic pH targeting and passive tumor targeting, enhanced efficacy by the synergistic effect	[141]
DPPC/Chol/DDAB (8:4:1, molar ratio)	PLL	Poly(ethylene glycol)-block-poly(L-aspartic acid) (PEG-b-PLD)	DOX and mitoxantrone	Good colloidal stability (>45 days), pH-sensitive, extended systemic circulation time, diminished burst release	[142]
DSPC/POPG/Chol (56:5:39, weight ratio)	Poly-L-arginine (PLA)	DXS	DOX	High drug-load retention, stable stored under room temperature after lyophilization	[143]
DSPC/Chol/POPG (56:39:5)	PLA	siRNA	DOX-loaded liposome, siRNA-loaded film	Extended serum half-life of 28 h, enhanced efficacy by a synergistic effect between SiRNA and doxorubicin	[144]
Soya lecithin (24.5 mg), Chol (11.5 mg), SA (2 mg)	PAH	PAA	PTX	Stable lyophilized formulation in simulated GI fluids, sustained release for 24 h, 4.07-fold increase in oral bioavailability compared to free drug, comparable antitumor efficacy with improved safety as opposed to i.v. Taxol®, target potential	[145]
Egg PC/Chol/SA (7:3:1, molar ratio)	PAH	PAA	Amoxicillin and metronidazole	Prolonged drug release in simulated gastric fluid, improved efficacy	[146]
DODAB	Galactomannan (GMC, a neutral polymer)	Xanthan (XAN)	Epidermal growth factor (EGF)	Up to 5 times the sustained release of EGF at a first-order rate of 0.005 min^{-1}	[147]
Chol/DSPC/POPG (2:6:2, mass ratio)	poly(β-amino ester)	HA	DOX	pH-triggered drug release, CD44 targeting, improved therapeutic effect and reduced side effects	[148]

Chol: cholesterol; DMPC: 1,2-dimyristoyl-*sn*-glycero-3-phosphocholine; DLPA: dilauroyl phosphatidic acid; DPPC: 1, 2-dipalmitoyl-*sn*-glycero-3-phosphocholine; DDAB: dimethyldioctadecyl-ammonium bromide; EYPC: egg yolk L-α-phosphatidylcholine; EYPG: egg yolk L-α-phosphatidyl-DL-glycerol; DOTAP: dioleoyl-3-trimethylammonium propane; DOPE: 1,2-Dioleoyl-*sn*-glycero-3-phosphoethanolamine; DSPC: 1,2-distearoyl-sn-glycero-3-phosphocholine; POPG: 1-palmitoyl-2-oleoyl-*sn*-glycero-3-phospho-(1′-rac-glycerol) sodium salt; DOPC: 1,2-dioleoyl-*sn*-glycero-3-phosphocholine; DODAB: dioctadecyl ammonium bromide; SA: stearyl amine.

In addition to the properties of polymers, the layer-by-layer assembly is also sensitive to processing parameters. For example, salt concentration and valence in the solution determine the ionization degree of the polyelectrolytes, the Debye length of charges, and the kinetics and thermodynamics of the assembly [115]. Other parameters, such as concentration of polymers in the solution, temperature, titration rate, as well as stirring speed, also play non-negligible roles in the coating process and should be optimized whenever necessary [115,132,138,149]. During the fabricating process, separating the coated particles and free polymers followed by a washing step to remove residual free polymers are essential after the coating of each layer [150].

Compared with liposomes coated with one layer of polymer, the thin multi-layer is more robust with greatly enhanced stability in resisting damages both in the biological environment and from surfactants, lyophilization, spay-drying, etc. [8,151]. The stiffness of the liposomal core, which can be modulated by incorporating cholesterol, directly influences the mechanical properties of the LbL liposomal system, giving rise to a longer elimination lifetime and higher tumor accumulation and penetration obtained with the compliant liposomes (DSPC with 40 mol% Chol) than those of the DSPC-liposomes [152]. Moreover, this multilayer provides more sites for drug encapsulation and regulates the release kinetics of encapsulated drugs to a more significant extent [142,153]. The improved release profile for low-stable drugs was obtained by anionic xanthan and cationic-galactomannan-coated cationic-DODAB liposomes for protein drug delivery. One layer of xanthan and galactomannan slowed down the release of encapsulated epidermal growth factor, which is five times slower than that of plain liposomes [147]. Although the number of layers is essential to developing stabilized formulation and to the pharmacokinetics of encapsulated drugs [140,142], the coverage of polymers in the first layer and the ratio of charged lipids on the vesicle controlled the release rate [119].

4.3. Cross-Linked-Polymer-Caged Liposomes

Chemical cross-linking of the polymers coated on the liposome can efficiently prevent dissociating of polymers and make liposomes more stable, but sometimes it is at the expense of controllable releasing of the payload. To address this problem, triggered release is particularly in demand. Lee et al. [116] prepared DPPC-DOPG-Chol-liposomes (51.4:3.6:45, molar ratio, whereby DOPG is the abbreviation of 1,2-dioleoyl-*sn*-glycero-3-phosphoglycerol) modified with cholesterol-poly(acrylic acid) conjugates, followed by cross-linking of PAA with 2,2′-(ethylenedioxy)-bis(ethylamine), forming a remarkably stable "polymer-caged liposome" that preserved the spherical configuration even after free-drying and rehydration, whereas un-crosslinked ones were not stable during long circulation (Figure 5d). More significantly, the residual carboxylate groups allow for the pH-sensitive release of the payload. Later, protease-triggered, polymer-caged liposomes were fabricated using a urokinase plasminogen activator (peptide GSGRSAGC) and poly(acrylic acid) graft copolymer, which was thereafter crosslinked with diamine [154]. The caged liposomes were stable under physiological conditions until interacting with tumor-specific protease and quickly releasing its contents. Polydopamine coating infers a surface with antifouling properties. Awasthi et al. [155] successed in crosslinking dopamine uniformly on liposomes under physiological conditions, in contrast to the traditional protocol performed under basic conditions, which yield unstable and non-uniform coatings. Implants coated with a stable polydopamine liposome are resistant to biofouling, which enables practical application of polydopamine-coated liposomes.

5. Targeting and Stimulus-Responsive Functionalization for Biomedical Applications

Liposomes that can target specific sites or/and are responsive to environmental stimulus are important to mediate liposome–target interaction and drug release, obtaining local, on-demand delivery. Selectively targeted, stimulus-responsive, and dual functionalized liposomes have attracted much attention as drug-delivery vehicles. Polymer-modified liposomal drug-delivery systems for specific disease and tissue targeting are of particular importance for therapeutic applications [156,157].

5.1. Targeting

Mucosal drug delivery [158] has enabled targeted delivery to the mucus layer with a prolonged local effect. Chitosan, acquired by partial deacetylation of chitin, is comprised of glucosamine and *N*-acetyl glucosamine linked by β-(1-4) glycosidic bonds. The primary amine groups on the chitosan backbone are protonated at a low pH, making chitosan molecules positively charged. More importantly, chitosan can bind to a negative mucus layer and is mucoadhesive, showing enhanced penetration across intestinal and nasal barriers and improved bioavailability of drugs at the diseased sites. For this reason, chitosan-coated liposomes have been examined for administration via intravenous, oral, ocular, and transdermal routes [159,160]. Studies have shown that liposomes coated with chitosan can penetrate through the intestinal mucosa after oral administration, without detaching from the liposome surfaces [161]; when complexed with sodium tripolyphosphate (TPP), chitosan formed a crosslinked coating layer for liposomes encapsulating quercetin, which increased bioavailability and optimized release of quercetin in intestine after oral administration [162].

Targeting tumor-associated compounds, such as CD44 and folic receptor, is crucial to enhance the therapeutic efficacy of anticancer liposomal formulations (Figure 3) [163]. HA, a major component of the extra-cellular matrix (ECM), is biocompatible and non-toxic, therefore, it has a wide application in biomaterials [164]. HA receptor CD44 is a transmembrane protein that maintains a low level in normal cells but is overexpressed in a number of solid tumors [165]. As HA is a targeting agent to cancer cells overexpressing CD44, HA–DPPE conjugates facilitate the recognition of modified liposomes by MiaPaCa2 cells expressing CD44, and the uptake increases with increasing molecular weight of HA from 4800 to 12,000 Da [166]. As HA is negatively charged under biological conditions due to the negative carboxylic residues, HA-coated liposomes show colloidal stability and no significant change in encapsulated drug for >3 months, in contrast to <1 month for the uncoated ones, possibly attributable to the polymer–liposome network [167]. Folate receptor is another tumor marker overexpressed in many cancers, such as ovarian, endometrial, and renal cancers [168]. A commonly used approach to target folate receptors is to conjugate folic acid, a high-affinity ligand, to a polymer via the gamma-carboxyl of folic acid. As a targeting ligand, folic acid (FA) shows unique advantages, such as non-immunogenic, good stability, high specificity, low price, and compatibility with organic solvents. It also has disadvantages, of which the hydrophobicity of folic acid is a big concern. Incorporating folate–PEG–lipid conjugates (FA–PEG–DSPE/DPPE/SA) into liposomes has proven to significantly promote folate receptor-mediated endocytosis, remarkably improve therapeutic effects, and reduce systemic toxicity [169].

The blood–brain barrier (BBB) rigorously blocks drugs from penetrating the brain. By introducing two targeting moieties, including the *D*-peptide ligand targeting nicotine acetylcholine receptors on the BBB and an integrin ligand targeting integrin on the blood–brain tumor barrier and glioma cells, to the modified liposomes encapsulating doxorubicin, a better anti-glioma effect along with prolonged median survival was observed for glioma-bearing nude mice than those treated by liposomes with none or one moiety; deep penetration of the formulation is still limited by high interstitial pressure and dense ECM in tumors [170].

5.2. Stimuli-Responsive Polymers

Triggered release of encapsulated therapeutic agents at the desired site is important to achieve high bioavailability and therapeutic efficacy. Specific fusion or destabilization of liposomes as responses to certain pathological changes between normal tissues and the diseased or target sites, or to the changes in environmental conditions between endosome and cytoplasm after uptake by cells through the endocytic pathway, can be utilized to enable effective controlled release and improved therapeutic efficacy of the payload. In combination with the above-mentioned polymer modification techniques, drug-delivery liposomes responsive to one or more stimuli, such as pH, temperature, light, redox, and specific enzymes, have been intensively studied and well-reviewed [171–175].

A reduction in pH has been reported for tumor tissues (pH 6.72–7.01 for human tumor xenograft lines) [176], inflammatory diseases (ca. 0.5 pH unit reduction) [177], or endo/lysosome (pH ~6.2 for early endosome, and 4.6–5.0 for lysosome) [178]. The change in pH can be utilized to modulate the release of encapsulated therapeutic agents from pH-sensitive liposomes by means of destabilization of liposomes or vesicle fusion. A brief summary of representative polymers for liposomal modification is listed in Table 2. Briefly, the strategies for designing polymer include: (1) protonation/deprotonation of charged groups triggered by a change in pH induces hydrophilicity/hydrophobicity transition and sometimes conformational switch of polymers; (2) pH-cleavable PEGylation (dePEGylation) by acid-labile linkers.

Table 2. pH-responsive polymers for the modification of liposomes for drug delivery.

Polymer	Responsive pH	Composition of Vesicles	Responsive Groups	Payload	TARGETING SITE	Properties	Ref.
			Polymers/Modified Polymers				
Octylamine-*graft*-poly (aspartic) (PASP-*g*-C8)	5.0	Lecithin/Chol/ PASP-*g*-C8 (48:12:x, mass ratio)	Carboxyl groups	Cytarabine (CYT)	Tumor cells	pH-induced destabilization of the liposomes, good biological stability, strong toxicity to tumor cells, and low effect on normal ones	[179]
Lipid-poly(2-ethylacrylic acid) (PEAA-C10)	4.5	PC/Chol/PEAA	Carboxyl group	Calcein	Potentially for tumor or localized infection	pH- and temperature-sensitive due to lipid-anchored PEAA and due to the introduction of diisopropylamide	[180]
MGlu-HA-C10, CHex-HA-C10	pKa = 5.37–6.70	EYPC/HA derivatives	Carboxyl groups	Doxorubicin (DOX)	Interior of cells	High molecular affinity to highly CD44-expressing cells and delivering drugs to the interior of cells as a result of pH-responsive membrane disruptive ability in endo/lysosomes	[181]
MGlu-HA and Chex-HA with anchor moieties (MGlu-HA-A14 and CHex-HA-A14)	-	EYPC/HA derivatives (7/3, *w/w*)	Carboxyl groups	A model antigenic protein ovalbumin (OVA)	Antigen-presenting cells (APCs), cytoplasm	Cytoplasmic delivery of OVA into dendritic cells, promoted Th1 cytokine production from these cells with CHex-HA-A	[182]
Succinylated poly(glycidol) (SucPG)	-	EYPC/SucPG (9:1, 8:2, and 7:3, mass ratio)	Carboxyl groups	Calcein	Cytoplasm	Transferring the content into cytoplasm by fusing with membranes of endosome and/or lysosome potentially with high stability and high efficiency	[183]
3-methyl-glutarylated hyperbranched poly(glycidol)s (MGlu-HPGs-C10)	6.5	EYPC/ polymer = 7/3, *w/w*	Carboxyl groups	Pyranine	Cytosol of DC2.4 cells	pH-sensitivity-inducing content release at mildly acidic pH, efficient drug-delivery to cytosol of DC2.4 cells	[184]
DSPE-PEG-$H_7K(R_2)_2$	6.8	DOPE/CHEMS/ DSPE-PEG or DSPE-PEG-$H_7K(R_2)_2$	H_7 sequence	DOX	Glioma	Tumor-specific pH-triggered DOX release under acidic conditions	[185]
DSPE-PEG_{2000}-TH	ca. 6.5 (pKa of the imidazole ring)	Chol/SPC/DSPE-PEG_{2000} or DSPE-PEG_{2000}-TH (33:59:2:6, molar ratio)	Imidazole ring in histidine	Paclitaxel (PTX)	Endoplasmic reticulum and Golgi apparatus, tumor cell	86.3% tumor inhibition rate in mice	[186]
DSPE-PEG_{2000}-STP	5.8	SPC/Chol/STP-PEG2000-DSPE/DOX (8:2:2:1, mass ratio)	-Lys-Asp-Glu-Glu-segment	DOX	Cytoplasm	Enhanced recognition ability and peneration by formation of α-helix at Lys-Asp-Glu-Glu-segment in the *N*-terminal in the presence of protons	[187]

Table 2. *Cont.*

R6H4-C18	6.4	SPC/Chol (20:1, mass ratio), 2.5 mol% R6H4-C18	Arginine and histidine	PTX	Tumor	Enhanced cellular uptake and intracellular drug delivery	[188]
pH-responsive block copolymer							
Stearoyl-PEG-poly(methacryloyl sulfadimethoxine) copolymer (stearoyl-PEG-PSDM)	7.0	mPEG-DSPE/stearoyl-PEG-PSDM/lipid	Sulfadimethoxine		Cancer	Stable in serum, undergoing rearrangement in tumor-like environment, high intracellular drug delivery	[189]
Poly(styrene-*co*-maleic acid) (PSMA)	pK_1: 5.27	DSPC/SMA (20:1, molar ratio)	Carboxylate groups pK1: 5.27		Cytoplasmic delivery	Configurational transition of the polymer below pK1 leading to disruptive lipid bilayer of erythrocytes, enhanced cytosolic delivery of encapsulated biomolecules through endosome destabilization together with stability in serum, excellent cytocompatibility, and efficient drug delivery than unmodified liposomes	[190]
Methoxy-poly(ethylene glycol)-*b*-poly(N-2-hydroxypropyl methacrylamide-co-histidine)-cholesterol [mPEG-P(HPMA-*g*-His)-Chol)]	5.0	mPEG-P(HPMA-*g*-His)-chol /DPPC (1:34, molar ratio)	Imidazole ring of histidine	DOX	Extracellular matrix (ECM) of tumor	ECM targeting, rapid drug release in an acidic environment, preferential tumor accumulation	[191]
PEG_m-$PDPA_n$-PEG_m triblock copolymers	ca. 6.2	HSPC or DOPC/Chol/ PEG_m-$PDPA_n$-PEG_m in various molar ratios	Tertiary amine groups	DOX	Tumor	pH-controllable drug release due to escape of the bola polymer from liposome at acidic pH as a result of hydrophobic to hydrophilic transition of the PDPA segment	[51]
C_7H_{15}-AZO-*b*-$PDPA_n$-*b*-mPEG	6.0	HSPC/DOPC/ Chol/C_7H_{15}-AZO-*b*-$PDPA_n$-*b*-mPEG, with different ratios	Tertiary amine groups	DOX	-	pH- and photo-dual responsive	[192]
dePEGylation							
mPEG-Hz-CHEMS	5.5 [193]	Soy PC/Chol/ mPEG2000-Hz-CHEMS/PTX (90:10:3:3)	Hydrazone	-	-	Prolonged circulation time and almost eliminated ABC phenomenon	[194]
PEG_B-Hz-DPPE	5.0	DOPE/DSPC/ CHEMS/Chol/ PEG_B-Hz-DPPE (4:2:2:2:0.5, molar ratio)	Acid labile hydrazide–hydrazone hybrid bond	Calcein/ gemcitabine	Tumor	Simultaneous long circulation and pH sensitivity, increased tumor aggregation	[195]
$mPEG_{2000}$-Hz-stearate (PHS)	<6.5	SPC/ cholesterol/PHS	Hydrazone bond	-	Tumor	Stronger pH sensitivity than that of PEG_{2000}-Hz-PE, superior cellular uptake and endosomal escape	[196]
$mPEG_{2000}$-Hz-Chol	5.5	S100PC/Chol/ mPEG2000-Hz-Chol (90:10:3)	Hydrazone	PTX	Breast cancer cells	Highly sensitive to mild acidic environment, accumulative drug release and enhanced cellular uptake at pH 5.5	[193]
PEG-diortho ester-distearoyl glycerol (POD)	5.5	POD/DOPE (1:9)	Diortho ester	ANTS and DPX	-	Stabilized liposome in serum and blood circulation, sensitive to acidic environment but stable in neutral pH	[197]

MGlu-HA: 3-methylglutarylated hyaluronic acid; Chex-HA: 2-carboxycyclohexane-1-carboxylated hyaluronic acid; TH: an engineered a-helical cell penetrating peptide AGYLLGHINLHHLAHL(Aib)HHIL-NH_2; PDPA: poly(2-(diisopropylamino) ethylmethacrylate; STP: a peptide SKDEEWHKNNFPLSP; ANTS: 8-aminonaphthalene-1,2,3-trisulfonic acid; DPX: *p*-xylenebis(pyridinium) bromide.

The pH-responsive homopolymer-bearing carboxyl groups, such as poly(aspartic), grafted with hydrophobic anchor octylamine (PASP-*g*-C8) [179], has been applied to induce destabilization and/or fusogenicity under weakly acidic conditions. Modification of widely investigated polymers with pH-sensitive moieties for the functionalization of liposomes could combine the functionality of both the polymer (such as long circulation for PEG) and pH sensitivity to the liposomal formulation. Such polymers include pH-sensitive PEG–lipid conjugates (DSPE-PEG-H7K(R2)2/TH/STP and stearoyl-poly(ethylene glycol)-poly(methacryloyl sulfadimethoxine) copolymer (stearoyl-PEG-PSDM) [185–187,189], HA derivatives bearing 3-methyl glutarylated (MGlu) units or 2-carboxycyclohexane-1-carboxylated (CHex) units (MGlu-HA or CHex-HA) [181], 3-methylglutarylated hyperbranched poly(glycidol) (MGlu-HPG) [184,198], etc. Liposome-coated MGlu-HA or CHex-HA not only exhibited a high cellular association to high CD44-expressing cells, but also delivered encapsulated drugs into cells via pH-responsive membrane-disruptive ability [181].

For copolymers bearing weakly charged groups and hydrophobic groups, the decreased ionization of the hydrophilic segments induces configuration changing from random coil to collapsed uncharged globular, which in turn changes the surface charge and aggregation of liposomes, as reflected by the zeta-potential and size distribution [190]. Such phenomena that hydrophilic-to-hydrophobic transition of polymers destabilizes liposomal formulation have been reported for poly(styrene-*co*-maleic acid) (PSMA, $pK_1 = 5.27$), which undergoes a conformational change from charged random coil to uncharged globular, as a result of the decreased degree of ionization in the carboxylate groups. The pK1 value of PSMA can be adjusted by the molecular weight of the polymer. Consequently, enhanced cytosolic delivery of encapsulated biomolecules through endosome destabilization together with stability in serum, excellent cytocompatibility, and more efficient drug delivery than unmodified liposomes were observed for the PSMA-modified DSPC liposomes [190]. A hydrophobic to hydrophilic transition was reported for the PDMA section of a bola triblock copolymer, PEG_m-$PDPA_n$-PEG_m. The bola polymer stabilizes liposome at normal pH but destabilizes it and promotes drug release under acidic conditions [51].

Stimulus-responsive dePEGylation is an attractive approach for triggered release (Figure 6). Although the stealth liposomes show a long circulating time and minimal payload leakage during circulation, they may diminish the fusogenic capacity of liposomes and hinder the release of encapsulated drugs at the diseased/target sites (PEG dilemma) [171,199]. To facilitate drug release at the desired location/enhance internalization of the nanocarriers into target cells, cleavage of PEG (dePEGylation) at the desired sites can be made using PEG-(stimuli-responsive linker)-lipid conjugates. Such linkers include not only pH-responsive diortho ester [197], vinyl ether [200,201], hydrazone or hydrazide–hydrazone [14,202], but also reducing agent-responsive disulfide [203] and enzyme-responsive peptides [204]. In addition to promoting extracellular/intercellular release, the dePEGylation approach exposes the liposomal surface, which may cause enhanced liposome–cellular interaction, restored fusogenicity of liposomes, and enablement of endosomal escape, as well as a lowered anti-PEG immune response [171].

Mild hyperthermia has been investigated as an effective method of enhancing local drug release. For thermo-sensitive polymers with a lower critical solution temperature (LCST) near body temperature, the temperature-induced configuration change can be utilized to manipulate drug release from liposomes. Poly(*N*-isopropylacrylamide) (PNIPAAm) is a prototype polymer exhibiting an LCST near 32 °C in an aqueous environment, above which temperature its polymer chain undergoes a coil-to-globule transition [205]. Therefore, PNIPAAm derivatives have been the most popular polymers for thermo-responsive drug delivery. The reported PNIPAAm derivatives and their corresponding LCST include $C_{12}H_{25}$–PNIPAAm–COOH conjugate (37 °C) [206], PNIPAAm-DSPE (34 °C in water and 29.8 °C in 0.01 M PBS, pH 7.4) [207], and p(NIPAAm-co-DMAAm)-DSPE (46.9 °C in water and 38.8 °C in PBS) [207]. As PNIPAAm is not biodegradable, poly(*N*-(2-hydroxypropyl)methacrylamide) (PHPMA) polymers have been studied as biodegradable alternatives [208]. Quick thermo-responsive polymer p(NIPAM-*r*-HPMA) (LCST 42 °C), synthesized by a reversible addition-fragmentation chain transfer (RAFT) technique, maintained the stability of liposomes at 37 °C but promoted 70% doxorubicin release within 1 min even at 42 °C with 1% polymer incorporated into the liposome [209].

Other reported thermo-sensitive polymers for liposome modification include a block copolymer of (2-ethoxy)ethoxyethyl vinyl ether (EOEOVE) with anchor group octadecyl vinyl ether (ODVE) (P(EOEOVE-*s*-ODVE)) [210], Pluronic F127 and its derivatives [211], etc.

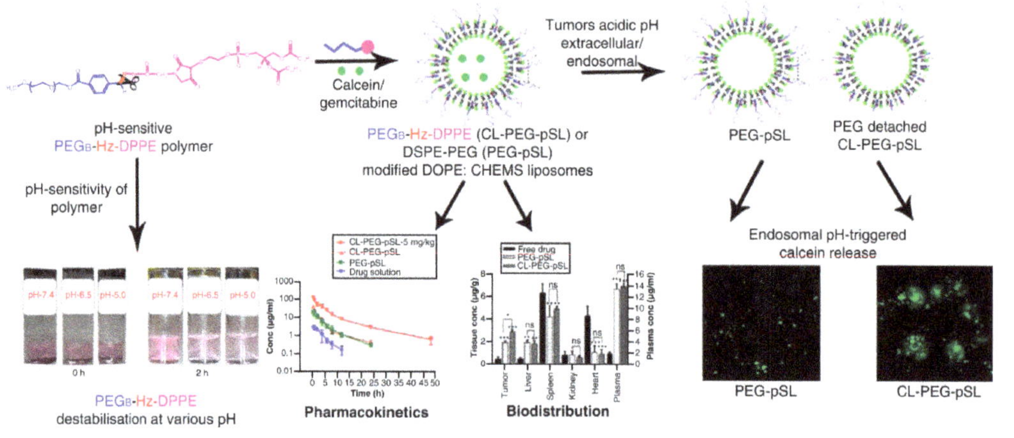

Figure 6. Liposomes modified with pH-sensitive PEG-Hz-DPPE polymers. DePEGylation was achieved by introducing a pH-sheddable hydrazide–hydrazone linker to the PEG–lipid conjugate. Under mild acidic environments, rapid endo/lysosomal escape and enhanced accumulation of drugs in model tumor cells show that cleavable PEGylation is an efficient strategy for cancer therapy. * $p < 0.05$; ** $p < 0.01$; *** $p < 0.001$ versus free drug. Adapted from Ref. [195]. Copyright © 2019, Future Medicine.

In addition to pH and temperature, stimuli such as light, redox, magnetic fields, and enzymes have also been reported to trigger drug release from liposomes modified with specific stimulus-responsive molecules [172,212]. Liposomes functionalized with a combination of more than one stimulus or combined stimuli and targeting have also been designed for more effective drug release [213].

6. Conclusions and Perspective

In summary, polymer-modified liposomes as drug-delivery carriers have found broad and promising applications by specific polymers. In addition to the clinically approved formulations, much more promising studies have been conducted at lab-scale. Some critical issues should be addressed to bring more liposomal drug-delivery systems into market. More efforts should be put into regulatory matters and scaling-up of complex formulations, sufficient and comprehensive in vitro and in vivo experiments, and a deeper understanding of the mechanism of action for encapsulated drugs.

Author Contributions: Conception, Y.C., X.D. and X.C.; writing—original draft preparation, Y.C.; writing—review and editing, Y.C., X.D. and X.C.; funding acquisition, Y.C. and X.C. All authors have read and agreed to the published version of the manuscript.

Funding: This work was supported by the "Pioneer" and "Leading Goose" R&D Program of Zhejiang from the Science Technology Department of Zhejiang Province, grant number 2022C03050, the Zhejiang Provincial Natural Science Foundation of China, grant number LY18H140001, and the National Natural Science Foundation of China, grant number 81400511. X. Chen is sponsored by the Zhejiang Provincial Program for the Cultivation of High-level Innovative Health Talents (2021).

Institutional Review Board Statement: Not applicable.

Informed Consent Statement: Not applicable.

Data Availability Statement: Not applicable.

Acknowledgments: The authors thank Weifeng Lin for his helpful comments on the conception and editing of the manuscript.

Conflicts of Interest: The authors declare no conflict of interest.

References

1. Allen, T.M.; Cullis, P.R. Drug delivery systems: Entering the mainstream. *Science* **2004**, *303*, 1818–1822. [CrossRef] [PubMed]
2. Bangham, A.D.; Horne, R.W. Negative staining of phospholipids and their structural modification by surface-active agents as observed in the electron microscope. *J. Mol. Biol.* **1964**, *8*, 660–668. [CrossRef]
3. van der Koog, L.; Gandek, T.B.; Nagelkerke, A. Liposomes and Extracellular Vesicles as Drug Delivery Systems: A Comparison of Composition, Pharmacokinetics, and Functionalization. *Adv. Healthc. Mater.* **2021**, *11*, e2100639. [CrossRef] [PubMed]
4. Cao, Y.; Ma, Y.; Tao, Y.; Lin, W.; Wang, P. Intra-Articular Drug Delivery for Osteoarthritis Treatment. *Pharmaceutics* **2021**, *13*, 2166. [CrossRef] [PubMed]
5. Barenholz, Y. Doxil®—The first FDA-approved nano-drug: Lessons learned. *J. Control. Release* **2012**, *160*, 117–134. [CrossRef]
6. Bulbake, U.; Doppalapudi, S.; Kommineni, N.; Khan, W. Liposomal Formulations in Clinical Use: An Updated Review. *Pharmaceutics* **2017**, *9*, 12. [CrossRef]
7. Beltrán-Gracia, E.; López-Camacho, A.; Higuera-Ciapara, I.; Velázquez-Fernández, J.B.; Vallejo-Cardona, A.A. Nanomedicine review: Clinical developments in liposomal applications. *Cancer Nanotechnol.* **2019**, *10*, 11. [CrossRef]
8. Chen, K.H.; Di Sabatino, M.; Albertini, B.; Passerini, N.; Kett, V.L. The effect of polymer coatings on physicochemical properties of spray-dried liposomes for nasal delivery of BSA. *Eur. J. Pharm. Sci.* **2013**, *50*, 312–322. [CrossRef]
9. Yang, K.J.; Son, J.; Jung, S.Y.; Yi, G.; Yoo, J.; Kim, D.K.; Koo, H. Optimized phospholipid-based nanoparticles for inner ear drug delivery and therapy. *Biomaterials* **2018**, *171*, 133–143. [CrossRef]
10. Lai, F.; Caddeo, C.; Manca, M.L.; Manconi, M.; Sinico, C.; Fadda, A.M. What's new in the field of phospholipid vesicular nanocarriers for skin drug delivery. *Int. J. Pharm.* **2020**, *583*, 119398. [CrossRef]
11. Werle, M.; Takeuchi, H. Chitosan-aprotinin coated liposomes for oral peptide delivery: Development, characterisation and in vivo evaluation. *Int. J. Pharm.* **2009**, *370*, 26–32. [CrossRef] [PubMed]
12. Lin, W.; Goldberg, R.; Klein, J. Poly-phosphocholination of liposomes leads to highly-extended retention time in mice joints. *J. Mater. Chem. B* **2022**. [CrossRef] [PubMed]
13. Das, M.; Huang, L. Liposomal Nanostructures for Drug Delivery in Gastrointestinal Cancers. *J. Pharmacol. Pharmacol. Exp. Ther.* **2019**, *370*, 647–656. [CrossRef] [PubMed]
14. Chen, Y.; Cheng, Y.; Zhao, P.; Zhang, S.; Li, M.; He, C.; Zhang, X.; Yang, T.; Yan, R.; Ye, P.; et al. Co-delivery of doxorubicin and imatinib by pH sensitive cleavable PEGylated nanoliposomes with folate-mediated targeting to overcome multidrug resistance. *Int. J. Pharm.* **2018**, *542*, 266–279. [CrossRef] [PubMed]
15. Ameselem, S.; Cohen, R.; Barenholz, Y. In vitro tests to predict in vivo performance of liposomal dosage forms. *Chem. Phys. Lipids* **1993**, *64*, 219–237. [CrossRef]
16. Mayer, L.D.; Tai, L.C.; Ko, D.S.; Masin, D.; Ginsberg, R.S.; Cullis, P.R.; Bally, M.B. Influence of vesicle size, lipid composition, and drug-to-lipid ratio on the biological activity of liposomal doxorubicin in mice. *Cancer Res.* **1989**, *49*, 5922–5930.
17. Un, K.; Sakai-Kato, K.; Oshima, Y.; Kawanishi, T.; Okuda, H. Intracellular trafficking mechanism, from intracellular uptake to extracellular efflux, for phospholipid/cholesterol liposomes. *Biomaterials* **2012**, *33*, 8131–8141. [CrossRef]
18. Smistad, G.; Jacobsen, J.; Sande, S.A. Multivariate toxicity screening of liposomal formulations on a human buccal cell line. *Int. J. Pharm.* **2007**, *330*, 14–22. [CrossRef]
19. Fang, J.; Nakamura, H.; Maeda, H. The EPR effect: Unique features of tumor blood vessels for drug delivery, factors involved, and limitations and augmentation of the effect. *Adv. Drug Deliv. Rev.* **2011**, *63*, 136–151. [CrossRef]
20. Maruyama, K. Intracellular targeting delivery of liposomal drugs to solid tumors based on EPR effects. *Adv. Drug Deliv. Rev.* **2011**, *63*, 161–169. [CrossRef]
21. Matsumura, Y.; Maeda, H. A New Concept for Macromolecular Therapeutics in Cancer Chemotherapy: Mechanism of Tumoritropic Accumulation of Proteins and the Antitumor Agent Smancs. *Cancer Res.* **1986**, *46*, 6387–6392. [PubMed]
22. Peer, D.; Karp, J.M.; Hong, S.; Farokhzad, O.C.; Margalit, R.; Langer, R. Nanocarriers as an emerging platform for cancer therapy. *Nat. Nanotechnol.* **2007**, *2*, 751–760. [CrossRef]
23. Castro, M.; Lindqvist, D. Liposome-mediated delivery of challenging chemicals to aid environmental assessment of Bioaccumulative (B) and Toxic (T) properties. *Sci. Rep.* **2020**, *10*, 9725. [CrossRef] [PubMed]
24. Zucker, D.; Marcus, D.; Barenholz, Y.; Goldblum, A. Liposome drugs' loading efficiency: A working model based on loading conditions and drug's physicochemical properties. *J. Control. Release* **2009**, *139*, 73–80. [CrossRef] [PubMed]
25. Eloy, J.O.; Claro de Souza, M.; Petrilli, R.; Barcellos, J.P.; Lee, R.J.; Marchetti, J.M. Liposomes as carriers of hydrophilic small molecule drugs: Strategies to enhance encapsulation and delivery. *Colloids Surf. B Biointerfaces* **2014**, *123*, 345–363. [CrossRef]
26. Li, T.; Cipolla, D.; Rades, T.; Boyd, B.J. Drug nanocrystallisation within liposomes. *J. Control. Release* **2018**, *288*, 96–110. [CrossRef]
27. Shah, S.; Dhawan, V.; Holm, R.; Nagarsenker, M.S.; Perrie, Y. Liposomes: Advancements and innovation in the manufacturing process. *Adv. Drug Deliv. Rev.* **2020**, *154–155*, 102–122. [CrossRef]

28. Zhao, L.; Temelli, F.; Curtis, J.M.; Chen, L. Preparation of liposomes using supercritical carbon dioxide technology: Effects of phospholipids and sterols. *Food Res. Int.* **2015**, *77*, 63–72. [CrossRef]
29. Shah, V.M.; Nguyen, D.X.; Patel, P.; Cote, B.; Al-Fatease, A.; Pham, Y.; Huynh, M.G.; Woo, Y.; Alani, A.W. Liposomes produced by microfluidics and extrusion: A comparison for scale-up purposes. *Nanomedicine* **2019**, *18*, 146–156. [CrossRef]
30. Akbarzadeh, A.; Rezaei-Sadabady, R.; Davaran, S.; Joo, S.W.; Zarghami, N.; Hanifehpour, Y.; Samiei, M.; Kouhi, M.; Nejati-Koshki, K. Liposome: Classification, preparation, and applications. *Nanoscale Res. Lett.* **2013**, *18*, 102. [CrossRef]
31. Ali, M.H.; Moghaddam, B.; Kirby, D.J.; Mohammed, A.R.; Perrie, Y. The role of lipid geometry in designing liposomes for the solubilisation of poorly water soluble drugs. *Int. J. Pharm.* **2013**, *453*, 225–232. [CrossRef] [PubMed]
32. Sur, S.; Fries, A.C.; Kinzler, K.W.; Zhou, S.; Vogelstein, B. Remote loading of preencapsulated drugs into stealth liposomes. *Proc. Natl. Acad. Sci. USA* **2014**, *111*, 2283–2288. [CrossRef] [PubMed]
33. Torchilin, V.P. Recent advances with liposomes as pharmaceutical carriers. *Nat. Rev. Drug Discov.* **2005**, *4*, 145–160. [CrossRef] [PubMed]
34. Lin, W.; Kampf, N.; Goldberg, R.; Driver, M.J.; Klein, J. Poly-phosphocholinated Liposomes Form Stable Superlubrication Vectors. *Langmuir* **2019**, *35*, 6048–6054. [CrossRef] [PubMed]
35. Caracciolo, G. Clinically approved liposomal nanomedicines: Lessons learned from the biomolecular corona. *Nanoscale* **2018**, *10*, 4167–4172. [CrossRef]
36. Cedervall, T.; Lynch, I.; Lindman, S.; Berggård, T.; Thulin, E.; Nilsson, H.; Dawson, K.A.; Linse, S. Understanding the nanoparticle–protein corona using methods to quantify exchange rates and affinities of proteins for nanoparticles. *Proc. Natl. Acad. Sci. USA* **2007**, *104*, 2050–2055. [CrossRef]
37. Comiskey, S.J.; Heath, T.D. Serum-induced leakage of negatively-charged liposomes at nanomolar lipid concentrations. *Biochemistry* **1990**, *29*, 3626–3631. [CrossRef]
38. Kelly, C.; Jefferies, C.; Cryan, S.A. Targeted liposomal drug delivery to monocytes and macrophages. *J. Drug Deliv.* **2011**, *2011*, 727241. [CrossRef]
39. Allen, T.M.; Hansen, C.; Rutledge, J. Liposomes with prolonged circulation times: Factors affecting uptake by reticuloendothelial and other tissues. *Biochim. Biophys. Acta Biomembr.* **1989**, *981*, 27–35. [CrossRef]
40. Gustafson, H.H.; Holt-Casper, D.; Grainger, D.W.; Ghandehari, H. Nanoparticle uptake: The phagocyte problem. *Nano Today* **2015**, *10*, 487–510. [CrossRef]
41. Takeuchi, H.; Kojima, H.; Yamamoto, H.; Kawashima, Y. Polymer coating of liposomes with a modified polyvinyl alcohol and their systemic circulation and RES uptake in rats. *J. Control. Release* **2000**, *68*, 195–205. [CrossRef]
42. Allen, T.M.; Everest, J.M. Effect of Liposome Size and Drug Release Properties on Pharmacokinetics of Encapsulaed Drug in Rats. *J. Pharmacol. Exp. Ther.* **1983**, *226*, 539–544. [PubMed]
43. Nel, A.E.; Madler, L.; Velegol, D.; Xia, T.; Hoek, E.M.; Somasundaran, P.; Klaessig, F.; Castranova, V.; Thompson, M. Understanding biophysicochemical interactions at the nano-bio interface. *Nat. Mater.* **2009**, *8*, 543–557. [CrossRef] [PubMed]
44. Gabizon, A.; Papahadjopoulos, D. Liposome formulations with prolonged circulation time in blood and enhanced uptake by tumors. *Proc. Natl. Acad. Sci. USA* **1988**, *85*, 6949–6953. [CrossRef]
45. Hadinoto, K.; Sundaresan, A.; Cheow, W.S. Lipid-polymer hybrid nanoparticles as a new generation therapeutic delivery platform: A review. *Eur. J. Pharm. Biopharm.* **2013**, *85*, 427–443. [CrossRef]
46. Mukherjee, A.; Waters, A.K.; Kalyan, P.; Achrol, A.S.; Kesari, S.; Yenugonda, V.M. Lipid-polymer hybrid nanoparticles as a next-generation drug delivery platform: State of the art, emerging technologies, and perspectives. *Int. J. Nanomed.* **2019**, *14*, 1937–1952. [CrossRef]
47. Heo, M.B.; Cho, M.Y.; Lim, Y.T. Polymer nanoparticles for enhanced immune response: Combined delivery of tumor antigen and small interference RNA for immunosuppressive gene to dendritic cells. *Acta Biomater.* **2014**, *10*, 2169–2176. [CrossRef]
48. Liechty, W.B.; Kryscio, D.R.; Slaughter, B.V.; Peppas, N.A. Polymers for drug delivery systems. *Annu. Rev. Chem. Biomol. Eng.* **2010**, *1*, 149–173. [CrossRef]
49. Liu, Y.; Xie, X.; Chen, H.; Hou, X.; He, Y.; Shen, J.; Shi, J.; Feng, N. Advances in next-generation lipid-polymer hybrid nanocarriers with emphasis on polymer-modified functional liposomes and cell-based-biomimetic nanocarriers for active ingredients and fractions from Chinese medicine delivery. *Nanomedicine* **2020**, *29*, 102237. [CrossRef]
50. Zhang, Y.; Mintzer, E.; Uhrich, K.E. Synthesis and characterization of PEGylated bolaamphiphiles with enhanced retention in liposomes. *J. Colloid Interface Sci.* **2016**, *482*, 19–26. [CrossRef]
51. Hao, W.; Han, X.; Shang, Y.; Xu, S.; Liu, H. Insertion of pH-sensitive bola-type copolymer into liposome as a "stability anchor" for control of drug release. *Colloids Surf. B Biointerfaces* **2015**, *136*, 809–816. [CrossRef] [PubMed]
52. Masuda, T.; Shimada, N.; Maruyama, A. Liposome-Surface-Initiated ARGET ATRP: Surface Softness Generated by "Grafting from" Polymerization. *Langmuir* **2019**, *35*, 5581–5586. [CrossRef] [PubMed]
53. Li, M.; Jiang, S.; Simon, J.; Passlick, D.; Frey, M.L.; Wagner, M.; Mailander, V.; Crespy, D.; Landfester, K. Brush Conformation of Polyethylene Glycol Determines the Stealth Effect of Nanocarriers in the Low Protein Adsorption Regime. *Nano Lett.* **2021**, *21*, 1591–1598. [CrossRef] [PubMed]
54. Labouta, H.I.; Gomez-Garcia, M.J.; Sarsons, C.D.; Nguyen, T.; Kennard, J.; Ngo, W.; Terefe, K.; Iragorri, N.; Lai, P.; Rinker, K.D.; et al. Surface-grafted polyethylene glycol conformation impacts the transport of PEG-functionalized liposomes through a tumour extracellular. *RSC Adv.* **2018**, *8*, 7697. [CrossRef]

55. Kenworthy, A.K.; Hristova, K.; Needham, D.; McIntosh, T.J. Range and magnitude of the steric pressure between bilayers containing phospholipids with covalently attached poly(ethylene glycol). *Biophys. J.* **1995**, *68*, 1921–1936. [CrossRef]
56. Erfani, A.; Seaberg, J.; Aichele, C.P.; Ramsey, J.D. Interactions between Biomolecules and Zwitterionic Moieties: A Review. *Biomacromolecules* **2020**, *21*, 2557–2573. [CrossRef]
57. Chen, S.; Li, L.; Zhao, C.; Zheng, J. Surface hydration: Principles and applications toward low-fouling/nonfouling biomaterials. *Polymer* **2010**, *51*, 5283–5293. [CrossRef]
58. Harris, J.M.; Chess, R.B. Effect of pegylation on pharmaceuticals. *Nat. Rev. Drug Discov.* **2003**, *2*, 214–221. [CrossRef]
59. Lee, J.H.; Lee, H.B.; Andrade, J.D. Blood compatibility of polyethylene oxide surfaces. *Prog. Polym. Sci.* **1995**, *20*, 1043–1079. [CrossRef]
60. Chen, S.; Yu, F.; Yu, Q.; He, Y.; Jiang, S. Strong Resistance of a Thin Crystalline Layer of Balanced Charged Groups to Protein Adsorption. *Langmuir* **2006**, *22*, 8186–8191. [CrossRef]
61. Gabizon, A.; Shmeeda, H.; Barenholz, Y. Pharmacokinetics of Pegylated Liposomal Doxorubicin. *Clin. Pharmacokinet.* **2003**, *42*, 419–436. [CrossRef] [PubMed]
62. Gabizon, A.; Catane, R.; Uziely, B.; Kaufman, B.; Safra, T.; Cohen, R.; Martin, F.; Huang, A.; Barenholz, Y. Prolonged Circulation Time and Enhanced Accumulation in Malignant Exudates of Doxorubicin Encapsulated in Polyethylene-glycol Coated Liposomes. *Cancer Res.* **1994**, *54*, 987–992. [PubMed]
63. Son, K.; Ueda, M.; Taguchi, K.; Maruyama, T.; Takeoka, S.; Ito, Y. Evasion of the accelerated blood clearance phenomenon by polysarcosine coating of liposomes. *J. Control. Release* **2020**, *322*, 209–216. [CrossRef] [PubMed]
64. Mohamed, M.; Abu Lila, A.S.; Shimizu, T.; Alaaeldin, E.; Hussein, A.; Sarhan, H.A.; Szebeni, J.; Ishida, T. PEGylated liposomes: Immunological responses. *Sci. Technol. Adv. Mater.* **2019**, *20*, 710–724. [CrossRef]
65. Garbuzenko, O.; Barenholz, Y.; Priev, A. Effect of grafted PEG on liposome size and on compressibility and packing of lipid bilayer. *Chem. Phys. Lipids* **2005**, *135*, 117–129. [CrossRef]
66. Hashizaki, K.; Taguchi, H.; Itoh, C.; Sakai, H.; Abe, M.; Saito, Y.; Ogawa, N. Effects of poly(ethylene glycol) (PEG) concentration on the permeability of PEG-grafted liposomes. *Chem. Pharm. Bull.* **2005**, *53*, 27–31. [CrossRef]
67. Kristensen, K.; Urquhart, A.J.; Thormann, E.; Andresen, T.L. Binding of human serum albumin to PEGylated liposomes: Insights into binding numbers and dynamics by fluorescence correlation spectroscopy. *Nanoscale* **2016**, *8*, 19726–19736. [CrossRef]
68. Kenworthy, A.K.; Simon, S.A.; McIntosh, T.J. Structure and phase behavior of lipid suspensions containing phospholipids with covalently attached poly(ethylene glycol). *Biophys. J.* **1995**, *68*, 1903–1920. [CrossRef]
69. Nunes, S.S.; de Oliveira Silva, J.; Fernandes, R.S.; Miranda, S.E.M.; Leite, E.A.; de Farias, M.A.; Portugal, R.V.; Cassali, G.D.; Townsend, D.M.; Oliveira, M.C.; et al. PEGylated versus Non-PEGylated pH-Sensitive Liposomes: New Insights from a Comparative Antitumor Activity Study. *Pharmaceutics* **2022**, *14*, 272. [CrossRef]
70. Orozco-Alcaraz, R.; Kuhl, T.L. Impact of membrane fluidity on steric stabilization by lipopolymers. *Langmuir* **2012**, *28*, 7470–7475. [CrossRef]
71. Papahadjopoulos, D.; Allen, T.M.; Gabizon, A.; Mayhew, E.; Matthay, K.; Huang, S.K.; Lee, K.D.; Woodle, M.C.; Lasic, D.D.; Redemann, C. Sterically stabilized liposomes: Improvements in pharmacokinetics and antitumor therapeutic efficacy. *Proc. Natl. Acad. Sci. USA* **1991**, *88*, 11460–11464. [CrossRef] [PubMed]
72. Chanan-Khan, A.; Szebeni, J.; Savay, S.; Liebes, L.; Rafique, N.M.; Alving, C.R.; Muggia, F.M. Complement activation following first exposure to pegylated liposomal doxorubicin (Doxil): Possible role in hypersensitivity reactions. *Ann Oncol.* **2003**, *14*, 1430–1437. [CrossRef] [PubMed]
73. Ishida, T.; Atobe, K.; Wang, X.; Kiwada, H. Accelerated blood clearance of PEGylated liposomes upon repeated injections: Effect of doxorubicin-encapsulation and high-dose first injection. *J. Control. Release* **2006**, *115*, 251–258. [CrossRef] [PubMed]
74. Ishida, T.; Ichihara, M.; Wang, X.; Kiwada, H. Spleen plays an important role in the induction of accelerated blood clearance of PEGylated liposomes. *J. Control. Release* **2006**, *115*, 243–250. [CrossRef]
75. Chen, E.; Chen, B.-M.; Su, Y.-C.; Chang, Y.-C.; Cheng, T.-L.; Barenholz, Y.; Roffler, S.R. Premature Drug Release from Polyethylene Glycol (PEG)-Coated Liposomal Doxorubicin via Formation of the Membrane Attack Complex. *ACS Nano* **2020**, *14*, 7808–7822. [CrossRef]
76. Chen, B.M.; Cheng, T.L.; Roffler, S.R. Polyethylene Glycol Immunogenicity: Theoretical, Clinical, and Practical Aspects of Anti-Polyethylene Glycol Antibodies. *ACS Nano* **2021**, *15*, 14022–14048. [CrossRef]
77. Yang, Q.; Jacobs, T.M.; McCallen, J.D.; Moore, D.T.; Huckaby, J.T.; Edelstein, J.N.; Lai, S.K. Analysis of Pre-existing IgG and IgM Antibodies against Polyethylene Glycol (PEG) in the General Population. *Anal. Chem.* **2016**, *88*, 11804–11812. [CrossRef]
78. Freire Haddad, H.; Burke, J.A.; Scott, E.A.; Ameer, G.A. Clinical Relevance of Pre-Existing and Treatment-Induced Anti-Poly(Ethylene Glycol) Antibodies. *Regen Eng. Transl. Med.* **2021**, 1–11. [CrossRef]
79. Vrieze, J.D. Pfizer's vaccine raises allergy concerns. *Science* **2021**, *317*, 10–11. [CrossRef]
80. Kierstead, P.H.; Okochi, H.; Venditto, V.J.; Chuong, T.C.; Kivimae, S.; Frechet, J.M.J.; Szoka, F.C. The effect of polymer backbone chemistry on the induction of the accelerated blood clearance in polymer modified liposomes. *J. Control. Release* **2015**, *213*, 1–9. [CrossRef]
81. Weber, C.; Voigt, M.; Simon, J.; Danner, A.-K.; Frey, H.; Mailänder, V.; Helm, M.; Morsbach, S.; Landfester, K. Functionalization of Liposomes with Hydrophilic Polymers Results in Macrophage Uptake Independent of the Protein Corona. *Biomacromolecules* **2019**, *20*, 2989–2999. [CrossRef] [PubMed]

82. Koide, H.; Asai, T.; Kato, H.; Ando, H.; Shiraishi, K.; Yokoyama, M.; Oku, N. Size-dependent induction of accelerated blood clearance phenomenon by repeated injections of polymeric micelles. *Int. J. Pharm.* **2012**, *432*, 75–79. [CrossRef] [PubMed]
83. Liu, M.; Chu, Y.; Liu, H.; Su, Y.; Zhang, Q.; Jiao, J.; Liu, M.; Ding, J.; Liu, M.; Hu, Y.; et al. Accelerated Blood Clearance of Nanoemulsions Modified with PEG-Cholesterol and PEG-Phospholipid Derivatives in Rats: The Effect of PEG-Lipid Linkages and PEG Molecular Weights. *Mol. Pharm.* **2020**, *17*, 1059–1070. [CrossRef] [PubMed]
84. Ishida, T.; Ichihara, M.; Wang, X.; Yamamoto, K.; Kimura, J.; Majima, E.; Kiwada, H. Injection of PEGylated liposomes in rats elicits PEG-specific IgM, which is responsible for rapid elimination of a second dose of PEGylated liposomes. *J. Control. Release* **2006**, *112*, 15–25. [CrossRef] [PubMed]
85. McSweeney, M.D.; Shen, L.; DeWalle, A.C.; Joiner, J.B.; Ciociola, E.C.; Raghuwanshi, D.; Macauley, M.S.; Lai, S.K. Pre-treatment with high molecular weight free PEG effectively suppresses anti-PEG antibody induction by PEG-liposomes in mice. *J. Control. Release* **2021**, *329*, 774–781. [CrossRef]
86. Li, C.; Zhao, X.; Wang, Y.; Yang, H.; Li, H.; Li, H.; Tian, W.; Yang, J.; Cui, J. Prolongation of time interval between doses could eliminate accelerated blood clearance phenomenon induced by pegylated liposomal topotecan. *Int. J. Pharm.* **2013**, *443*, 17–25. [CrossRef]
87. McSweeney, M.D.; Price, L.S.L.; Wessler, T.; Ciociola, E.C.; Herity, L.B.; Piscitelli, J.A.; DeWalle, A.C.; Harris, T.N.; Chan, A.K.P.; Saw, R.S.; et al. Overcoming anti-PEG antibody mediated accelerated blood clearance of PEGylated liposomes by pre-infusion with high molecular weight free PEG. *J. Control. Release* **2019**, *311–312*, 138–146. [CrossRef]
88. Mima, Y.; Abu Lila, A.S.; Shimizu, T.; Ukawa, M.; Ando, H.; Kurata, Y.; Ishida, T. Ganglioside inserted into PEGylated liposome attenuates anti-PEG immunity. *J. Control. Release* **2017**, *250*, 20–26. [CrossRef]
89. Moghimi, S.M.; Hamad, I.; Andresen, T.L.; Jorgensen, K.; Szebeni, J. Methylation of the phosphate oxygen moiety of phospholipid-methoxy(polyethylene glycol) conjugate prevents PEGylated liposome-mediated complement activation and anaphylatoxin production. *FASEB J.* **2006**, *20*, 2591–2593. [CrossRef]
90. Nag, O.K.; Yadav, V.R.; Hedrick, A.; Awasthi, V. Post-modification of preformed liposomes with novel non-phospholipid poly(ethylene glycol)-conjugated hexadecylcarbamoylmethyl hexadecanoic acid for enhanced circulation persistence in vivo. *Int. J. Pharm.* **2013**, *446*, 119–129. [CrossRef]
91. Xu, H.; Wang, K.Q.; Deng, Y.H.; Chen, D.W. Effects of cleavable PEG-cholesterol derivatives on the accelerated blood clearance of PEGylated liposomes. *Biomaterials* **2010**, *31*, 4757–4763. [CrossRef] [PubMed]
92. Shimizu, T.; Abu Lila, A.S.; Fujita, R.; Awata, M.; Kawanishi, M.; Hashimoto, Y.; Okuhira, K.; Ishima, Y.; Ishida, T. A hydroxyl PEG version of PEGylated liposomes and its impact on anti-PEG IgM induction and on the accelerated clearance of PEGylated liposomes. *Eur. J. Pharm. Biopharm.* **2018**, *127*, 142–149. [CrossRef] [PubMed]
93. Liu, S.; Jiang, S. Chemical conjugation of zwitterionic polymers protects immunogenic enzyme and preserves bioactivity without polymer-specific antibody response. *Nano Today* **2016**, *11*, 285–291. [CrossRef]
94. Lila, A.S.A.; Nawata, K.; Shimizu, T.; Ishida, T.; Kiwada, H. Use of polyglycerol (PG), instead of polyethylene glycol (PEG), prevents induction of the accelerated blood clearance phenomenon against long-circulating liposomes upon repeated administration. *Int. J. Pharm.* **2013**, *456*, 235–242. [CrossRef] [PubMed]
95. Liu, M.; Li, J.; Zhao, D.; Yan, N.; Zhang, H.; Liu, M.; Tang, X.; Hu, Y.; Ding, J.; Zhang, N.; et al. Branched PEG-modification: A new strategy for nanocarriers to evade of the accelerated blood clearance phenomenon and enhance anti-tumor efficacy. *Biomaterials* **2022**, *283*, 121415. [CrossRef]
96. Nag, O.K.; Yadav, V.R.; Croft, B.; Hedrick, A.; Awasthi, V. Liposomes modified with superhydrophilic polymer linked to a nonphospholipid anchor exhibit reduced complement activation and enhanced circulation. *J. Pharm. Sci.* **2015**, *104*, 114–123. [CrossRef]
97. Papi, M.; Caputo, D.; Palmieri, V.; Coppola, R.; Palchetti, S.; Bugli, F.; Martini, C.; Digiacomo, L.; Pozzi, D.; Caracciolo, G. Clinically approved PEGylated nanoparticles are covered by a protein corona that boosts the uptake by cancer cells. *Nanoscale* **2017**, *9*, 10327–10334. [CrossRef]
98. Wu, J.; Zhao, C.; Hu, R.; Lin, W.; Wang, Q.; Zhao, J.; Bilinovich, S.M.; Leeper, T.C.; Li, L.; Cheung, H.M.; et al. Probing the weak interaction of proteins with neutral and zwitterionic antifouling polymers. *Acta Biomater.* **2014**, *10*, 751–760. [CrossRef]
99. Li, B.; Yuan, Z.; Hung, H.C.; Ma, J.; Jain, P.; Tsao, C.; Xie, J.; Zhang, P.; Lin, X.; Wu, K.; et al. Revealing the Immunogenic Risk of Polymers. *Angew. Chem. Int. Ed. Engl.* **2018**, *57*, 13873–13876. [CrossRef]
100. Cao, Z.; Zhang, L.; Jiang, S. Superhydrophilic zwitterionic polymers stabilize liposomes. *Langmuir* **2012**, *28*, 11625–11632. [CrossRef]
101. Li, Y.; Liu, R.; Yang, J.; Shi, Y.; Ma, G.; Zhang, Z.; Zhang, X. Enhanced retention and anti-tumor efficacy of liposomes by changing their cellular uptake and pharmacokinetics behavior. *Biomaterials* **2015**, *41*, 1–14. [CrossRef] [PubMed]
102. Chen, M.; Briscoe, W.H.; Armes, S.P.; Klein, J. Lubrication at Physiological Pressures by Polyzwitterionic Brushes. *Science* **2009**, *323*, 1698–1701. [CrossRef] [PubMed]
103. Cao, Y.; Klein, J. Lipids and lipid mixtures in boundary layers: From hydration lubrication to osteoarthritis. *Curr. Opin. Colloid Interface Sci.* **2022**, *58*, 101559. [CrossRef]
104. Lin, W.; Klein, J. Recent Progress in Cartilage Lubrication. *Adv. Mater.* **2021**, *33*, e2005513. [CrossRef] [PubMed]

105. Huang, H.; Zhang, C.; Crisci, R.; Lu, T.; Hung, H.C.; Sajib, M.S.J.; Sarker, P.; Ma, J.; Wei, T.; Jiang, S.; et al. Strong Surface Hydration and Salt Resistant Mechanism of a New Nonfouling Zwitterionic Polymer Based on Protein Stabilizer TMAO. *J. Am. Chem. Soc.* **2021**, *143*, 16786–16795. [CrossRef]
106. Liu, Q.; Li, W.; Wang, H.; Newby, B.M.; Cheng, F.; Liu, L. Amino Acid-Based Zwitterionic Polymer Surfaces Highly Resist Long-Term Bacterial Adhesion. *Langmuir* **2016**, *32*, 7866–7874. [CrossRef]
107. Ederth, T.; Lerm, M.; Orihuela, B.; Rittschof, D. Resistance of Zwitterionic Peptide Monolayers to Biofouling. *Langmuir* **2019**, *35*, 1818–1827. [CrossRef]
108. Romberg, B.; Oussoren, C.; Snel, C.J.; Carstens, M.G.; Hennink, W.E.; Storm, G. Pharmacokinetics of poly(hydroxyethyl-l-asparagine)-coated liposomes is superior over that of PEG-coated liposomes at low lipid dose and upon repeated administration. *Biochim. Biophys. Acta Biomembr.* **2007**, *1768*, 737–743. [CrossRef]
109. Jain, P.; Hung, H.C.; Lin, X.; Ma, J.; Zhang, P.; Sun, F.; Wu, K.; Jiang, S. Poly(ectoine) Hydrogels Resist Nonspecific Protein Adsorption. *Langmuir* **2017**, *33*, 11264–11269. [CrossRef]
110. Date, T.; Nimbalkar, V.; Kamat, J.; Mittal, A.; Mahato, R.I.; Chitkara, D. Lipid-polymer hybrid nanocarriers for delivering cancer therapeutics. *J. Control. Release* **2018**, *271*, 60–73. [CrossRef]
111. De Leo, V.; Milano, F.; Agostiano, A.; Catucci, L. Recent Advancements in Polymer/Liposome Assembly for Drug Delivery: From Surface Modifications to Hybrid Vesicles. *Polymers* **2021**, *13*, 1027. [CrossRef] [PubMed]
112. Tenchov, R.; Bird, R.; Curtze, A.E.; Zhou, Q. Lipid Nanoparticles-From Liposomes to mRNA Vaccine Delivery, a Landscape of Research Diversity and Advancement. *ACS Nano* **2021**, *15*, 16982–17015. [CrossRef] [PubMed]
113. Gasperini, A.A.; Puentes-Martinez, X.E.; Balbino, T.A.; Rigoletto Tde, P.; Correa Gde, S.; Cassago, A.; Portugal, R.V.; de La Torre, L.G.; Cavalcanti, L.P. Association between cationic liposomes and low molecular weight hyaluronic acid. *Langmuir* **2015**, *31*, 3308–3317. [CrossRef] [PubMed]
114. Park, J.H.; Cho, H.J.; Yoon, H.Y.; Yoon, I.S.; Ko, S.H.; Shim, J.S.; Cho, J.H.; Park, J.H.; Kim, K.; Kwon, I.C.; et al. Hyaluronic acid derivative-coated nanohybrid liposomes for cancer imaging and drug delivery. *J. Control. Release* **2014**, *174*, 98–108. [CrossRef] [PubMed]
115. Correa, S.; Boehnke, N.; Deiss-Yehiely, E.; Hammond, P.T. Solution Conditions Tune and Optimize Loading of Therapeutic Polyelectrolytes into Layer-by-Layer Functionalized Liposomes. *ACS Nano* **2019**, *13*, 5623–5634. [CrossRef]
116. Lee, S.-M.; Chen, H.; Dettmer, C.M.; O'Halloran, T.V.; Nguyen, S.T. Polymer-Caged Lipsomes: A pH-Responsive Delivery System with High Stability. *J. Am. Chem. Soc.* **2007**, *129*, 15096–15097. [CrossRef]
117. Hasan, M.; Ben Messaoud, G.; Michaux, F.; Tamayol, A.; Kahn, C.J.F.; Belhaj, N.; Linder, M.; Arab-Tehrany, E. Chitosan-coated liposomes encapsulating curcumin: Study of lipid–polysaccharide interactions and nanovesicle behavior. *RSC Adv.* **2016**, *6*, 45290–45304. [CrossRef]
118. Hamedinasab, H.; Rezayan, A.H.; Mellat, M.; Mashreghi, M.; Jaafari, M.R. Development of chitosan-coated liposome for pulmonary delivery of N-acetylcysteine. *Int. J. Biol. Macromol.* **2020**, *156*, 1455–1463. [CrossRef]
119. Fujimoto, K.; Toyoda, T.; Fukui, Y. Preparation of Bionanocapsules by the Layer-by-Layer Deposition of Polypeptides onto a Liposome. *Macromolecules* **2007**, *40*, 5122–5128. [CrossRef]
120. Takeuchi, H.; Kojima, H.; Yamamoto, H.; Kawashima, Y. Evaluation of circulation profiles of liposomes coated with hydrophilic polymers having different molecular weights in rats. *J. Control. Release* **2001**, *75*, 83–91. [CrossRef]
121. Mertins, O.; Dimova, R. Insights on the interactions of chitosan with phospholipid vesicles. Part II: Membrane stiffening and pore formation. *Langmuir* **2013**, *29*, 14552–14559. [CrossRef] [PubMed]
122. Fang, N.; Chan, V.; Mao, H.-Q.; Leong, K.W. Interactions of Phospholipid Bilayer with Chitosan: Effect of Molecular Weight and pH. *Biomacromolecules* **2001**, *2*, 1161–1168. [CrossRef] [PubMed]
123. Mady, M.M.; Darwish, M.M.; Khalil, S.; Khalil, W.M. Biophysical studies on chitosan-coated liposomes. *Eur. Biophys. J.* **2009**, *38*, 1127–1133. [CrossRef] [PubMed]
124. Schlenoff, J.B. Zwitteration: Coating surfaces with zwitterionic functionality to reduce nonspecific adsorption. *Langmuir* **2014**, *30*, 9625–9636. [CrossRef] [PubMed]
125. Wagner, J.; Dillenburger, M.; Simon, J.; Oberlander, J.; Landfester, K.; Mailander, V.; Ng, D.Y.W.; Mullen, K.; Weil, T. Amphiphilic dendrimers control protein binding and corona formation on liposome nanocarriers. *Chem. Commun. (Camb.)* **2020**, *56*, 8663–8666. [CrossRef]
126. Park, S.I.; Lee, E.O.; Kim, J.W.; Kim, Y.J.; Han, S.H.; Kim, J.D. Polymer-hybridized liposomes anchored with alkyl grafted poly(asparagine). *J. Colloid Interface Sci.* **2011**, *364*, 31–38. [CrossRef]
127. Borges, J.; Mano, J.F. Molecular interactions driving the layer-by-layer assembly of multilayers. *Chem. Rev.* **2014**, *114*, 8883–8942. [CrossRef]
128. Correa, S.; Boehnke, N.; Barberio, A.E.; Deiss-Yehiely, E.; Shi, A.; Oberlton, B.; Smith, S.G.; Zervantonakis, I.; Dreaden, E.C.; Hammond, P.T. Tuning Nanoparticle Interactions with Ovarian Cancer through Layer-by-Layer Modification of Surface Chemistry. *ACS Nano* **2020**, *14*, 2224–2237. [CrossRef]
129. Zhao, S.; Caruso, F.; Dähne, L.; Decher, G.; De Geest, B.G.; Fan, J.; Feliu, N.; Gogotsi, Y.; Hammond, P.T.; Hersam, M.C.; et al. The Future of Layer-by-Layer Assembly: A Tribute to ACS Nano Associate Editor Helmuth Möhwald. *ACS Nano* **2019**, *13*, 6151–6169. [CrossRef]

130. Alkekhia, D.; Hammond, P.T.; Shukla, A. Layer-by-Layer Biomaterials for Drug Delivery. *Annu. Rev. Biomed. Eng.* **2020**, *22*, 1–24. [CrossRef]
131. Fukui, Y.; Fujimoto, K. The preparation of sugar polymer-coated nanocapsules by the layer-by-layer deposition on the liposome. *Langmuir* **2009**, *25*, 10020–10025. [CrossRef] [PubMed]
132. Chun, J.-Y.; Choi, M.-J.; Min, S.-G.; Weiss, J. Formation and stability of multiple-layered liposomes by layer-by-layer electrostatic deposition of biopolymers. *Food Hydrocoll.* **2013**, *30*, 249–257. [CrossRef]
133. Ruano, M.; Mateos-Maroto, A.; Ortega, F.; Ritacco, H.; Rubio, J.E.F.; Guzman, E.; Rubio, R.G. Fabrication of Robust Capsules by Sequential Assembly of Polyelectrolytes onto Charged Liposomes. *Langmuir* **2021**, *37*, 6189–6200. [CrossRef] [PubMed]
134. Ghostine, R.A.; Markarian, M.Z.; Schlenoff, J.B. Asymmetric growth in polyelectrolyte multilayers. *J. Am. Chem. Soc.* **2013**, *135*, 7636–7646. [CrossRef] [PubMed]
135. Kashcooli, Y.; Park, K.; Bose, A.; Greenfield, M.; Bothun, G.D. Patchy Layersomes Formed by Layer-by-Layer Coating of Liposomes with Strong Biopolyelectrolytes. *Biomacromolecules* **2016**, *17*, 3838–3844. [CrossRef]
136. Chen, M.X.; Li, B.K.; Yin, D.K.; Liang, J.; Li, S.S.; Peng, D.Y. Layer-by-layer assembly of chitosan stabilized multilayered liposomes for paclitaxel delivery. *Carbohydr. Polym.* **2014**, *111*, 298–304. [CrossRef]
137. Haidar, Z.S.; Hamdy, R.C.; Tabrizian, M. Protein release kinetics for core-shell hybrid nanoparticles based on the layer-by-layer assembly of alginate and chitosan on liposomes. *Biomaterials* **2008**, *29*, 1207–1215. [CrossRef]
138. Haidar, Z.S.; Hamdy, R.C.; Tabrizian, M. Biocompatibility and safety of a hybrid core-shell nanoparticulate OP-1 delivery system intramuscularly administered in rats. *Biomaterials* **2010**, *31*, 2746–2754. [CrossRef]
139. Xian, J.; Zhong, X.; Gu, H.; Wang, X.; Li, J.; Li, J.; Wu, Y.; Zhang, C.; Zhang, J. Colonic Delivery of Celastrol-Loaded Layer-by-Layer Liposomes with Pectin/Trimethylated Chitosan Coating to Enhance Its Anti-Ulcerative Colitis Effects. *Pharmaceutics* **2021**, *13*, 2005. [CrossRef]
140. Hermal, F.; Frisch, B.; Specht, A.; Bourel-Bonnet, L.; Heurtault, B. Development and characterization of layer-by-layer coated liposomes with poly(L-lysine) and poly(L-glutamic acid) to increase their resistance in biological media. *Int. J. Pharm.* **2020**, *586*, 119568. [CrossRef]
141. Dreaden, E.C.; Kong, Y.W.; Morton, S.W.; Correa, S.; Choi, K.Y.; Shopsowitz, K.E.; Renggli, K.; Drapkin, R.; Yaffe, M.B.; Hammond, P.T. Tumor-Targeted Synergistic Blockade of MAPK and PI3K from a Layer-by-Layer Nanoparticle. *Clin. Cancer Res.* **2015**, *21*, 4410–4419. [CrossRef] [PubMed]
142. Ramasamy, T.; Haidar, Z.S.; Tran, T.H.; Choi, J.Y.; Jeong, J.-H.; Shin, B.S.; Choi, H.-G.; Yong, C.S.; Kim, J.O. Layer-by-layer assembly of liposomal nanoparticles with PEGylated polyelectrolytes enhances systemic delivery of multiple anticancer drugs. *Acta Biomater.* **2014**, *10*, 5116–5127. [CrossRef] [PubMed]
143. Correa, S.; Choi, K.Y.; Dreaden, E.C.; Renggli, K.; Shi, A.; Gu, L.; Shopsowitz, K.E.; Quadir, M.A.; Ben-Akiva, E.; Hammond, P.T. Highly scalable, closed-loop synthesis of drug-loaded, layer-by-layer nanoparticles. *Adv. Funct. Mater.* **2016**, *26*, 991–1003. [CrossRef]
144. Deng, Z.J.; Morton, S.W.; Ben-Akiva, E.; Dreaden, E.C.; Shopsowitz, K.E.; Hammond, P.T. Layer-by-Layer Nanoparticles for Systemic Codelivery of an Anticancer Drug and siRNA for Potential Triple-Negative Breast Cancer Treatment. *ACS Nano* **2013**, *7*, 9571–9584. [CrossRef] [PubMed]
145. Jain, S.; Kumar, D.; Swarnakar, N.K.; Thanki, K. Polyelectrolyte stabilized multilayered liposomes for oral delivery of paclitaxel. *Biomaterials* **2012**, *33*, 6758–6768. [CrossRef]
146. Jain, P.; Jain, S.; Prasad, K.N.; Jain, S.K.; Vyas, S.P. Polyelectrolyte coated multilayered liposomes (nanocapsules) for the treatment of Helicobacter pylori infection. *Mol. Pharm.* **2009**, *6*, 593–603. [CrossRef]
147. Kaminski, G.A.; Sierakowski, M.R.; Pontarolo, R.; Santos, L.A.; de Freitas, R.A. Layer-by-layer polysaccharide-coated liposomes for sustained delivery of epidermal growth factor. *Carbohydr. Polym.* **2016**, *140*, 129–135. [CrossRef]
148. Men, W.; Zhu, P.; Dong, S.; Liu, W.; Zhou, K.; Bai, Y.; Liu, X.; Gong, S.; Zhang, S. Layer-by-layer pH-sensitive nanoparticles for drug delivery and controlled release with improved therapeutic efficacy in vivo. *Drug Deliv.* **2020**, *27*, 180–190. [CrossRef]
149. Liu, W.; Liu, J.; Liu, W.; Li, T.; Liu, C. Improved physical and in vitro digestion stability of a polyelectrolyte delivery system based on layer-by-layer self-assembly alginate-chitosan-coated nanoliposomes. *J. Agric. Food Chem.* **2013**, *61*, 4133–4144. [CrossRef]
150. Yan, Y.; Bjornmalm, M.; Caruso, F. Assembly of Layer-by-Layer Particles and Their Interactions with Biological Systems. *Chem. Mater.* **2014**, *26*, 452–460. [CrossRef]
151. Lai, W.F.; Wong, W.T.; Rogach, A.L. Molecular Design of Layer-by-Layer Functionalized Liposomes for Oral Drug Delivery. *ACS Appl. Mater. Interfaces* **2020**, *12*, 43341–43351. [CrossRef] [PubMed]
152. Kong, S.M.; Costa, D.F.; Jagielska, A.; Van Vliet, K.J.; Hammond, P.T. Stiffness of targeted layer-by-layer nanoparticles impacts elimination half-life, tumor accumulation, and tumor penetration. *Proc. Natl. Acad. Sci. USA* **2021**, *118*, e2104826118. [CrossRef] [PubMed]
153. Correa, S.; Dreaden, E.C.; Gu, L.; Hammond, P.T. Engineering nanolayered particles for modular drug delivery. *J. Control. Release* **2016**, *240*, 364–386. [CrossRef] [PubMed]
154. Basel, M.T.; Shrestha, T.B.; Troyer, D.L.; Bossmann, S.H. Protease-sensitive, polymer-caged liposomes: A method for making highly targeted liposomes using triggered release. *ACS Nano* **2011**, *5*, 2162–2175. [CrossRef]
155. Awasthi, A.K.; Gupta, S.; Thakur, J.; Gupta, S.; Pal, S.; Bajaj, A.; Srivastava, A. Polydopamine-on-liposomes: Stable nanoformulations, uniform coatings and superior antifouling performance. *Nanoscale* **2020**, *12*, 5021–5030. [CrossRef]

156. Mohanty, A.; Uthaman, S.; Park, I.K. Utilization of polymer-lipid hybrid nanoparticles for targeted anti-cancer therapy. *Molecules* **2020**, *25*, 4377. [CrossRef]
157. Yuba, E. Development of functional liposomes by modification of stimuli-responsive materials and their biomedical applications. *J. Mater. Chem. B* **2020**, *8*, 1093. [CrossRef]
158. Shaikh, R.; Raj Singh, T.R.; Garland, M.J.; Woolfson, A.D.; Donnelly, R.F. Mucoadhesive drug delivery systems. *J. Pharm. Bioallied Sci.* **2011**, *3*, 89–100. [CrossRef]
159. Alavi, S.; Haeri, A.; Dadashzadeh, S. Utilization of chitosan-caged liposomes to push the boundaries of therapeutic delivery. *Carbohydr. Polym.* **2017**, *157*, 991–1012. [CrossRef]
160. Ways, T.M.M.; Lau, W.M.; Khutoryanskiy, V.V. Chitosan and Its Derivatives for Application in Mucoadhesive Drug Delivery Systems. *Polymers* **2018**, *10*, 267. [CrossRef]
161. Thongborisute, J.; Takeuchi, H.; Yamamoto, H.; Kawashima, Y. Visualization of the penetrative and mucoadhesive properties of chitosan and chitosan-coated liposomes through the rat intestine. *J. Liposome Res.* **2006**, *16*, 127–141. [CrossRef] [PubMed]
162. Caddeo, C.; Diez-Sales, O.; Pons, R.; Carbone, C.; Ennas, G.; Puglisi, G.; Fadda, A.M.; Manconi, M. Cross-linked chitosan/liposome hybrid system for the intestinal delivery of quercetin. *J. Colloid Interface Sci.* **2016**, *461*, 69–78. [CrossRef] [PubMed]
163. Sudimack, J.; Lee, R.J. Targeted drug delivery via the folate receptor. *Adv. Drug Deliv. Rev.* **2000**, *41*, 147–162. [CrossRef]
164. Dovedytis, M.; Liu, Z.J.; Bartlett, S. Hyaluronic acid and its biomedical applications: A review. *Eng. Regen.* **2020**, *1*, 102–113. [CrossRef]
165. Chen, C.; Zhao, S.; Karnad, A.; Freeman, J.W. The biology and role of CD44 in cancer progression: Therapeutic implications. *J. Hematol. Oncol.* **2018**, *11*, 64. [CrossRef]
166. Arpicco, S.; Lerda, C.; Dalla Pozza, E.; Costanzo, C.; Tsapis, N.; Stella, B.; Donadelli, M.; Dando, I.; Fattal, E.; Cattel, L.; et al. Hyaluronic acid-coated liposomes for active targeting of gemcitabine. *Eur. J. Pharm. Biopharm.* **2013**, *85*, 373–380. [CrossRef]
167. Manca, M.L.; Castangia, I.; Zaru, M.; Nacher, A.; Valenti, D.; Fernandez-Busquets, X.; Fadda, A.M.; Manconi, M. Development of curcumin loaded sodium hyaluronate immobilized vesicles (hyalurosomes) and their potential on skin inflammation and wound restoring. *Biomaterials* **2015**, *71*, 100–109. [CrossRef]
168. Garin-Chesa, P.; Campbell, I.; Saigo, P.; Lewis, J.; Old, L.; Rettig, W. Trophoblast and ovarian cancer antigen LK26. Sensitivity and specificity in immunopathology and molecular identification as a folate-binding protein. *Am. J. Path.* **1993**, *142*, 557–567.
169. Kumar, P.; Huo, P.; Liu, B. Formulation Strategies for Folate-Targeted Liposomes and Their Biomedical Applications. *Pharmaceutics* **2019**, *11*, 381. [CrossRef]
170. Wei, X.; Gao, J.; Zhan, C.; Xie, C.; Chai, Z.; Ran, D.; Ying, M.; Zheng, P.; Lu, W. Liposome-based glioma targeted drug delivery enabled by stable peptide ligands. *J. Control. Release* **2015**, *218*, 13–21. [CrossRef]
171. Romberg, B.; Hennink, W.E.; Storm, G. Sheddable coatings for long-circulating nanoparticles. *Pharm. Res.* **2008**, *25*, 55–71. [CrossRef] [PubMed]
172. Lee, Y.; Thompson, D.H. Stimuli-responsive liposomes for drug delivery. *Wiley Interdiscip. Rev. Nanomed. Nanobiotechnol.* **2017**, *9*, e1450. [CrossRef] [PubMed]
173. Abri Aghdam, M.; Bagheri, R.; Mosafer, J.; Baradaran, B.; Hashemzaei, M.; Baghbanzadeh, A.; de la Guardia, M.; Mokhtarzadeh, A. Recent advances on thermosensitive and pH-sensitive liposomes employed in controlled release. *J. Control. Release* **2019**, *315*, 1–22. [CrossRef] [PubMed]
174. Dou, Y.; Li, C.; Li, L.; Guo, J.; Zhang, J. Bioresponsive drug delivery systems for the treatment of inflammatory diseases. *J. Control. Release* **2020**, *327*, 641–666. [CrossRef] [PubMed]
175. Kong, L.; Campbell, F.; Kros, A. DePEGylation strategies to increase cancer nanomedicine efficacy. *Nanoscale Horiz* **2019**, *4*, 378–387. [CrossRef]
176. Volk, T.; Jähde, E.; Fortmeyer, H.P.; Glüsenkamp, K.H.; Rajewsky, M.F. pH in human tumour xenografts: Effect of intravenous administration of glucose. *Br. J. Cancer* **1993**, *68*, 492–500. [CrossRef]
177. Punnia-Moorthy, A. Evaluation of pH changes in inflammation of the subcutaneous air pouch lining in the rat, induced by carrageenan, dextran and Staphylococcus aureus. *J. Oral Pathol.* **1987**, *16*, 36–44. [CrossRef]
178. Scott, C.C.; Gruenberg, J. Ion flux and the function of endosomes and lysosomes: pH is just the start: The flux of ions across endosomal membranes influences endosome function not only through regulation of the luminal pH. *Bioessays* **2011**, *33*, 103–110. [CrossRef]
179. Shen, X.; Su, H. In vitro stability and cytotoxicity analysis of liposomes anchored with octylamine-*graft*-poly (aspartic). *RSC Adv.* **2016**, *6*, 58034–58045. [CrossRef]
180. Lu, T.; Wang, Z.; Ma, Y.; Zhang, Y.; Chen, T. Influence of polymer size, liposomal composition, surface charge, and temperature on the permeability of pH-sensitive liposomes containing lipid-anchored poly(2-ethylacrylic acid). *Int. J. Nanomed.* **2012**, *7*, 4917–4926. [CrossRef]
181. Miyazaki, M.; Yuba, E.; Hayashi, H.; Harada, A.; Kono, K. Hyaluronic Acid-Based pH-Sensitive Polymer-Modified Liposomes for Cell-Specific Intracellular Drug Delivery Systems. *Bioconjug. Chem.* **2018**, *29*, 44–55. [CrossRef] [PubMed]
182. Miyazaki, M.; Yuba, E.; Hayashi, H.; Harada, A.; Kono, K. Development of pH-Responsive Hyaluronic Acid-Based Antigen Carriers for Induction of Antigen-Specific Cellular Immune Responses. *ACS Biomater. Sci. Eng.* **2019**, *5*, 5790–5797. [CrossRef] [PubMed]

183. Kono, K.; Igawa, T.; Takagishi, T. Cytoplasmic delivery of calcein mediated by liposomes modified with a pH-sensitive poly(ethylene glycol) derivative. *Biochim. Biophys. Acta* **1997**, *1325*, 143–154. [CrossRef]
184. Yuba, E.; Harada, A.; Sakanishi, Y.; Kono, K. Carboxylated hyperbranched poly(glycidol)s for preparation of pH-sensitive liposomes. *J. Control. Release* **2011**, *149*, 72–80. [CrossRef]
185. Shi, K.; Li, J.; Cao, Z.; Yang, P.; Qiu, Y.; Yang, B.; Wang, Y.; Long, Y.; Liu, Y.; Zhang, Q.; et al. A pH-responsive cell-penetrating peptide-modified liposomes with active recognizing of integrin alphavbeta3 for the treatment of melanoma. *J. Control. Release* **2015**, *217*, 138–150. [CrossRef]
186. Zhang, Q.; Tang, J.; Fu, L.; Ran, R.; Liu, Y.; Yuan, M.; He, Q. A pH-responsive alpha-helical cell penetrating peptide-mediated liposomal delivery system. *Biomaterials* **2013**, *34*, 7980–7993. [CrossRef]
187. Han, Q.; Wang, W.; Jia, X.; Qian, Y.; Li, Q.; Wang, Z.; Zhang, W.; Yang, S.; Jia, Y.; Hu, Z. Switchable Liposomes: Targeting-Peptide-Functionalized and pH-Triggered Cytoplasmic Delivery. *ACS Appl. Mater. Interfaces* **2016**, *8*, 18658–18663. [CrossRef]
188. Jiang, T.; Zhang, Z.; Zhang, Y.; Lv, H.; Zhou, J.; Li, C.; Hou, L.; Zhang, Q. Dual-functional liposomes based on pH-responsive cell-penetrating peptide and hyaluronic acid for tumor-targeted anticancer drug delivery. *Biomaterials* **2012**, *33*, 9246–9258. [CrossRef]
189. Bersani, S.; Vila-Caballer, M.; Brazzale, C.; Barattin, M.; Salmaso, S. pH-sensitive stearoyl-PEG-poly(methacryloyl sulfadimethoxine) decorated liposomes for the delivery of gemcitabine to cancer cells. *Eur. J. Pharm. Biopharm.* **2014**, *88*, 670–682. [CrossRef]
190. Banerjee, S.; Sen, K.; Pal, T.K.; Guha, S.K. Poly(styrene-co-maleic acid)-based pH-sensitive liposomes mediate cytosolic delivery of drugs for enhanced cancer chemotherapy. *Int. J. Pharm.* **2012**, *436*, 786–797. [CrossRef]
191. Chiang, Y.T.; Lo, C.L. pH-responsive polymer-liposomes for intracellular drug delivery and tumor extracellular matrix switched-on targeted cancer therapy. *Biomaterials* **2014**, *35*, 5414–5424. [CrossRef] [PubMed]
192. Zhang, X.; Lei, B.; Wang, Y.; Xu, S.; Liu, H. Dual-Sensitive On-Off Switch in Liposome Bilayer for Controllable Drug Release. *Langmuir* **2019**, *35*, 5213–5220. [CrossRef] [PubMed]
193. Chen, D.; Jiang, X.; Huang, Y.; Zhang, C.; Ping, Q. pH-sensative mPEG-Hz-cholesterol conjugates as a liposome delivery system. *J. Bioact. Compat. Polym.* **2010**, *25*, 527–542. [CrossRef]
194. Chen, D.; Liu, W.; Shen, Y.; Mu, H.; Zhang, Y.; Liang, R.; Wang, A.; Sun, K.; Fu, F. Effects of a novel pH-sensitive liposome with cleavable esterase-catalyzed and pH-responsive double smart mPEG lipid derivative on ABC phenomenon. *Int. J. Nanomed.* **2011**, *6*, 2053–2061. [CrossRef]
195. Kanamala, M.; Palmer, B.D.; Jamieson, S.M.; Wilson, W.R.; Wu, Z. Dual pH-sensitive liposomes with low pH-triggered sheddable PEG for enhanced tumor-targeted drug delivery. *Nanomedicine* **2019**, *14*, 1971–1989. [CrossRef]
196. Ding, Y.; Sun, D.; Wang, G.L.; Yang, H.G.; Xu, H.F.; Chen, J.H.; Xie, Y.; Wang, Z.Q. An efficient PEGylated liposomal nanocarrier containing cell-penetrating peptide and pH-sensitive hydrazone bond for enhancing tumor-targeted drug delivery. *Int. J. Nanomed.* **2015**, *10*, 6199–6214. [CrossRef]
197. Guo, X.; Szoka, F.C.J. Steric stabilization of fusogenic liposomes by a low-pH sensitive PEG-diortho ester-lipid conjugate. *Bioconjug. Chem.* **2001**, *12*, 291–300. [CrossRef]
198. Yoshizaki, Y.; Yuba, E.; Sakaguchi, N.; Koiwai, K.; Harada, A.; Kono, K. Potentiation of pH-sensitive polymer-modified liposomes with cationic lipid inclusion as antigen delivery carriers for cancer immunotherapy. *Biomaterials* **2014**, *35*, 8186–8196. [CrossRef]
199. Hatakeyama, H.; Akita, H.; Harashima, H. The polyethyleneglycol dilemma: Advantage and disadvantage of PEGylation of liposomes for systemic genes and nucleic acids delivery to tumors. *Biol. Pharm. Bull.* **2013**, *36*, 892–899. [CrossRef]
200. Shin, J.; Shum, P.; Thompson, D.H. Acid-triggered release via dePEGylation of DOPE liposomes containing acid-labile vinyl ether PEG-lipids. *J. Control. Release* **2003**, *91*, 187–200. [CrossRef]
201. Shin, J.; Shum, P.; Grey, J.; Fujiwara, S.; Malhotra, G.S.; Gonzalez-Bonet, A.; Hyun, S.H.; Moase, E.; Allen, T.M.; Thompson, D.H. Acid-labile mPEG-vinyl ether-1,2-dioleylglycerol lipids with tunable pH sensitivity: Synthesis and structural effects on hydrolysis rates, DOPE liposome release performance, and pharmacokinetics. *Mol. Pharm.* **2012**, *9*, 3266–3276. [CrossRef] [PubMed]
202. Kanamala, M.; Palmer, B.D.; Wilson, W.R.; Wu, Z. Characterization of a smart pH-cleavable PEG polymer towards the development of dual pH-sensitive liposomes. *Int. J. Pharm.* **2018**, *548*, 288–296. [CrossRef] [PubMed]
203. Kirpotin, D.; Hong, K.; Mullah, N.; Papahadjopoulos, D.; Zalipsky, S. Liposomes with detachable polymer coating: Destabilization and fusion of dioleoylphosphatidylethanolamine vesicles triggered by cleavage of surface-grafted poly(ethylene glycol). *FEBS Lett.* **1996**, *388*, 115–118. [CrossRef]
204. Hatakeyama, H.; Akita, H.; Kogure, K.; Oishi, M.; Nagasaki, Y.; Kihira, Y.; Ueno, M.; Kobayashi, H.; Kikuchi, H.; Harashima, H. Development of a novel systemic gene delivery system for cancer therapy with a tumor-specific cleavable PEG-lipid. *Gene Ther.* **2007**, *14*, 68–77. [CrossRef] [PubMed]
205. Wu, C.; Zhou, S. First Observation of the Molten Globule State of a Single Homopolymer Chain. *Phys. Rev. Lett.* **1996**, *30*, 3053. [CrossRef]
206. Pippa, N.; Meristoudi, A.; Pispas, S.; Demetzos, C. Temperature-dependent drug release from DPPC:C12H25-PNIPAM-COOH liposomes: Control of the drug loading/release by modulation of the nanocarriers' components. *Int. J. Pharm.* **2015**, *485*, 374–382. [CrossRef]
207. Xi, L.; Li, C.; Wang, Y.; Gong, Y.; Su, F.; Li, S. Novel Thermosensitive Polymer-Modified Liposomes as Nano-Carrier of Hydrophobic Antitumor Drugs. *J. Pharm. Sci.* **2020**, *109*, 2544–2552. [CrossRef]

208. Paasonen, L.; Romberg, B.; Storm, G.; Yliperttula, M.; Urtti, A.; Hennink, W.E. Temperature-sensitive poly(*N*-(2-hydroxypropyl) methacrylamide mono/dilactate)-coated liposomes for triggered contents release. *Bioconjug. Chem.* **2007**, *18*, 2131–2136. [CrossRef]
209. Mo, Y.; Du, H.; Chen, B.; Liu, D.; Yin, Q.; Yan, Y.; Wang, Z.; Wan, F.; Qi, T.; Wang, Y.; et al. Quick-Responsive Polymer-Based Thermosensitive Liposomes for Controlled Doxorubicin Release and Chemotherapy. *ACS Biomater. Sci. Eng.* **2019**, *5*, 2316–2329. [CrossRef]
210. Kono, K.; Ozawa, T.; Yoshida, T.; Ozaki, F.; Ishizaka, Y.; Maruyama, K.; Kojima, C.; Harada, A.; Aoshima, S. Highly temperature-sensitive liposomes based on a thermosensitive block copolymer for tumor-specific chemotherapy. *Biomaterials* **2010**, *31*, 7096–7105. [CrossRef]
211. Wang, M.; Kim, J.-C. Light- and temperature-responsive liposomes incorporating cinnamoyl Pluronic F127. *Int. J. Pharm.* **2014**, *468*, 243–249. [CrossRef] [PubMed]
212. Fouladi, F.; Steffen, K.J.; Mallik, S. Enzyme-Responsive Liposomes for the Delivery of Anticancer Drugs. *Bioconjug. Chem.* **2017**, *28*, 857–868. [CrossRef] [PubMed]
213. Chen, M.; Amerigos, J.C.K.; Su, Z.; Guissi, N.E.I.; Xiao, Y.; Zong, L.; Ping, Q. Folate Receptor-Targeting and Reactive Oxygen Species-Responsive Liposomal Formulation of Methotrexate for Treatment of Rheumatoid Arthritis. *Pharmaceutics* **2019**, *11*, 582. [CrossRef] [PubMed]

pharmaceutics MDPI

Article

The Preparation of a Novel Poly(Lactic Acid)-Based Sustained H_2S Releasing Microsphere for Rheumatoid Arthritis Alleviation

Yue Yu [1], Zhou Wang [1], Qian Ding [1], Xiangbin Yu [2], Qinyan Yang [1], Ran Wang [1], Yudong Fang [1], Wei Qi [1], Junyi Liao [1], Wei Hu [1] and Yizhun Zhu [1,*]

[1] State Key Laboratory of Quality Research in Chinese Medicine & School of Pharmacy, Macau University of Science and Technology, Macau SAR 999078, China; 1709853fct30001@student.must.edu.mo (Y.Y.); 1709853jct30002@student.must.edu.mo (Z.W.); 1909853qct30001@student.must.edu.mo (Q.D.); 1909853ucw30006@student.must.edu.mo (Q.Y.); 1809853pct30001@student.must.edu.mo (R.W.); 1909853scw30001@student.must.edu.mo (Y.F.); wqi@must.edu.mo (W.Q.); 1809853gct20004@student.must.edu.mo (J.L.); 1909853xct30001@student.must.edu.mo (W.H.)

[2] School of Pharmacy, Fujian Medical University, Fuzhou 350108, China; yxb4666@fjmu.edu.cn

* Correspondence: yzzhu@must.edu.mo; Tel.: +86-853-8897-2880

Citation: Yu, Y.; Wang, Z.; Ding, Q.; Yu, X.; Yang, Q.; Wang, R.; Fang, Y.; Qi, W.; Liao, J.; Hu, W.; et al. The Preparation of a Novel Poly(Lactic Acid)-Based Sustained H_2S Releasing Microsphere for Rheumatoid Arthritis Alleviation. *Pharmaceutics* **2021**, *13*, 742. https://doi.org/10.3390/pharmaceutics13050742

Academic Editors: Ana Isabel Fernandes, Angela Faustino Jozala and Thierry Vandamme

Received: 30 March 2021
Accepted: 23 April 2021
Published: 18 May 2021

Publisher's Note: MDPI stays neutral with regard to jurisdictional claims in published maps and institutional affiliations.

Abstract: Rheumatoid arthritis (RA) is a chronic, inflammatory autoimmune disease that mainly erodes joints and surrounding tissues, and if it is not treated in time, it can cause joint deformities and loss of function. S-propargyl-cysteine (SPRC) is an excellent endogenous hydrogen sulfide donor which can relieve the symptoms of RA through the promotion of H_2S release via the CSE/H_2S pathway in vivo. However, the instant release of H_2S in vivo could potentially limit its further clinical use. To solve this problem, in this study, a SPRC-loaded poly(lactic acid) (PLA) microsphere (SPRC@PLA) was prepared, which could release SPRC in vitro in a sustained manner, and further promote sustained in vivo H_2S release. Furthermore, its therapeutical effect on RA in rats was also studied. A spherical-like SPRC@PLA was successfully prepared with a diameter of approximately 31.61 μm, yielding rate of 50.66%, loading efficiency of 6.10% and encapsulation efficiency of 52.71%. The SPRC@PLA showed significant prolonged in vitro SPRC release, to 4 days, and additionally, an in vivo H_2S release around 3 days could also be observed. In addition, a better therapeutical effect and prolonged administration interval toward RA rats was also observed in the SPRC@PLA group.

Keywords: S-propargyl-cysteine; poly(lactic acid); endogenous hydrogen sulfide; water-in-oil-in-water; rheumatoid arthritis

1. Introduction

Rheumatoid arthritis (RA) is a chronic, inflammatory autoimmune disease that mainly erodes joints and surrounding tissues [1–4] and if it is not treated in time, it can cause joint deformities and loss of function. It is often accompanied by tissue and organ injury, including cardiovascular and lung [5–7]. The pathogenesis of RA is still not clear, therefore, an ideal drug has not been found to completely cure this type of disease [8,9]. At present, the treatment of RA is mainly based on non-steroidal anti-inflammatory drugs, glucocorticoids, traditional anti-rheumatic drugs, and biological agents for improving the condition of the disease [10–12]. However, the specific treatment of RA is still a dilemma in modern medicine.

Poly(lactic acid) (PLA) is produced by the polymerization of lactic acid. Because of its excellent properties such as good biocompatibility and degradability, it has been widely studied since it was discovered [13–16]. The initial raw material of PLA is plant starch, which produces extremely low pollution during the production process, and can also be completely decomposed into CO_2 and H_2O after use and utilized by nature [17,18]. Due to its excellent performance, PLA has been recognized to be a new type of green and environmentally friendly polymer material. Because of its biodegradability, PLA can be mixed with specific drugs to produce microparticles [19]. When these microparticles reach the action site, they slowly decompose into CO_2 and H_2O, and the drug is gradually released at the corresponding action site, therefore, improving the therapeutic index [13,14,20,21].

Hydrogen sulfide (H_2S) has always been considered to be a poisonous gas with a smell similar to rotten eggs, and it is produced in large quantities in some polluted environments [22]. With the deepening of research, recent studies have found that H_2S is also an important physiological gas molecule and is considered to be the third gasotransmitter after nitric oxide (NO) and carbon monoxide (CO) [23,24]. Endogenous H_2S is produced via the catalyzation of cystathionine pyridoxal-5-phosphate dependent enzymes, including cystathionine-β-synthase (CBS), cystathionine-y-lyase (CSE), and 3-mercaptopyruvate sulfurtransferase (3-MST). In human blood, the concentration of H_2S at normal physiological levels is about 40 μM, and the local concentration in the brain can reach more than 100 μM. As a gas signal molecule, H_2S could reduce high glucose-induced myocardial injury [25] or kidney injury [26], however, the half-life of direct administration of H_2S is too short, and it is also difficult to precisely control the dosage. Therefore, it is of great significance to study a series of H_2S donor which could be used as a CSE substrate to further release H_2S in a relatively slow manner [27,28]. S-allyl-cysteine (SAC) is an extract in garlic, which could reduce the area of myocardial infarction by regulating the level of H_2S in ischemic myocardial tissue [29,30]. According to the structure of SAC, our group synthesized a compound called S-propargyl-cysteine (SPRC, also known as ZYZ-802) [31–33], which is a compound with a similar structure to SAC (Figure 1). Our previous study found that SPRC could be used as a new type of H_2S donor for ischemia-hypoxic cell models and the treatment of coronary artery ligation rat myocardial infarction models [32,34]. In addition, SPRC could also exert its neuroprotective effect through its anti-inflammatory effect [35,36]. Recent studies have also shown that SPRC could treat rheumatoid arthritis in rats by regulating endogenous H_2S [31,37,38]. However, the instant release of H_2S by SPRC might prevent its clinical use, hence, how to achieve a sustained release of H_2S in vivo through SPRC remains to be a challenging problem.

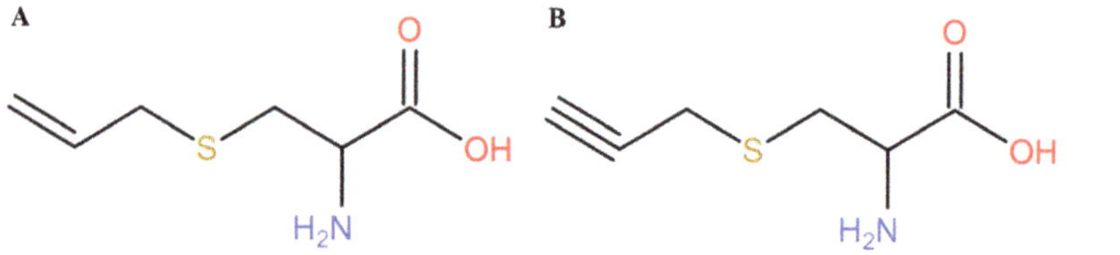

Figure 1. The chemical structure of (**A**) S-allyl-cysteine (SAC) and (**B**) S-propargyl-cysteine (SPRC).

In this study, we aim to solve the problem that SPRC might prompt the H_2S in an instant manner, a SPRC-loaded PLA-based microsphere was successfully prepared (SPRC@PLA), which showed sustained release of SPRC in vitro, therefore, elevating the plasma H_2S concentration for almost 3 days. Through this long elevation period, the administration interval for treating RA has also been increased as compared with that determined in a previous study [31].

2. Materials and Methods

2.1. Materials

Poly(lactic acid) (PLA) polymer, with Mw around 10,000~18,000 Da and viscosity of 0.16~0.24 was purchased from Evonik Industries (AG, Essen, Germany). SPRC was synthesized, as previously reported [39,40]. Poly(vinyl alcohol) (PVA), with MW around 25,000 Da, and 88% mole hydrolyzed, was purchased from Polysciences (Warrington, PA, USA). Elisa kit of TNF-α, IL-1β, IL-6, and IL-10 were purchased from MultiSciences

(Hangzhou, Zhejiang, China). Complete Freund's adjuvant (CFA), monobromobimane (MBB), diethylenetriaminepentaacetic acid (DTPA), dichloromethane (DCM), and acetonitrile were purchased from Macklin Industrial Corporation (Shanghai, China).

2.2. The Preparation of SPRC-Loaded Poly(Lactic Acid) (PLA) Microsphere (SPRC@PLA)

A double emulsion evaporation method (W1/O/W2) was followed with slight modification [41]. First, 50 mg of SPRC was dissolved in 1 mL of distilled water to prepare the inner water phase (W1). Meanwhile, the oil phase (O), which was various amounts of PLA dissolved in 12 mL of DCM, was also prepared. Then, the W1 was dispersed in O, with further emulsification through an Ultraturrax T25 high-speed homogenizer (IKA, Staufen, Germany) at 9000~12,000 rpm for 5 min to prepare the primary water-in-oil emulsion (W1/O). Then, the W1/O was dispersed in 100 mL of 0.5% (*w*/*w*) PVA solution with a paddle agitation at 800 rpm for 4 h, until the evaporation of organic solvent. Then, particles were collected through filtration via sieve with 200 mesh, intended to remove the potential bulk shape microspheres, and washed three times with distilled water to remove the excess residual PVA and SPRC on the surface. Finally, the obtained particles were lyophilized overnight to obtain the SPRC@PLA. Table 1 showed the detailed information of the different formulations.

Table 1. The formulations of different SPRC-loaded poly (lactic acid) (PLA) microspheres (SPRC@PLAs).

Formulations	SPRC	W1	PLA	DCM	HS	W2
F-1	50 mg	1 mL	400 mg	12 mL	12,000 rpm	100 mL
F-2	50 mg	1 mL	800 mg	12 mL	12,000 rpm	100 mL
F-3	50 mg	1 mL	1200 mg	12 mL	12,000 rpm	100 mL
F-4	50 mg	1 mL	800 mg	12 mL	9000 rpm	100 mL
F-5	50 mg	1 mL	800 mg	12 mL	15,000 rpm	100 mL

W1 is the distilled water volume, HS is the homogenization speed, and W2 is the PVA volume.

2.3. The Production Yeild of SPRC@PLA

The percentage of production yield (PY) was calculated using the following equation:

$$PY\ (\%) = (W_{SPRC@PLA})/(W_{PLA} + W_{SPRC}), \quad (1)$$

where W is the weight of corresponding component.

2.4. The Quantification of SPRC

The loaded drug (SPRC) was quantified by HPLC method, as reported with little modification [42]. Briefly, an Agilent 1200 series HPLC system (Santa Clara, CA, USA) was used to detect SPRC samples from physicochemical properties. A reversed-phase HPLC column (Agilent C18 column, 250 mm × 4.6 mm, 5 μm) was used. The mobile phase was chosen as acetonitrile and water. The detection wavelength was set as 220 nm. The gradient procedure was as follows: 0–1 min, 3% acetonitrile; 1–2 min, 3–15% acetonitrile; 2–5 min, 15–25% acetonitrile; 5–7 min, 25% acetonitrile; 7–10 min, 25–30% acetonitrile The wavelength of SPRC was determined as 220 nm, the flow rate was 0.5 $mL{\cdot}min^{-1}$, the column temperature was set as 35 °C, and the sample injection volume was 20 μL.

2.5. The Morphology Study of SPRC@PLA

Samples were firstly dispersed in distilled water, and a Microtrac S3500 (Montgomeryville, PA, USA) was used for the measurement of particle size and size distribution. A Phenom Pro Desktop SEMS-3400 scanning electron microscope (Thermo Fisher Scientific Inc., Waltham, MA, USA) was conducted to observe the morphology of SPRC@PLA. Samples were gold coated before examination.

2.6. The Encapsulation Efficiency of SPRC@PLA

The loading efficiency (LE) and encapsulation efficiency (EE) were determined by dissolving 50 mg of SPRC@PLA in 3 mL of DCM with further extract SPRC with 5 mL distilled water and analyzed using a 1290 Infinity II LC System (Agilent Technologies, Inc., Santa Clara, CA, USA). LE and EE were calculated using the following equations:

$$\text{LE }(\%) = (W_{\text{SPRCi}} - W_{\text{SPRCs}})/W_{\text{SPRC@PLA}} \quad (2)$$

$$\text{EE }(\%) = (W_{\text{SPRCi}} - W_{\text{SPRCs}})/W_{\text{SPRCi}} \quad (3)$$

where W_{SPRCi} is the weight of SPRC initially fed, W_{SPRCs} is the weight of SPRC in supernatant, and $W_{\text{SPRC@PLA}}$ is the weight of SPRC@PLA.

2.7. The SPRC Release In Vitro

The in vitro releasing experiment was conducted, using the method as reported with little modification [43]. First, 50 mg of differently prepared SPRC@PLA was dispersed in vials filled with 3 mL of PBS buffer (pH = 7.4, 37 °C) and placed in a shaker bath with a constant shaking speed of 100 rpm and temperature at 37 °C (Clifton Shaking Bath NE5, Nikel Electro Ltd., Weston-super-Mare, UK). Then, 0.5 mL of the samples were taken out, and then the same volume of PBS was refilled at predetermined intervals, and samples were analyzed using a 1290 Infinity II LC System (Agilent Technologies Inc., Santa Clara, CA, USA).

2.8. The Measurement of H_2S Release In Vivo

The concentration of H_2S was measured, as reported with little modification [44], and the schematic for detection of H_2S in vivo is shown in Figure 2. Briefly, 15 μL of serum sample, 25 μL of MBB acetonitrile solution, and 35 μL of 0.3% DTPA containing Tris-HCl buffer (pH 9.5) were mixed and incubated in a hypoxia incubator for 30 min. Subsequently, 25 μL of sulfosalicylic acid was added to stop the reaction, and then centrifugated at 12,000 rpm for 10 min. Finally, 30 μL of supernatant, 267 μL of acetonitrile, and 3 μL of internal standard (hydrocortisone methanol solution) were mixed and analyzed with LC-MS.

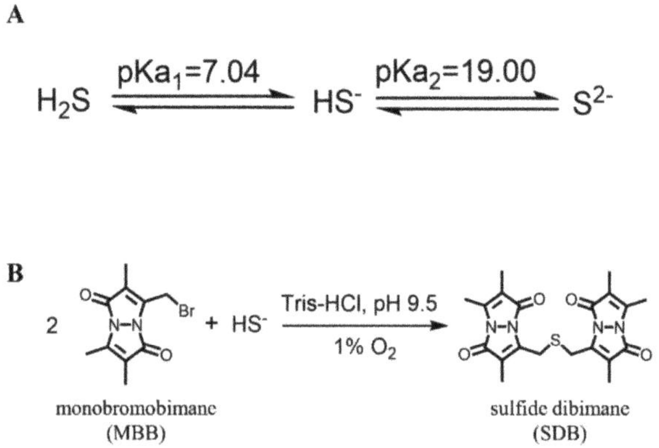

Figure 2. The mechanism for the detection of H_2S. (**A**) The acid dissociation constant of H_2S; (**B**) the mechanism of monobromobimane (MBB) reaction with HS^- to produce SDB in an alkaline and hypoxia environment.

Samples were analyzed using an Agilent 1200 series HPLC system (Agilent Technologies Inc., Santa Clara, CA, USA) coupled with an Agilent 6460 Triple Quadrupole (Agilent Technologies Inc., Santa Clara, CA, USA). A ZORBAX Eclipse Plus 95 C18, 2.1 × 50 mm, 1.8 μm column (Agilent Technologies Inc., Santa Clara, CA, USA) was used and temperature was set at 35 °C. The mobile phase consisted of water (A) and acetonitrile (B) and the gradient delivery was as follows: at 0–0.5 min, 5% B; 0.5–0.6 min, 5–20% B; 0.6–5.0 min, 20–47.5% B; 5.0–5.1 min, 47.5–95% B; 5.1–6.0 min, 95% B, at a flow rate of 0.3 mL·min^{-1}. The mass spectrometer was operated in positive ion mode. The scan type chosen was MRM with gas temperature at 325 °C and gas flow at 10 L·min^{-1}. Scan time was 500 ms and start-stop mass was 100~1000. The sample injection volume was 5 μL.

2.9. The SPRC@PLA Promoted H_2S Release In Vivo

The Animal Care and Use Committee of Municipal Affairs Bureau of Macau approved all studies described herein (approval number AL010/DICV/SIS/2018, 23 June 2018), and the experiment was conducted under the guidance of the *NIH Guide for the Care and Use of Laboratory Animals* (8th edition). The neonatal Sprague-Dawley (SD) rats were purchased from the University of Hong Kong.

Samples of SPRC powder and SPRC@PLA were dissolved or dispersed in saline for subcutaneous injection, each sample contained the same amount of SPRC, and the amounts used were calculated through the weight of the rats (100 mg·kg^{-1}). The rats' serum was collected at predetermined times (0, 0.5, 1, 1.5, 2, 3, 6, 12, 24, 48, and 72 h) into heparin sodium tubes and analyzed. Each group contained 3 rats.

2.10. SPRC@PLA Showed Anti-Inflmmation Effect towards Rheumatoid Arthritis

The AIA rat model was established via the injection of CFA (10 mg·mL^{-1}), according to the manufacturer's instructions. In total, 30 rats were randomly divided into four groups as follows: Control group (n = 5), no intervention; AIA group (n = 5), injection of 100 μL of CFA; SPRC group (n = 5), after injection of 100 μL of CFA, further subcutaneous injected with 2 mL of SPRC solution every 3 days for 30 days; SPRC@PLA group (n = 5), after injection of 100 μL of CFA, further subcutaneous injected with 2 mL of SPRC@PLA suspension every 3 days for 30 days (the amounts of SPRC used were all equivalent to 100 mg·kg^{-1} of SPRC.)

The paw volume was measured using a UGO Basile 7140 plethysmometer (Ugo Basile, Gemonio VA, Italy) and body weight was measured at the 0, 5th, 15th, 20th, 25th, and 30th day post the injection of CFA. The arthritis index was scored (Table 2) from 0 to 4 per limb, with 0 = no sign of inflammation and 1~4 = increasing degrees of inflammation, and a maximum score of 16 per rat.

Table 2. The arthritis scoring system.

Arthritis Score	Degree of Inflammation
0	No erythema and swelling
1	Erythema and mild swelling confined to the tarsals or ankle joint
2	Erythema and mild swelling extending from the ankle to the tarsals
3	Erythema and moderate swelling extending from the ankle to metatarsal joints
4	Erythema and severe swelling encompassing the ankle, foot, and digits; ankylosis of the limb might be present

At day 30, a blood sample was collected from rats in each group, the pro-inflammatory cytokine levels (TNF-α, IL-1β, and IL-6) and anti-inflammatory cytokine (IL-10) level in serum were measured using ELISA kits, according to the manufacturer's instructions.

2.11. Statistical Analysis

Statistical analyses of samples were performed using IBM SPSS Statistics Base (V22, IBM, Armonk, NY, USA.) and GraphPad Prism (V8, GraphPad Software, San Diego, CA, USA). Each experiment was performed at least three times. The data are expressed as the mean ± SD. Statistical significance was determined using a one-way analysis of variance (ANOVA) test, unless otherwise stated, $p < 0.05$ was considered to be significant.

3. Results

3.1. The Characterization of SPRC@PLA

First, the influence of PLA was investigated. As shown in Table 3, with an increase in the amount of PLA used, a decreasing trend of LE and an increasing trend of EE could be observed. The influence of the amount of PLA used on particle size was also investigated. The particle size showed an increasing trend with an increase in the amount of PLA used. While interestingly, there is no significant influence on PY.

Table 3. The influence of the amount of PLA used (n = 3, mean ± SD).

Samples	PLA	PY	LE	EE	Particle Size
F-1	400 mg	(49.81 ± 0.61)%	(10.14 ± 0.57)%	(44.94 ± 2.34)%	(13.28 ± 1.90) μm
F-2	800 mg	(50.66 ± 0.55)%	(6.10 ± 0.27)%	(52.71 ± 2.16)%	(31.61 ± 2.01) μm
F-3	1200 mg	(49.45 ± 0.55)%	(4.44 ± 0.20)%	(55.04 ± 2.19)%	(51.60 ± 2.07) μm

PY, production yield; LE, loading efficiency; EE, encapsulation efficiency.

The influence of homogenization speed was also investigated. As shown in Table 4, with an increase in homogenization speed, the LE and EE both showed an increasing trend while conversely, the particle size showed a decreasing trend. Interestingly, the PY still showed no significant change with an increase in homogenization speed.

Table 4. The influence of homogenization speed (n = 3, mean ± SD).

Samples	HS	PY	LE	EE	Particle Size
F-4	9000 rpm	(50.18 ± 0.68)%	(5.25 ± 0.36)%	(45.05 ± 3.45)%	(47.78 ± 2.84) μm
F-2	12,000 rpm	(50.66 ± 0.55)%	(6.10 ± 0.27)%	(52.71 ± 2.16)%	(31.61 ± 2.01) μm
F-5	15,000 rpm	(49.79 ± 0.69)%	(7.05 ± 0.20)%	(57.52 ± 2.54)%	(20.39 ± 2.72) μm

Where the HS: homogenization speed; the PY: production yield; LE: loading efficiency; EE: encapsulation efficiency.

The in vitro release profiles from F-1 to F-5 were also investigated for the selection of the optimized formulations, and the results are shown in Figure 3. SPRC might dissolve extremely fast in PBS due to its high hydrophilicity. However, a significantly prolonged in vitro release period could be observed in F-1 to F-5 as compared with the SPRC group, which was up to almost 4 days. F-3 and F-4 both showed an incomplete cumulative release potential due to the larger size usually accompanied with a relatively sustained release manner. In addition, F-1, F-2, and F-5 all showed a sustained and complete release within 96 h. By combining the in vitro release results with the particle size, it could be deduced that particle size might play a vital role in the property of in vitro release.

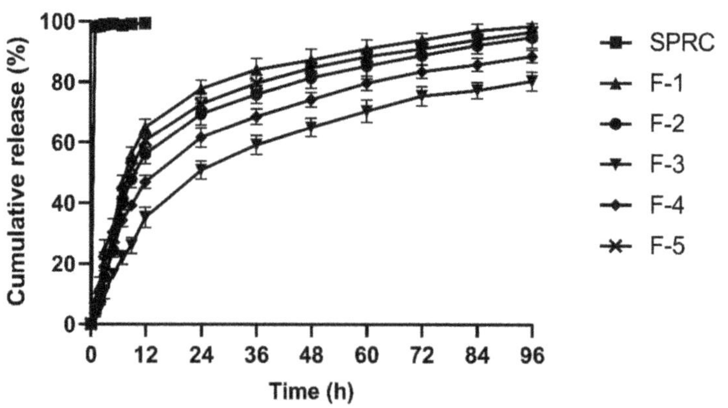

Figure 3. The in vitro release of SPRC from SPRC@PLA in PBS (n = 3, mean ± SD).

F-1 to F-5 showed a similar PY, which indicated that neither the amount of PLA used, nor the homogenization speed could influence the PY of the prepared SPRC@PLA. Normally, for subcutaneous injection, micro-sized particles with a range between 20 to 100 μm [45] are generally used, since, on the one hand, it usually has sufficient size to incorporate enough active pharmaceutical ingredient, and, on the other hand, sizes between this range are normally suitable, and therefore do not induce inflammation in the injection area. Hence, although F-1 and F-5 both showed a sustained and complete release of SPRC, for further in vivo study, F-1 and F-5 were not selected.

Above all, F-2 was chosen as the optimized formulation for further study due to its high EE, stable PY, relative monodispersed particle size, as well as its sustained and complete release in vitro. The SEM of F-2 is shown in Figure 4. For a convenient expression, F-2 is denoted as SPRC@PLA for the remainder of this paper.

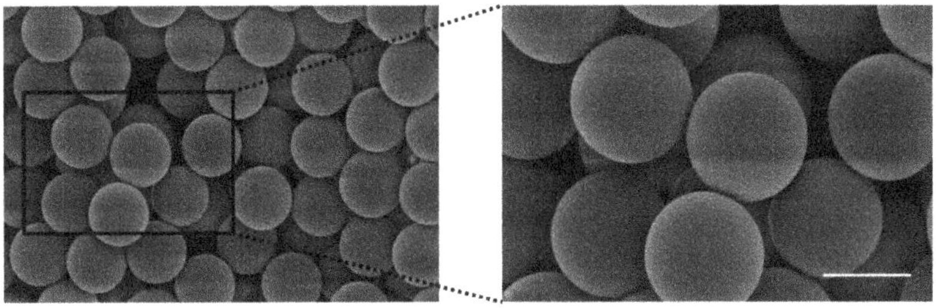

Figure 4. The SEM of SPRC@PLA microspheres (scale bar = 20 μm).

3.2. *The Elevation of Plasma H_2S Concentration by Supplementations*

Generally, H_2S is unstable, and can exist as the mixed state of hydrogen sulfide (H_2S), hydrogen sulfide anion (HS^-), and sulfide anion (S^{2-}) under physiological conditions (Figure 1A). It has been reported [46,47] that H_2S, HS^-, or S^{2-} could react quickly with MBB to produce a relatively stable SDB in a Tris-HCl buffer (pH 9.5) under 1% oxygen (Figure 1B). It would be much easier to detect the SDB rather than the H_2S in vivo. Herein, the LC-MS was adopted for the measurement of SDB in vivo, which could indirectly reflect the equal amount of H_2S in vivo. Two peaks, as shown in Figure 5A, indicated effective separation of SDB (Peak 1) and internal standard (Peak 2). Then, the calibration curve was calculated with a concentration range from 0.625 to 20 μM, (Figure 5B) which indicated a good linear correlation of this method. The SPR promoted H_2S release in vivo in a fast manner, while SPRC@PLA sustained the elevated plasma H_2S concentration, as shown in Figure 5C. Instantaneous H_2S production and metabolism could be observed within 6 h after a single injection of SPRC solution. Differently, SPRC@PLA slowly elevated the plasma H_2S concentration, which was potentially induced by the sustained SPRC release from SPRC@PLA.

3.3. *Supplementations Increased the Expression of CSE*

The SPRC has been reported to be able to promote the H_2S release in vivo through the CSE/H_2S signaling pathway, according to our previous studies [6,7], and the CSE mainly distributed in heart and liver [48–51]. The expression of CSE in the heart and liver were investigated and the increased expression could be found in both SPRC and SPRC@PLA groups. The SPRC@PLA group showed a higher expression of CSE than the SPRC group both in heart and liver, mainly because of the sustained release of SPRC from SPRC@PLA (Figure 6).

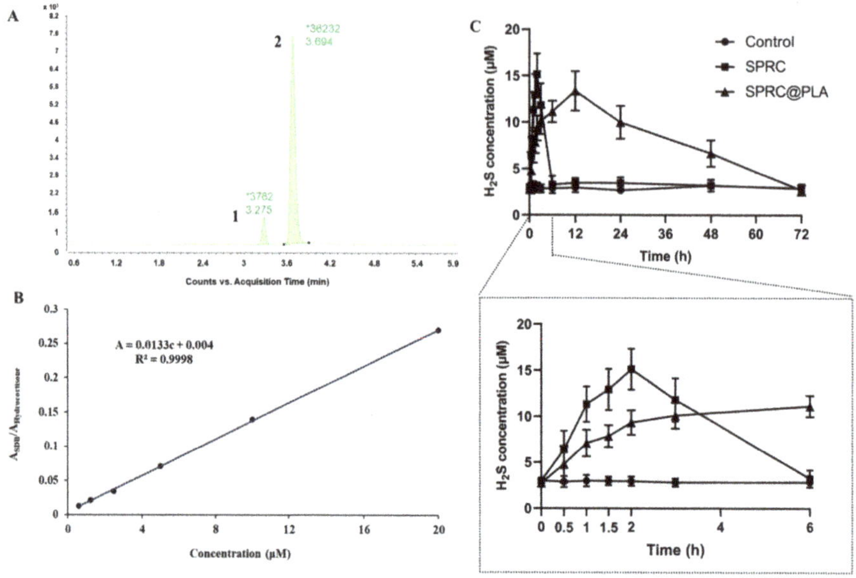

Figure 5. The detection of endogenous H_2S via LC-MS. (**A**) The chromatography of SDB, peak 1/SDB, peak 2/hydrocortisone (internal standard); (**B**) the calibration curve of SDB in different concentration (0.625~20 µM); (**C**) the 3-day endogenous H_2S concentration changes in plasma after a single injection of SPRC or SPRC@PLA. Dosage of 100 mg kg^{-1} was calculated according to rats' body weight (n = 3, mean ± SD).

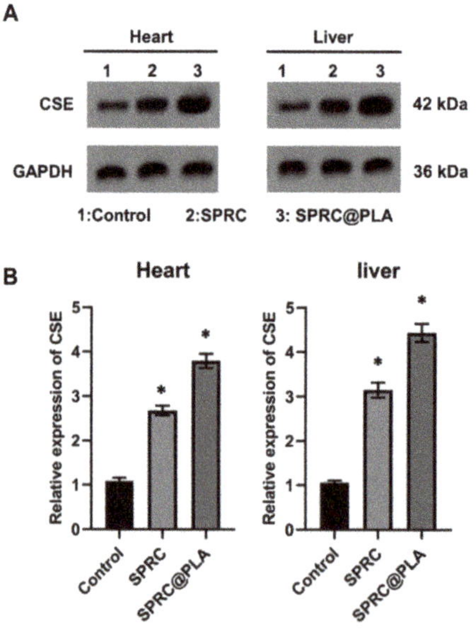

Figure 6. (**A**) The expression of CSE in hearts and liver of rats determined by Western blot and (**B**) the relative expression fold changes. GAPDH was used as a loading control and (*) indicated significant different as compared with the control group (n = 5, mean ± SD).

3.4. *Supplementations Inhibited the Paw Swollen in AIA Rats*

As shown in Figure 7, the paw swollen was calculated through the paw volume and arthritis index, while before the 10th day, no significant increase of these parameters could be observed. However, after 10 days, an instant and dramatic increase of paw volume and arthritis index could be observed in the AIA model group, while the SPRC group showed the same trend, which indicated a low therapeutical effect of the SPRC group. Conversely, the SPRC@PLA group showed significant inhibition of both paw volume and arthritis index.

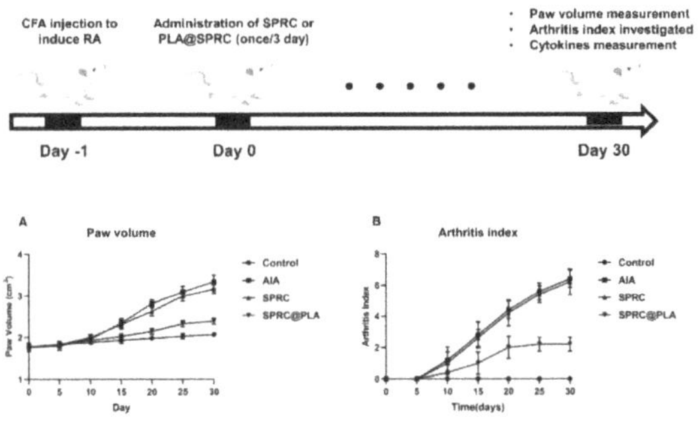

Figure 7. The (**A**) paw volume was measured by plethysmometer, and the (**B**) arthritis index were assessed using the arthritis scoring system to evaluate the severity of swollen symptoms (*n* = 5, mean ± SD).

As illustrated in Figure 8, SPRC showed a negligible anti-inflammatory effect in AIA rats as compared with the model group, while a dramatic decrease in pro-inflammatory cytokines and an increase in anti-inflammatory cytokines could be observed in the SPRC@PLA group.

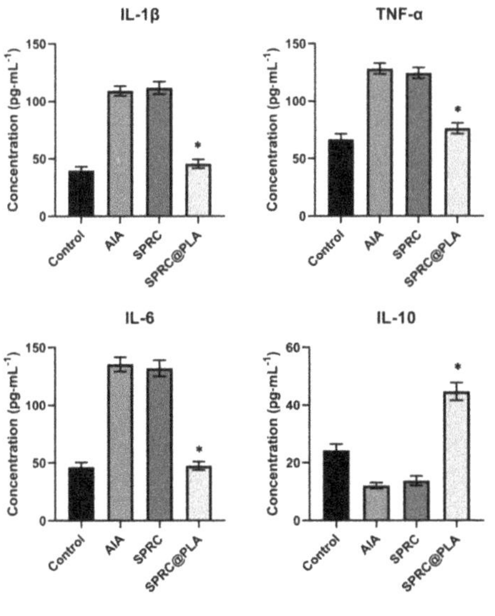

Figure 8. The pro-inflammatory cytokine levels of IL-1β, TNF-α, and IL-6, and anti-inflammatory cytokine level of IL-10 in rats were measured. * indicated a significant different as compared with the AIA model group (*n* = 5, mean ± SD).

4. Conclusions

In summary, in this study, SPRC@PLA, a spherical-like microsphere, with a diameter of approximately 30 μm was successfully prepared via the W1/O/W2 emulsification method. In addition, SPRC@PLA showed sustained in vitro SPRC release up to 4 days, and this prolonged in vitro release also promoted in vivo H_2S release in a sustained manner for 3 days with a single injection. In addition, a once per three-day injection of SPRC@PLA showed good therapeutical effect towards AIA, which increased the administration intervals as compared with those in our previous study [31].

Author Contributions: Conceptualization, Z.W. and Y.Y.; methodology, Y.Y. and X.Y.; software, R.W.; investigation, Q.D., W.H., and W.Q.; data curation, R.W., Y.F., and J.L.; writing—original draft preparation, Y.Y. and Q.Y.; writing—review and editing, Y.Z. and R.W.; supervision, Y.Z.; project administration, Y.Z.; funding acquisition, Y.Z. All authors have read and agreed to the published version of the manuscript.

Funding: This research was funded by the Macau Science and Technology Development fund (067/2018/A2, 033/2017/AMJ, 0007/2019/AKP, and 0052/2020/A), and the National Natural Science Foundation of China (grant no. 81973320) to Yi Zhun Zhu.

Institutional Review Board Statement: The Animal Care and Use Committee of Municipal Affairs Bureau of Macau approved all studies described herein (approval number AL010/DICV/SIS/2018), and the experiment was conducted under the guidance of the *NIH Guide for the Care and Use of Laboratory Animals* (8th edition).

Data Availability Statement: Data can be received from the authors upon reasonable request.

Conflicts of Interest: The authors declare no conflict of interest.

References

1. Guo, Q.; Wang, Y.; Xu, D.; Nossent, J.; Pavlos, N.J.; Xu, J. Rheumatoid arthritis: Pathological mechanisms and modern pharmacologic therapies. *Bone Res.* **2018**, *6*, 1–14. [CrossRef]
2. McInnes, I.B.; Schett, G. The Pathogenesis of Rheumatoid Arthritis. *N. Engl. J. Med.* **2011**, *365*, 2205–2219. [CrossRef]
3. Kim, E.J.; Seo, J.B.; Yu, J.S.; Lee, S.; Lim, J.S.; Choi, J.U.; Lee, C.-M.; Rashan, L.; Kim, K.H.; Cho, Y.-C. Anti-Inflammatory Effects of a Polyphenol, Catechin-7,4′-O-Digallate, from Woodfordia uniflora by Regulating NF-κB Signaling Pathway in Mouse Macrophages. *Pharmaceutics* **2021**, *13*, 408. [CrossRef] [PubMed]
4. Ferreira-Silva, M.; Faria-Silva, C.; Viana Baptista, P.; Fernandes, E.; Ramos Fernandes, A.; Corvo, M.L. Liposomal Nanosystems in Rheumatoid Arthritis. *Pharmaceutics* **2021**, *13*, 454. [CrossRef]
5. Olson, A.L.; Swigris, J.J.; Sprunger, D.B.; Fischer, A.; Fernandez-Perez, E.R.; Solomon, J.; Murphy, J.; Cohen, M.; Raghu, G.; Brown, K.K. Rheumatoid arthritis-interstitial lung disease-associated mortality. *Am. J. Respir. Crit. Care Med.* **2011**, *183*, 372–378. [CrossRef] [PubMed]
6. Crowson, C.S.; Liao, K.P.; Davis, J.M.; Solomon, D.H.; Matteson, E.L.; Knutson, K.L.; Hlatky, M.A.; Gabriel, S.E. Rheumatoid arthritis and cardiovascular disease. *Am. Heart J.* **2013**, *166*, 622–628.e1. [CrossRef]
7. Gremese, E.; Ferraccioli, G. The metabolic syndrome: The crossroads between rheumatoid arthritis and cardiovascular risk. *Autoimmun. Rev.* **2011**, *10*, 582–589. [CrossRef]
8. Birch, J.T.; Bhattacharya, S. Emerging trends in diagnosis and treatment of rheumatoid arthritis. *Prim. Care Clin. Off. Pract.* **2010**, *37*, 779–792. [CrossRef] [PubMed]
9. Burmester, G.R.; Pope, J.E. Novel treatment strategies in rheumatoid arthritis. *Lancet* **2017**, *389*, 2338–2348. [CrossRef]
10. Kotak, S.; Mardekian, J.; Horowicz-Mehler, N.; Shah, A.; Burgess, A.; Kim, J.; Gemmen, E.; Boyd, H.; Koenig, A. Impact of Etanercept Therapy on Disease Activity and Health-Related Quality of Life in Moderate Rheumatoid Arthritis Patients Population from a National British Observational Cohort. *Value Health* **2015**, *18*, 817–823. [CrossRef] [PubMed]
11. Smolen, J.S.; Aletaha, D.; McInnes, I.B. Rheumatoid arthritis. *Lancet* **2016**, *388*, 2023–2038.e1. [CrossRef]
12. Lee, D.M.; Weinblatt, M.E. Rheumatoid arthritis. *Lancet* **2001**, *358*, 903–911. [CrossRef]
13. Brzeziński, M.; Kost, B.; Wedepohl, S.; Socka, M.; Biela, T.; Calderón, M. Stereocomplexed PLA microspheres: Control over morphology, drug encapsulation and anticancer activity. *Colloids Surf. B Biointerfaces* **2019**, *184*, 110544. [CrossRef]
14. Anderson, J.M.; Shive, M.S. Biodegradation and biocompatibility of PLA and PLGA microspheres. *Adv. Drug Deliv. Rev.* **1997**, *28*, 5–24. [CrossRef]
15. Ayad, C.; Libeau, P.; Lacroix-Gimon, C.; Ladavière, C.; Verrier, B. LipoParticles: Lipid-Coated PLA Nanoparticles Enhanced In Vitro mRNA Transfection Compared to Liposomes. *Pharmaceutics* **2021**, *13*, 377. [CrossRef] [PubMed]
16. Gangapurwala, G.; Vollrath, A.; De San Luis, A.; Schubert, U.S. PLA/PLGA-Based Drug Delivery Systems Produced with Supercritical CO2—A Green Future for Particle Formulation? *Pharmaceutics* **2020**, *12*, 1118. [CrossRef]

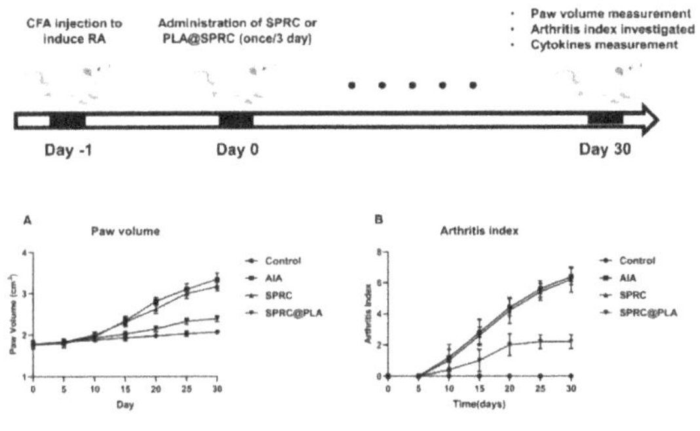

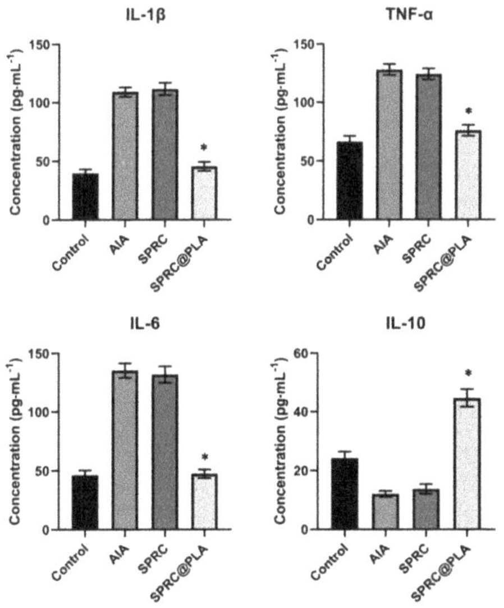

17. Singhvi, M.S.; Zinjarde, S.S.; Gokhale, D.V. Polylactic acid: Synthesis and biomedical applications. *J. Appl. Microbiol.* **2019**, *127*, 1612–1626. [CrossRef]
18. Kumari, A.; Kumar, V.; Yadav, S.K. Plant extract synthesized PLA nanoparticles for controlled and sustained release of Quercetin: A green approach. *PLoS ONE* **2012**, *7*, e41230. [CrossRef]
19. Lee, B.K.; Yun, Y.; Park, K. PLA micro- and nano-particles. *Adv. Drug Deliv. Rev.* **2016**, *107*, 176–191. [CrossRef]
20. Tian, Y.; Xu, J.; Li, Y.; Zhao, R.; Du, S.; Lv, C.; Wu, W.; Liu, R.; Sheng, X.; Song, Y.; et al. MicroRNA-31 Reduces Inflammatory Signaling and Promotes Regeneration in Colon Epithelium, and Delivery of Mimics in Microspheres Reduces Colitis in Mice. *Gastroenterology* **2019**, *156*, 2281–2296.e6. [CrossRef]
21. Zhang, C.; Yang, L.; Wan, F.; Bera, H.; Cun, D.; Rantanen, J.; Yang, M. Quality by design thinking in the development of long-acting injectable PLGA/PLA-based microspheres for peptide and protein drug delivery. *Int. J. Pharm.* **2020**, *585*, 119441. [CrossRef] [PubMed]
22. Wu, D.; Wang, H.; Teng, T.; Duan, S.; Ji, A.; Li, Y. Hydrogen sulfide and autophagy: A double edged sword. *Pharmacol. Res.* **2018**, *131*, 120–127. [CrossRef]
23. Kumar, M.; Sandhir, R. Hydrogen Sulfide in Physiological and Pathological Mechanisms in Brain. *CNS Neurol. Disord. Drug Targets* **2018**, *17*, 654–670. [CrossRef] [PubMed]
24. Olas, B. Hydrogen sulfide in signaling pathways. *Clin. Chim. Acta* **2015**, *439*, 212–218. [CrossRef]
25. Zhao, H.L.; Wu, B.Q.; Luo, Y.; Zhang, W.Y.; Hao, Y.L.; Liang, J.J.; Fang, F.; Liu, W.; Chen, X.H. Exogenous hydrogen sulfide ameliorates high glucose-induced myocardial injury & inflammation via the CIRP-MAPK signaling pathway in H9c2 cardiac cells. *Life Sci.* **2018**, *208*, 315–324. [CrossRef] [PubMed]
26. Chen, Y.; Jin, S.; Teng, X.; Hu, Z.; Zhang, Z.; Qiu, X.; Tian, D.; Wu, Y. Hydrogen sulfide attenuates LPS-induced acute kidney injury by inhibiting inflammation and oxidative stress. *Oxid. Med. Cell. Longev.* **2018**, *2018*, 6717212. [CrossRef] [PubMed]
27. Zaorska, E.; Tomasova, L.; Koszelewski, D.; Ostaszewski, R.; Ufnal, M. Hydrogen sulfide in pharmacotherapy, beyond the hydrogen sulfide-donors. *Biomolecules* **2020**, *10*, 323. [CrossRef]
28. Powell, C.R.; Dillon, K.M.; Matson, J.B. A review of hydrogen sulfide (H2S) donors: Chemistry and potential therapeutic applications. *Biochem. Pharmacol.* **2018**, *149*, 110–123. [CrossRef] [PubMed]
29. Shin, C.C.; Moore, P.K.; Zhu, Y.Z. S-allylcysteine mediates cardioprotection in an acute myocardial infarction rat model via a hydrogen sulfide-mediated pathway. *Am. J. Physiol. Heart Circ. Physiol.* **2007**, *293*, H2693–H2701. [CrossRef]
30. Yue, L.J.; Zhu, X.Y.; Li, R.S.; Chang, H.J.; Gong, B.; Tian, C.C.; Liu, C.; Xue, Y.X.; Zhou, Q.; Xu, T.S.; et al. S-allyl-cysteine sulfoxide (alliin) alleviates myocardial infarction by modulating cardiomyocyte necroptosis and autophagy. *Int. J. Mol. Med.* **2019**, *44*, 1943–1951. [CrossRef]
31. Wu, W.J.; Jia, W.W.; Liu, X.H.; Pan, L.L.; Zhang, Q.Y.; Yang, D.; Shen, X.Y.; Liu, L.; Zhu, Y.Z. S-propargyl-cysteine attenuates inflammatory response in rheumatoid arthritis by modulating the Nrf2-ARE signaling pathway. *Redox Biol.* **2016**, *10*, 157–167. [CrossRef] [PubMed]
32. Liang, Y.H.; Shen, Y.Q.; Guo, W.; Zhu, Y.Z. SPRC protects hypoxia and re-oxygenation injury by improving rat cardiac contractile function and Intracellular calcium handling. *Nitric Oxide Biol. Chem.* **2014**, *41*, 113–119. [CrossRef]
33. MA, K.; Liu, Y.; Zhu, Q.; Liu, C.-h.; Duan, J.L.; Tan, B.K.H.; Zhu, Y.Z. H2S donor, S-propargyl-cysteine, increases CSE in SGC-7901 and cancer-induced mice: Evidence for a novel anti-cancer effect of endogenous H2S? *PLoS ONE* **2011**, *6*, e20525. [CrossRef] [PubMed]
34. Wang, Q.; Wang, X.L.; Liu, H.R.; Rose, P.; Zhu, Y.Z. Protective effects of cysteine analogues on acute myocardial ischemia: Novel modulators of endogenous H2S production. *Antioxid. Redox Signal.* **2010**, *12*, 1155–1165. [CrossRef] [PubMed]
35. Gong, Q.H.; Wang, Q.; Pan, L.L.; Liu, X.H.; Xin, H.; Zhu, Y.Z. S-Propargyl-cysteine, a novel hydrogen sulfide-modulated agent, attenuates lipopolysaccharide-induced spatial learning and memory impairment: Involvement of TNF signaling and NF-κB pathway in rats. *Brain. Behav. Immun.* **2011**, *25*, 110–119. [CrossRef]
36. Gong, Q.H.; Pan, L.L.; Liu, X.H.; Wang, Q.; Huang, H.; Zhu, Y.Z. S-propargyl-cysteine (ZYZ-802), a sulphur-containing amino acid, attenuates beta-amyloid-induced cognitive deficits and pro-inflammatory response: Involvement of ERK1/2 and NF-κB pathway in rats. *Amino Acids* **2011**, *40*, 601–610. [CrossRef] [PubMed]
37. Wu, W.; Qin, M.; Jia, W.; Huang, Z.; Li, Z.; Yang, D.; Huang, M.; Xiao, C.; Long, F.; Mao, J.; et al. Cystathionine-γ-lyase ameliorates the histone demethylase JMJD3-mediated autoimmune response in rheumatoid arthritis. *Cell. Mol. Immunol.* **2019**, *16*, 694–705. [CrossRef] [PubMed]
38. Jia, W.; Wu, W.; Yang, D.; Xiao, C.; Su, Z.; Huang, Z.; Li, Z.; Qin, M.; Huang, M.; Liu, S.; et al. Histone demethylase JMJD3 regulates fibroblast-like synoviocyte-mediated proliferation and joint destruction in rheumatoid arthritis. *FASEB J.* **2018**, *32*, 4031–4042.e6. [CrossRef]
39. Zheng, Y.; Liu, H.; Ma, G.; Yang, P.; Zhang, L.; Gu, Y.; Zhu, Q.; Shao, T.; Zhang, P.; Zhu, Y.; et al. Determination of S-propargyl-cysteine in rat plasma by mixed-mode reversed-phase and cation-exchange HPLC-MS/MS method and its application to pharmacokinetic studies. *J. Pharm. Biomed. Anal.* **2011**, *54*, 1187–1191. [CrossRef]
40. Tran, B.H.; Huang, C.; Zhang, Q.; Liu, X.; Lin, S.; Liu, H.; Wang, S.; Zhu, Y.Z. Cardioprotective effects and pharmacokinetic properties of a controlled release formulation of a novel hydrogen sulfide donor in rats with acute myocardial infarction. *Biosci. Rep.* **2015**, *35*, 1–12. [CrossRef]

41. Liu, R.; Ma, G.H.; Wan, Y.H.; Su, Z.G. Influence of process parameters on the size distribution of PLA microcapsules prepared by combining membrane emulsification technique and double emulsion-solvent evaporation method. *Colloids Surfaces B Biointerfaces* **2005**, *45*, 144–153. [CrossRef]
42. Ma, G.; Zhang, L.; Zhang, P.; Bao, X.; Zhou, N.; Shi, Q.; Zheng, Y.; Liu, H.; Bu, F.; Zhang, Y.; et al. Physicochemical characteristics and gastrointestinal absorption behaviors of S-propargyl-cysteine, a potential new drug candidate for cardiovascular protection and antitumor treatment. *Xenobiotica* **2015**, *45*, 322–334. [CrossRef]
43. Juhász, Á.; Ungor, D.; Berta, K.; Seres, L.; Csapó, E. Spreadsheet-based nonlinear analysis of in vitro release properties of a model drug from colloidal carriers. *J. Mol. Liq.* **2021**, *328*, 115405. [CrossRef]
44. Zhu, Y.Z.; Zhong, J.W.; Ho, P.; Yoke, Y.L.; Yi, C.Z.; Shan, H.H.; Chee, S.T.; Whiteman, M.; Lu, J.; Moore, P.K. Hydrogen sulfide and its possible roles in myocardial ischemia in experimental rats. *J. Appl. Physiol.* **2007**, *102*, 261–268. [CrossRef] [PubMed]
45. Bragagni, M.; Beneitez, C.; Martín, C.; De La Ossa, D.H.P.; Mura, P.A.; Gil-Alegre, M.E. Selection of PLA polymers for the development of injectable prilocaine controlled release microparticles: Usefulness of thermal analysis. *Int. J. Pharm.* **2013**, *441*, 468–475. [CrossRef]
46. Shen, X.; Chakraborty, S.; Dugas, T.R.; Kevil, C.G. Hydrogen sulfide measurement using sulfide dibimane: Critical evaluation with electrospray ion trap mass spectrometry. *Nitric Oxide Biol. Chem.* **2014**, *41*, 97–104. [CrossRef]
47. Shen, X.; Pattillo, C.B.; Pardue, S.; Bir, S.C.; Wang, R.; Kevil, C.G. Measurement of plasma hydrogen sulfide in vivo and in vitro. *Free Radic. Biol. Med.* **2011**, *50*, 1021–1031. [CrossRef]
48. Tran, B.H.; Yu, Y.; Chang, L.; Tan, B.; Jia, W.; Xiong, Y.; Dai, T.; Zhong, R.; Zhang, W.; Le, V.M.; et al. A novel liposomal S-propargyl-cysteine: A sustained release of hydrogen sulfide reducing myocardial fibrosis via TGF-β1/smad pathway. *Int. J. Nanomed.* **2019**, *14*, 10061–10077. [CrossRef] [PubMed]
49. Sidhapuriwala, J.N.; Hegde, A.; Ang, A.D.; Zhu, Y.Z.; Bhatia, M. Effects of s-propargyl-cysteine (sprc) in caerulein-induced acute pancreatitis in mice. *PLoS ONE* **2012**, *7*, e32574. [CrossRef]
50. Xin, H.; Wang, M.; Tang, W.; Shen, Z.; Miao, L.; Wu, W.; Li, C.; Wang, X.; Xin, X.; Zhu, Y.Z. Hydrogen Sulfide Attenuates Inflammatory Hepcidin by Reducing IL-6 Secretion and Promoting SIRT1-Mediated STAT3 Deacetylation. *Antioxid. Redox Signal.* **2016**, *24*, 70–83. [CrossRef]
51. Wang, M.; Xin, H.; Tang, W.; Li, Y.; Zhang, Z.; Fan, L.; Miao, L.; Tan, B.; Wang, X.; Zhu, Y.Z. AMPK Serves as a Therapeutic Target Against Anemia of Inflammation. *Antioxid. Redox Signal.* **2017**, *27*, 251–268. [CrossRef] [PubMed]

pharmaceutics

Article

Optimization and Development of Selective Histone Deacetylase Inhibitor (MPT0B291)-Loaded Albumin Nanoparticles for Anticancer Therapy

Athika Darumas Putri [1], Pai-Shan Chen [2], Yu-Lin Su [1], Jia-Pei Lin [1], Jing-Ping Liou [1] and Chien-Ming Hsieh [1,*]

1 School of Pharmacy, College of Pharmacy, Taipei Medical University, Taipei 11031, Taiwan; d301108007@tmu.edu.tw (A.D.P.); m301107002@tmu.edu.tw (Y.-L.S.); linjpjpjp@gmail.com (J.-P.L.); jpl@tmu.edu.tw (J.-P.L.)

2 Graduate Institute of Toxicology, College of Medicine, National Taiwan University, Taipei 10617, Taiwan; paishanchen@ntu.edu.tw

* Correspondence: cmhsieh@tmu.edu.tw; Tel.: +886-2-27361661 (ext. 6111)

Abstract: Histone deacetylase (HDAC) inhibitors have emerged as a new class of antitumor agent for various types of tumors. MPT0B291, a novel selective inhibitor of HDAC6, demonstrated significant antiproliferative activity in various human cancer cell types. However, MPT0B291 has very low water solubility, which limits its clinical use for cancer therapy. In the current study, MPT0B291 was encapsulated in human serum albumin (HSA), and its anticancer activities were investigated. Nanoparticles (NPs) were prepared using two-stage emulsification resulting in 100~200-nm NPs with a fine size distribution (polydispersity index of <0.3). The in vitro drug release profiles of MPT0B291-loaded HSA NPs presented sustained-release properties. The cytotoxic effect on MIA PaCa-2 human pancreatic carcinoma cells was found to be similar to MPT0B291-loaded HSA NPs and the free-drug group. The albumin-based formulation provided a higher maximum tolerated dose than that of a drug solution with reduced toxicity toward normal cells. Furthermore, in vivo pharmacokinetic studies demonstrated an effective increase (5~8-fold) in the bioavailability of NPs containing MPT0B291 loaded in HSA compared to the free-drug solution with an extended circulation time ($t_{1/2}$) leading to significantly enhanced efficacy of anticancer treatment.

Keywords: albumin nanoparticle; MPT0B291; high-pressure homogenizer; histone deacetylase

Citation: Putri, A.D.; Chen, P.-S.; Su, Y.-L.; Lin, J.-P.; Liou, J.-P.; Hsieh, C.-M. Optimization and Development of Selective Histone Deacetylase Inhibitor (MPT0B291)-Loaded Albumin Nanoparticles for Anticancer Therapy. *Pharmaceutics* **2021**, *13*, 1728. https://doi.org/10.3390/pharmaceutics13101728

Academic Editors: Ana Isabel Fernandes and Angela Faustino Jozala

Received: 12 September 2021
Accepted: 12 October 2021
Published: 19 October 2021

1. Introduction

Histone acetyltransferases (HATs) and histone deacetylases (HDACs) are known to simultaneously regulate both intracellular and extracellular responses toward epigenetic modifications by respectively executing the acetylation and deacetylation of lysine residues at the amino terminals of histones [1,2]. However, overexpression and atypical recruitment of HDACs for acetyl-group removal that occurs at their promoter sites raises the possibility of an imbalance in acetylation-deacetylation processes [3–5]. Aberrant deacetylation due to the HDAC mechanism was also found in non-histone proteins, such as p53, which initiated a mutation of p53 [6]. Consequently, targeting HDACs is considered an important strategy in developing anticancer agents.

Inhibition of HDACs has garnered potential interest in anticancer development as it induces cell-cycle arrest and cell apoptosis, and decreases cancer metastasis [7]. Several recently developed HDAC inhibitors, such as deacetylase-trichostatin A (TSA) and deacetylase-suberoylanilide hydroxamic acid (SAHA), showed excellent results in suppressing cancer cell growth [8–10].

Among various mammalian HDAC isozymes, HDAC6 is unique for being restricted to the cytoplasm and possessing two catalytic domains along with a ubiquitin-binding site [11]. One of the domains, CD2, induces deacetylation of the α-tubulin region of microtubules. Therefore, targeting HDAC6 could be a prospective cancer immunotherapy, as inhibition of its site showed improvement in tumorigenesis, through reducing histone hypoacetylation and increasing tumor-suppressor genes [12–14].

MPT0B291, an azaindolysulfonamide (shown in Figure 1), was developed as an HDAC6 inhibitor and is currently being studied for applications in clinical treatments. Compared to SAHA, MPT0B291 is considered a promising anticancer drug candidate due to its higher selectivity of HDAC inhibition, low toxicity, and broader spectrum of anticancer activity [14,15]. Despite this significant therapeutic potential, MPT0B291 has very low water solubility, which directly impacts its pharmacokinetics (PKs) and ultimately limits its clinical use. In addition, the poor aqueous solubility of MPT0B291 hinders its formulation for parenteral delivery.

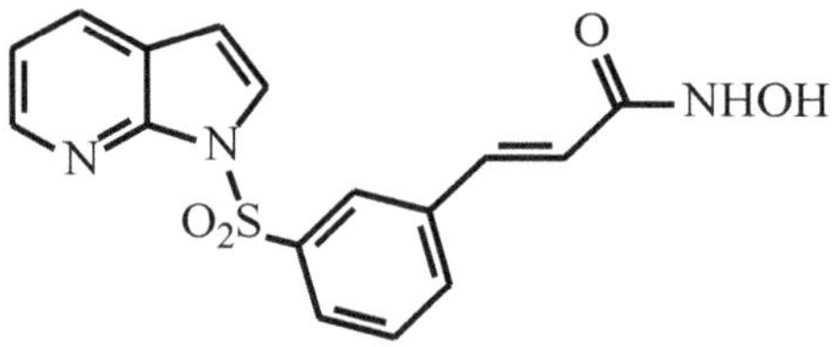

Figure 1. Chemical structure of MPT0B291, with molecular weight 343.36 g/mol.

Utilization of nanoparticles (NPs) for drug delivery and therapy has been developing for decades. NPs' fundamental characteristic of a high surface-to-volume ratio permits interaction with a greater surface area in comparison to that of larger particles with a similar volume [16]. This unique advantage in drug development enhances the drug-loading capacity and stability, and in a more feasible way enables the incorporation of ligands (i.e., either hydrophilic or hydrophobic molecules). Protein-based carriers have been extensively applied owing to their potential advantages over synthetic carriers, including low toxicity, high drug-binding capacity, marked uptake by target cells, easy preparation, and scaling-up capability [17,18].

Among successful drug nanocarriers that are now established, albumin-bound NPs have opened up an avenue as an effective nanocarrier in cancer therapeutics [19]. Albumin can closely and reversibly bind to hydrophobic paclitaxel through noncovalent bonds to enable in vivo transport and release of transported substances and has become a natural carrier of hydrophobic substances [20–22]. It can also provide improved efficacy and tolerability compared to cremophor-based paclitaxel solutions [23,24]. Using albumin as a nanocarrier is essential to disguise the active loaded drugs from unselective uptake by immune cells. The use of the first albumin-bound NPs to facilitate delivery of the anticancer drug, paclitaxel, has garnered tremendous interest, as they are able to increase the stability of the colloidal solution (Abraxane®). Three essential pathways, known as 'tumor-feeding mechanisms', corroborate the importance of albumin as a drug nanocarrier. High permeability of tumor neo-vessels permits more macronutrients, including albumin, to leak inside the tumor area than that seen with normal tissues, implying indirect contact of the co-loaded cytotoxic species which use albumin as the template core. Second, albumin trapped within a tumor is slowly digested due to the impaired lymphatic drainage which can lead to efficient targeting or effective binding of the co-loaded species with the targeted receptor. Third, the albumin-activated gp60 route allows albumin transcytosis to bind to the gp60 receptor on vascular endothelial cells [25].

Therefore, in the present study, we aimed to develop, characterize, and optimize novel nanocarrier formulations of MPT0B291 with the relatively inexpensive, commercially available, safe, and biocompatible human serum albumin (HSA). MPT0B291-loaded HSA NPs (MPT0B291-HSA NPs) were prepared, and their size distribution, morphology, and loading and encapsulation efficiencies were examined. The in vitro cytotoxicity of the optimized formulation was assessed against the Mia PACA-2 cell line. Finally, in vivo PK studies were performed to investigate whether albumin encapsulation could prolong the elimination half-life and improve the intravenous bioavailability of MPT0B291.

2. Materials and Methods

MPT0B291 was synthesized in our own laboratory (Taipei, Taiwan) [15]. BSF (20%) human albumin solution (≥96.0%, CSL Behring, Melbourne, Australia), soybean lecithin (Lipoid S100) (Lipoid, Ludwigshafen am Rhein, Germany), Bio-Rad protein assay dye reagent concentrate (Bio-Rad Laboratories, Hercules, CA, USA), bovine serum albumin, (BSA; Sigma-Aldrich Chemie, Steinheim, Germany), methanol, ethanol, acetonitrile, chloroform, Tween 80 (Merck, Darmstadt, Germany), dimethyl sulfoxide (Echo, Miaoli, Taiwan), formic acid, (Sigma-Aldrich Chemie), and trifluoroacetic acid (Riedel-de Haën, RdH Laborchemikalien, Seelze, Germany) were procured commercially. All organic solvents mentioned above were of analytical grade. Sodium phosphate monobasic (Sigma-Aldrich Laborchemikalien, Seelze, Germany), sodium phosphate dibasic, anhydrous (J.T. Baker, Phillipsburg, NJ, USA), Dulbecco's modified Eagle medium (DMEM), fetal bovine serum (FBS), horse serum, penicillin-streptomycin solution, 0.25% Trypsin-2.21 mM EDTA 1×, Matrigel® matrix basement membrane (Corning, Manassas, VA, USA), and thiazolyl blue tetrazolium bromide (Alfa Aesar, Lancashire, UK) were purchased commercially. Male Sprague-Dawley rats at 8 weeks of age and female fox chase SCID mice at 4 weeks of age were purchased from BioLASCO Taiwan (Yilan, Taiwan). All other chemicals and solvents used in this study were of fine analytical grade.

2.1. Preparation of MPT0B291-Loaded Albumin NPs

MPT0B291-HSA NPs were prepared by an emulsion-solvent evaporation method using a high-pressure homogenizer. Briefly, mixtures of MPT0B291 (30 mg) and soybean lecithin (135 mg) were dissolved in 800 μL of chloroform/ethanol (9:1). The solution was heated in an ultrasonic bath to 50 °C until the drug had completely dissolved. The drug-containing solution was then added to the albumin aqueous solution (1% *v*/*v*) with 5 min of sonication under 30% or 50% amplitude (ultrasonic oscillation; VCX 750, frequency: 20 kHz, Sonics and Materials, Newtown, CT, USA). The first emulsion was obtained followed by high-pressure homogenization (NanoLyzer-N2, Cogene, Hsinchu, Taiwan). A homogenization pressure (15,000 and 20,000 psi) was applied to the emulsion, and the number of homogenization cycles (10, 20, 30, and 40 cycles) was also optimized. The emulsion was subjected to various homogenization cycles, then passed through the homogenizer valve, and collected through a connecting tube at the base of the assembly, thus forming nano-sized emulsion droplets. Following high-pressure homogenization, the resulting solution was transferred to a round-bottomed flask and subjected to rotary evaporation (R-114, Buchi, Switzerland) under low vacuum (500 mmHg) for 25 min at 50 °C in order to ensure that the organic solvent was completely removed. The evaporated NPs were then filtered with 0.2 μm-regenerated cellulose (RC) membrane filter to remove impurities and unbound drugs. Finally, the NPs were freeze-dried (FDS-2, Taipei, Taiwan) using trehalose as cryoprotectant and stored at 4 °C for further experiments. A 3% trehalose solution was employed to stabilize the HSA NPs as well as to prevent the protein from denaturation during the lyophilization process and provide protection for long-term storage [26,27].

2.2. Particle Size, Size Distribution, Zeta Potential, and Surface Morphology

The particle size, size distribution, and zeta potential of the HSA NPs and MPT0B291-HSA NPs were measured by dynamic light scattering (DLS) using a Malvern Zetasizer NanoZS (Malvern Instruments, Worcestershire, UK). Samples were diluted with deionized water and measured at a scattering angle of 90° and temperature of 25 °C. The polydispersity index (PDI) gave an estimate of the size distribution of the HSA-NPs. The zeta potential was measured with a zeta potential analyzer using electrophoretic laser Doppler anemometry (Malvern Instruments, Worcestershire, UK). In addition, the shape and surface morphology of the MPT0B291-HAS NPs were further examined by transmission electron microscopy (TEM) (HT7700, Hitachi, Tokyo, Japan). Samples were diluted 50× with distilled water, and the NPs were stained with the heavy metal salt, uranyl acetate (2 *w*/*w*%), prior to imaging. A sample was prepared by placing a drop of the HSA NPs on a carbon-coated copper grid under suitable conditions.

2.3. Encapsulation Efficiency (EE) and Drug Loading (DL) of MPT0B291-HSA NPs

The drug concentration was initially determined by high-performance liquid chromatography (HPLC) using a Shimadzu-20AD system (Kyoto, Japan). The HPLC system was equipped with an XBridge C18 column (particle size 5 µm, 4.6 × 150 mm). A mixture of 0.043 M ammonium acetate and acetonitrile (45:55, *v*/*v*) was used as the mobile phase at a flow rate of 1 mL/min at 40 °C. The column effluent was monitored using an ultraviolet detector (UV-975, Jasco, Tokyo, Japan) at a wavelength of 265 nm, and the HPLC method was validated to have an acceptable coefficient of variation for accuracy and precision, which met the criteria of ±15% [28].

The drug content of MPT0B291-HSA NPs was determined via a literature search, which is briefly summarized as follows [29]. To release the drug content from the NPs, the MPT0B291-HSA NPs were diluted in acetonitrile and sonicated for 15 min. The supernatant obtained after centrifugation at 10,000 rpm for 5 min was then injected into the HPLC system to quantify the amount of MPT0B291 at 265 nm. The equations used for calculating the DL (%) and EE (%) are as follows:

$$\text{Encapsulation efficiency (EE, \%)} = \frac{W_{(\text{Total drug added}-\text{free non}-\text{encapsulated drug})}}{W_{\text{Total drug added}}} \times 100\% \quad (1)$$

and

$$\text{Drug loading (DL, \%)} = \frac{W_{(\text{initial drug added}-\text{free non}-\text{encapsulated drug})}}{W_{\text{nanoparticles content}}} \times 100\% \quad (2)$$

2.4. Stability of MPT0B291-HSA NPs

The MPT0B291-HSA NPs were reconstituted in water, and their sizes were measured by DLS at regular time intervals. In addition, the total drug concentrations were evaluated after 7 days of storage at 4 °C.

2.5. In Vitro Drug-Release Behavior

To investigate the kinetics of MPT0B291 release from MPT0B291-HSA NPs, a suspension of MPT0B291-HSA NPs containing 0.25 mg/mL of MPT0B291 was transferred to a dialysis bag with a molecular weight cutoff (MWCO) of 6000~8000 Da. The dialysis bag was subsequently placed into 25 mL of release medium (PBS) containing 1% *v*/*v* Tween 80. The temperature was maintained at 37.0 ± 0.5 °C, and the medium was stirred at a speed of 100 rpm. MPT0B291 which had been dissolved in propylene glycol (free MPT0B291; 0.25 mg/mL) was used as a control and was treated in the same manner. During a period of 48 h, the surrounding environment was maintained by replacing 2 mL of the release medium with an equal volume of fresh medium at regular intervals. The extraction solution was solubilized in 500 µL of acetonitrile and assayed by HPLC.

2.6. Cell Viability Assay

The cytotoxicity of the MPT0B291-HSA NPs was determined in MIA PaCa-2 cells using MTT assays. Briefly, MIA PaCa-2 cells were seeded (5×10^3 cells/well) in 96-well culture plates. After 24 h of incubation in a humidified incubator at 37 °C with 5% CO_2, the medium of adherent cells was replaced with serum-free culture medium and incubated with 200 µL of serial dilutions of HSA-NPs (0.01~1000 µg/mL) and MPT0B291-HSAX NPs (0.0050 µg/mL). After another 24 h, 100 µL of MTT (500 µg/mL in PBS, pH 7.4) was added and incubated at 37 °C for 2 h. The medium was then removed, and 100 µL of DMSO was added to each well to dissolve the crystals. The optical density (OD) was measured at

540 nm using a microplate reader (Cytation™ 3 Cell Imaging Multi-Mode Reader, BioTek, Winooski, VT, USA). The cell survival rate was calculated as follows:

$$\text{Cell survival rate } (\%) = \frac{\text{Absorbance value of test solution group}}{\text{Absorbance value of blank solution group}} \times 100\% \quad (3)$$

2.7. Maximum Tolerated Dose (MTD)

The MTD studies for the MPT0B291 solution and MPT0B291-HSA NPs were carried out in healthy Balb/c female mice. The single-dose study was conducted using healthy female mice with four animals per group. Two groups of mice received an i.v. injection of 50, 75, or 150 mg/kg body weight (BW) of MPT0B291 and 0, 75, 150, or 200 mg/kg BW of MPT0B291-HSA NPs through the tail vein. The MTD was defined as the allowed median BW loss of approximately 15% of the control and causing neither death due to toxic effects nor remarkable changes in general signs within 1 week of administration [30].

2.8. In Vivo PK Study

Male Sprague-Dawley rats (250 ± 15 g) were divided into two groups (with four rats per group). Rats were fasted for 12 h with free access to water, and then intravenously treated with the MPT0B291 solution (dissolved in propylene glycol) or MPT0B291-HSA NPs (relative to the MTP0B219 concentration of 5 mg/kg BW). Blood samples (approximately 0.5 mL) were collected in a heparinized tube at 5 min, 15 min, 30 min, 1 h, 2 h, 4 h, 6 h, 8 h, 12 h, and 24 h after drug administration. All collected blood samples were centrifuged at 4000 rpm and 4 °C for 10 min, and supernatant plasma samples were obtained and frozen at −80 °C for further analysis.

Quantitative analysis of MPT0B291 in rat plasma by an ultra-precision liquid chromatographic tandem mass spectroscopic (UPLC-MS/MS) method was performed using an Agilent 1290 Infinity II LC System (Agilent, Wilmington, DE, USA) coupled with an Agilent 6470 triple quadrupole LC/MS system (Agilent Technologies, Santa Clara, CA, USA). Optimized chromatographic separation of MPT0B291 was conducted with an ACQUITY UPLC BEH C18 column (1.7 µm, 2.1 × 100 mm; Waters, Milford, MA, USA) at an oven temperature of 40 °C. The mobile phase was 0.1% (*v*/*v*) formic acid in water (mobile phase A) and acetonitrile containing 0.1% (*v*/*v*) formic acid (mobile phase B) with gradient elution at a flow rate of 0.3 mL/min. All analytical procedures were evaluated with positive electrospray ionization (ESI). The LC gradient was programmed in linear steps as follows: 0~0.5 min, 5% mobile phase B (*v*/*v*); 0.5~1 min, 5% mobile phase B to 100% mobile phase B (*v*/*v*); 1~2.8 min, 100% mobile phase B; 2.8~3 min, 100% mobile phase B to 5% mobile phase B (*v*/*v*); and 3~4 min, 5% mobile phase B (*v*/*v*). Quantification was achieved using the multiple reaction monitoring (MRM) mode at m/z 344.1 → 91.0 for MPT0B291. The following PK parameters were determined: the area under the concentration-time curve (AUC), maximum peak concentration (Cmax), time of maximum peak concentration (Tmax), and mean residence time (MRT). These parameters were determined by DAS software vers. 2.0. All data are presented as mean ± standard deviation (SD).

2.9. Statistical Analysis

All data were sourced from multiple batches and expressed as the mean ± SD unless specifically stated. Student's *t*-test or a one-way analysis of variance (ANOVA) was performed for the statistical evaluation of data. Differences between groups were considered statistically significant when the probability (p) was <0.01.

3. Results and Discussion

3.1. Optimization and Preparation of HSA NPs

3.1.1. Effect of the Energy Output of Ultrasonication

The fact that there is an enhanced permeability retention (EPR) effect around the tumor area is well-established, a higher accumulation rate of blood-circulating proteins including albumin would also be predicted [31]. Therefore, limiting the NPs to a sufficiently small size, within or <250 nm along with a uniform particle distribution (with an expected polydispersity index (PDI) of <0.30), to facilitate prolonged NP circulation and penetration into tumor tissues via an EPR effect is critical. It is also important to note that using a higher albumin concentration for preparation of albumin NPs would be anticipated to initiate higher levels of disulfide bonds formation leading to increased particle size and a greater likelihood of protein aggregation [32–34]. Further, higher particle size might affect the lower volume-to-surface ratio of the NPs, in turn decreasing drug loading during drug-NPs preparation and cellular uptake in vivo [35–38]. Lomis and co-worker [33] observed that 1% of albumin would be appropriate as the starting concentration of HSA NPs processed through HPH [33]. Therefore, 1% albumin was selected in this study for the preparation of HSA NPs and MPT0B291-HSA NPs. The HSA NPs were prepared by a two-step emulsification method (sonication and homogenization). Optimizing HSA NPs' preparation is a complex process due to the wide range of parameters involved in controlling their size. In this study, we investigated the influences of the sonication amplitude and homogenization process on the average diameter of HSA NPs. As shown in Figure 2, two different energy inputs (30% and 50% sonication amplitudes), followed by various homogenization cycle numbers (10, 20, 30, and 40), under 20,000 psi of homogenization pressure, were investigated to understand their effects on the size distribution of HSA NPs. An improved dispersion was found with a 30% amplitude of sonication regardless of the homogenization cycles, while a slightly larger particle size and wider particle size distribution were found when using a 50% sonication amplitude.

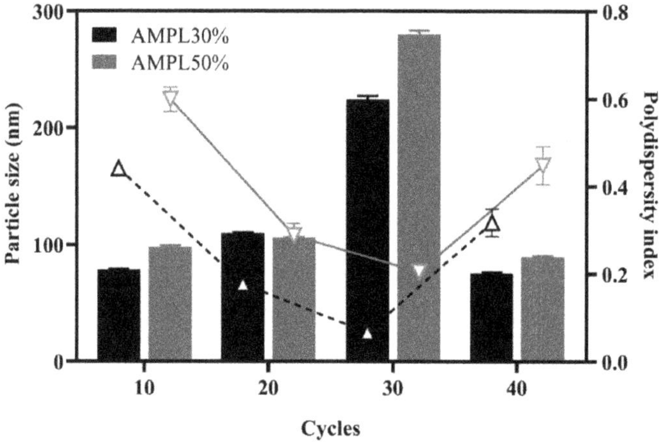

Figure 2. Effects of different amplitudes (AMPLs) of ultrasonication and different cycles of high-pressure homogenization on the particle size and size distribution. Column: particle size (nm); line: polydispersity index. Each point represents the mean ± SD. Error bars represent the standard deviation ($n = 3$).

In general, a higher ultrasonication amplitude would be expected to create a higher frequency of collisions between droplets and to further decrease the duration required to achieve a minimum emulsion droplet size. Fragmentation of the dispersed phase by ultrasonic radiation is mainly caused by a cavitation effect generating shear stress, local high pressure, and increased temperature [39]. A higher energy output can generate a more significant cavitation effect [40] which ultimately reduces the diameter of NPs. However, the activity of a hydrophobic drug counterpart involved in non-covalently bonding formation may have been interrupted by use of higher energy during the ultrasonication process. In the current study, applying a high amount of energy may have resulted in further instability of the formulation leading to particle aggregation. Ineffective promotion of a uniform distribution of particle sizes was found in groups formed with a 50% amplitude. It can be concluded that using a high sonication amplitude appeared to have a negative impact on the particle sizes obtained by the two-step emulsification method.

3.1.2. Effect of the Number of Homogenization Cycles and Pressure

High-pressure homogenization (HPH) is widely acknowledged to promote stable cross-linking of albumin through disulfide bonds in the binding of albumin NPs to paclitaxel (i.e., nab-Paclitaxel) [41]. In this study, HPH was utilized to enhance process emulsification in the second stage to facilitate smaller particle sizes and generate a more-homogeneous size distribution of NPs. With a fixed MPT0B291/HSA ratio following ultrasonication with the amplitude set to 30% for 5 min, the influence of homogenization pressures (15,000 and 20,000 psi) and various cycle numbers (10~40 cycles) were evaluated to study their impacts on the stability of NP formation and the size distribution at a fixed MPT0B291/HSA ratio. In Figure 3, the particle size increased with an increase in HPH cycles from 0 to 40 cycles when 15,000 psi was applied as the homogenization pressure. When utilizing 20,000 psi of homogenization pressure, the particle size increased between 10 and 30 cycles but then dramatically decreased to less than 100 nm. The smallest particle diameter (75.8 ± 0.86 nm) was obtained at a homogenization pressure of 20,000 psi with 40 cycles. Mohan and Narsimhan found that a higher turbulent intensity could lead to higher coalescence efficiencies and higher rates of collision between drops due to the larger turbulent forces, thus resulting in a higher coalescence rate [42]. In this case, a higher pressure of 20,000 psi seemed to affect the efficiency of the emulsifying properties leading to a higher coalescence rate after the homogenizing valve.

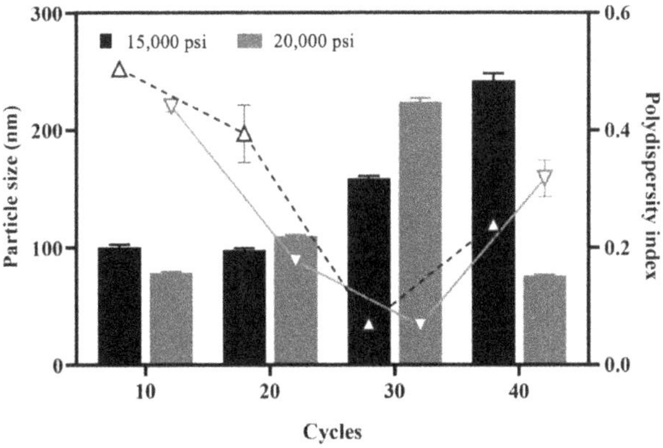

Figure 3. Effects of different pressures of high-pressure homogenization at different cycles on the particle size and size distribution. Column: particle size (nm); line: polydispersity index. Each point represents the mean ± SD. Error bars represent the standard deviation (n = 3).

The PDI decreased with an increase in homogenization cycles from 10 to 30 regardless of the homogenization pressure and reached the lowest point at 30 cycles with homogenization pressures of both 15,000 and 20,000 psi. However, when the number of cycles increased to 40, the PDI inversely increased for both homogenization pressures. The increased size observed with an increasing number of cycles may have been caused by the coalescence of very small droplets passing through the HPH valve at elevated pressures. Our results indicated that the homogenization pressure did not markedly influence the droplet size distribution, whereas the number of homogenization cycles was more influential on the particle size and size distribution in this study. Increasing the number of homogenization cycles can improve the homogeneity of the population by eliminating the few remaining large particles and reducing the PDI [43]. Although the pressure did not have a direct effect on the NP size when the NPs were prepared by HPH, increasing the number of homogenization cycles combined with the applied pressure led to a greater reduction in particle size, as shown in the case of 20,000 psi and 40 cycles. Several important factors influence the quality of NPs produced by homogenization. By increasing the applied homogenization pressure and the number of homogenization cycles, the HSA NPs were repeatedly subjected to high shear, which further reduced the size of the droplets to nano-sized droplets [44]. In summary, even when the mean diameter of the NPs reached an optimum, additional homogenization cycles could be used to reduce the PDI. Therefore, a further optimization of the HPH conditions is necessary during the development of HSA NP formulations. In this study, 20,000 psi was set to obtain smaller-sized NPs for further experiments.

3.1.3. Effect of the Ratio of Dispersed Phase (DP) to Continuous Phase (CP)

The ratio of the DP to the CP is one of the critical factors in preparing HSA NPs during the HPH processes. Thus, different DP/CP ratios of 0.1/30, 0.375/30, and 0.8/30 were evaluated to study their impacts on MPT0B291-HSA NP formulation with HPH processes. MPT0B291-HSA NPs were obtained from the ultrasonic oscillation with a fixed amplitude of 30%, followed by HPH utilizing 20 cycles of homogenization at 20,000 psi. As shown in Figure 4, with an increasing DP/CP ratio from 0.1/30 to 0.8/3, particles sizes of HSA NPs were reduced regardless of the number of cycles. A larger particle size and wider size distribution were found at the DP/CP ratio of 0.1/30 with either 10 or 20 of homogenization cycles. This might be due to the CP containing a large amount of water resulting in faster coalescence of droplets. In other words, an emulsified state might not properly form at lower fractions of the DP. Particle sizes at DP/CP ratios of 0.375/30 and 0.8/30 were both within our requirements (<200 nm), while the PDI was slightly higher for the 0.8/30 DP/CP ratio. Large aggregates were found in samples prepared using the 0.8/30 DP/CP ratio. This suggested that the DP could not be homogeneously dispersed into the CP when the DP fraction was too high. Therefore, a DP/CP ratio of 0.375/30 was selected as an optimal parameter for forming a relatively stable dispersion system.

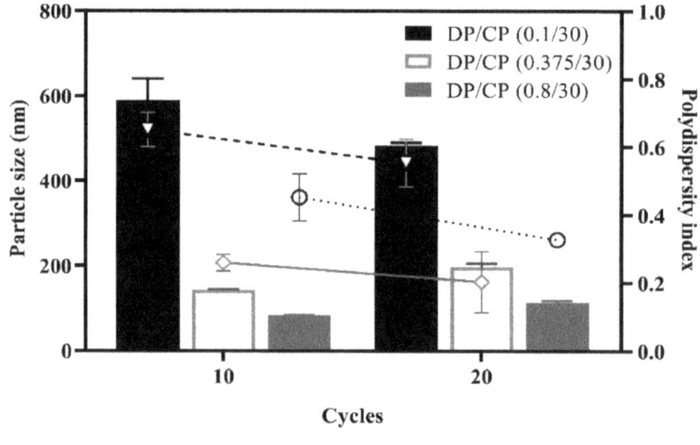

Figure 4. Effects of different ratios of the dispersed phase (DP) and continuous phase (CP) and different cycles of high-pressure homogenization on the particle size and size distribution. Column: particle size (nm); line: polydispersity index. Each point represents the mean ± SD. Error bars represent the standard deviation (n = 3).

3.2. Characterization of Albumin NPs and MPT0B291-HSA NPs

After determining optimal sonication and HPH conditions, the particle size and PDI of the optimized MPT0B291-HSA NPs were measured with a Zetasizer laser particle size analyzer. In addition, the morphology of the preparation was characterized by TEM using negative staining. Table 1 shows that the prepared MPT0B291-HSA NPs had an average hydrodynamic diameter of 136.3 ± 4.51 nm with a good PDI of 0.24, suggesting homogeneous distribution (monodisperse) of the NPs size within the acceptable range of protein-based nanomaterials [45–47]. Additionally, a value of less than 5% for the coefficient of variation for the particle size from multiple batches (3.3%) was noted, indicating a high reproducibility of the formulation. The particle size of MPT0B291-HSA NPs increased upon lecithin addition during MPT0B291-HSA NP formation. Incorporating lecithin was useful to maintain the final particle charge, as it is substantially correlated with the isoelectric point of soybean lecithin of 6.7 [45,46]. A similar approach was also used in other studies comprising egg yolk-lecithin and albumin to coat docetaxel in NP preparations [47,48]. The negative charge helps maintain the stability of the NPs in vivo. To further define the morphology of the formulated NPs, a TEM study was conducted. TEM images (Figure 5) showed that the morphology of the optimized MPT0B291-HSA NPs were spherical and evenly distributed with no obvious aggregations. These results agreed with the DLS data. The lyophilized powder of MPT0B291-HSA NPs also displayed good redispersibility when nanosuspensions were reconstituted with deionized water.

Table 1. Characterization of MPT0B291-loaded human serum albumin (HSA) nanoparticles (NPs). Each point represents the mean ± SD. Error bars represent the standard deviation (n = 3).

	Particle Size (nm)	PDI	Zeta Potential (mV)	EE (%)	DL (%)	Albumin Recovery (%)	Ratio of Albumin to Drug
MPT0B291-HSA NPs	136.3 ± 4.51	0.241 ± 0.077	−1.87 ± 0.133	92.0 ± 1.11	5.97 ± 0.07	95.0 ± 1.24	9.6

Abbreviations: PDI, polydispersity index; EE, encapsulation efficiency; DL, drug loading.

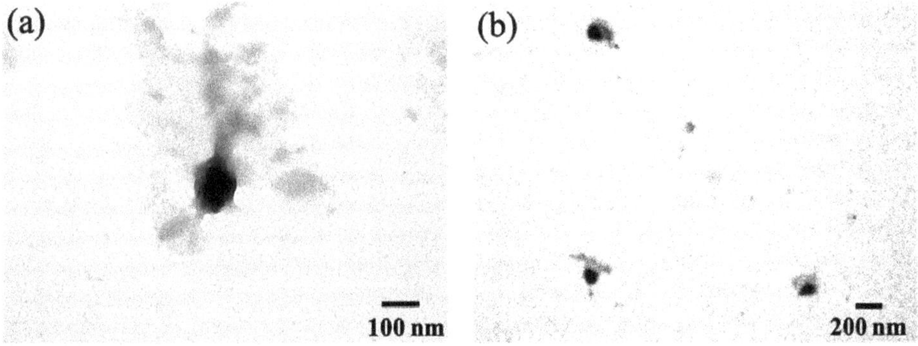

Figure 5. Transmission electron microscopic (TEM) images of MPT0B291-human serum albumin (HSA) nanoparticles (NPs). Scale bars represent 100 (**a**) and 200 nm (**b**).

The encapsulation efficiency (EE) and drug loading (DL) of MPT0B291-HSA NPs were 92.0 ± 1.11% and 5.97 ± 0.07%, respectively. Although there were no other NP products for comparison, these data suggest that MPT0B291 was effectively loaded into the HSA NPs. Their EE and DL values were almost equal to other anticancer drug-loaded NPs, which might fit future in vivo requirements.

Further, a Bradford assay was utilized to measure the protein recovery rate. As shown in Table 1, the recovery rate of albumin was 95.0 ± 1.24. The ratio of protein to drug recovered was 9.6 which is close to the original ratio of albumin to the drug (10:1). This result indicates no excessive loss of albumin during NP preparation.

3.3. Stability Studies of MPT0B291-HSA NPs

The stability of MPT0B291-HSA NPs stored at 4 °C was evaluated based on maintaining the particle size and drug content. Figure 6 shows that MPT0B291-HSA NPs remained almost intact during 4 weeks of storage (with a particle size of <200 nm). The PDI of the MPT0B291-HSA NP dispersion also remained <0.3 during the 4 weeks of storage. In terms of the drug content after reconstitution of MPT0B291-human serum albumin (HSA) nanoparticles (NPs), 3.70 ± 1.98% of the drug loss was found after 1 week of storage at 4 °C. These results emphasized that the self-assembly of albumin could emerge as an ideal template for drug payloads without an additional chemical crosslinker. This suggests that MPT0B291-HSA NPs can be expected to be stable in vitro as no apparent aggregation or drug loss was observed during the experimental period. In addition, the powder and colloidal dispersion forms of MPT0B291-HSA NPs were almost the same as those before lyophilization (data not shown), indicating that our MPT0B291-HSA NPs will be robust when applied to a pharmaceutical process.

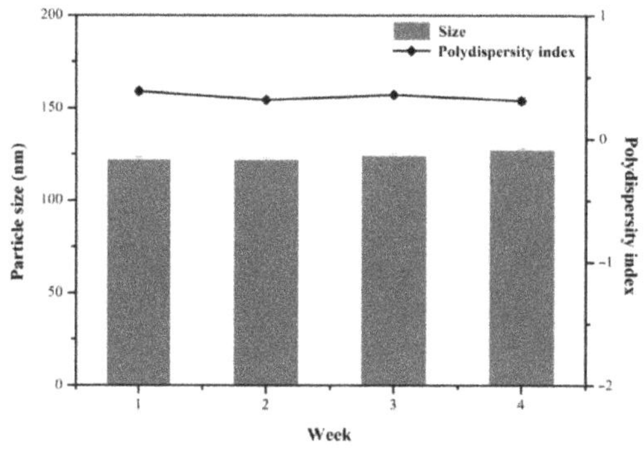

Figure 6. Particle size and size distribution of MPT0B291-human serum albumin (HSA) nanoparticles (NPs) stored at 4 °C for 4 weeks after reconstitution. Each point represents the mean ± SD. Error bars represent the standard deviation (n = 3).

3.4. In Vitro Drug Release

Drug-release profiles of 0.25 mg/mL MPT0B291 from HSA NPs and solution (propylene glycol) at 37 °C were studied in triplicate. The amount of MPT0B291 released from the NP solution at fixed intervals over a period of 48 h was determined and compared to the free MPT0B291 dissolved in propylene glycol, as shown in Figure 7. Approximately 60% of the drug was released within 48 h from MPT0B291-HSA NPs, showing that a significantly sustained release profile was found from MPT0B291-HSA NPs. Meanwhile, free MPT0B291 was rapidly released (60% within 1 h) and the complete release (nearly 100%) of the drug occurred within 8 h. The sustained-release property of MPT0B291-HSA NPs in vitro arises from the high affinity between MPT0B291 and albumin, in which the albumin further acts as a protective layer for the drug from immediate diffusion into the system, enabling the MPT0B291 to be released more stably and continuously, which might allow for the continuous targeting of cancer cells in vivo. In consequence, this would provide an effective method, devoid of side effects, which was precisely the advantage of the NP delivery system.

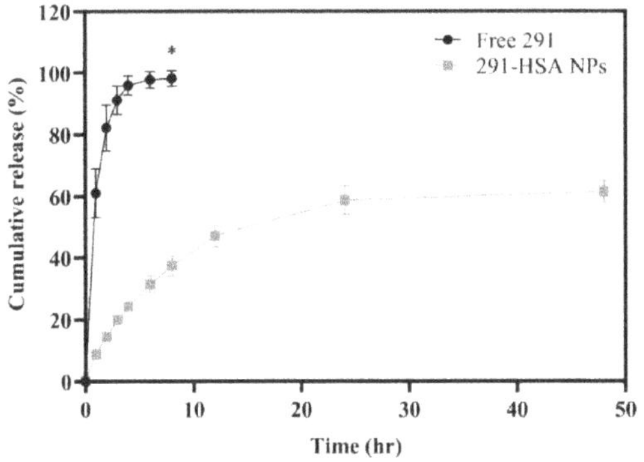

Figure 7. In vitro drug-release profiles of free MPT0B291 and MPT0B291-human serum albumin (HSA) nanoparticles (NPs) in pH 7.4 phosphate buffer containing 1% Tween 80 at 37 °C. Data shown are the mean ± SD (n = 3). * $p < 0.0001$ when free MPT0B291 was compared to MPT0B291-HSA NPs at 8 h.

3.5. In Vitro Cytotoxicity Test

The cytotoxicity of free MPT0B291 and MPT0B291-HSA NPs was investigated by MTT assays with Mia Paca-2 cells. As shown in Figure 8a, drug-free HSA NPs exhibited only a negligible cytotoxic effect, suggesting their potential suitability as drug carriers [49]. In Figure 8b and Supplementary Table S1, survival rates of Mia Paca-2 cells in different concentrations of free MPT0B291 were similar to those in MPT0B291-HSA NPs. Further, the values of the 50% inhibitory concentration (IC_{50}) of free MPT0B291 and MPT0B291-HSA NPs after 24 h of exposure were determined as 4.71 and 4.28 μM, respectively (Supplementary Table S1). These results indicated that MPT0B291-HSA NPs indeed had antiproliferative activity against Mia Paca-2 cells. The nearly identical cytotoxic activities exhibited by MPT0B291-HSA NPs and MPT0B291 at equal concentrations indicated that the use of HSA-NPs as a drug vehicle did not affect the anticancer effect of MPT0B291, while maintaining similar anticancer activities in vitro but with lower cytotoxicity.

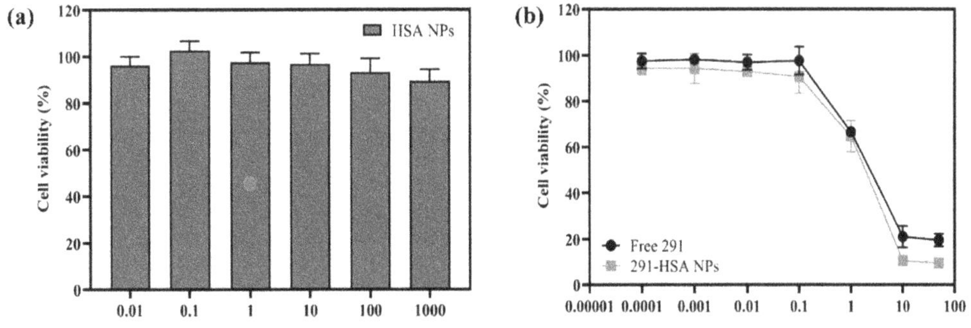

Figure 8. Cell viability of blank human serum albumin (HSA) nanoparticles (NPs) in Mia Paca-2 cells (**a**) and comparison of the cell viability of free MPT0B291 and MPT0B291-HSA NPs in Mia Paca-2 cells (**b**). Each point represents the mean ± SD. Error bars represent the standard deviation (n = 3).

3.6. Maximum Tolerated Dose (MTD)

Mice were treated with MPT0B291-HSA NPs and free MPT0B291 to establish the MTD. According to the results (Figure 9), none of the mice that received injections experienced significant weight loss. Studies showed that after a single i.v. dose of 150 mg/kg BW of the MPT0B291 solution, one mouse was found dead after 24 h and another one also died on the following day. Therefore, the MTD of MPT0B291 solution administered was approximately 75 mg/kg BW by the i.v. route. On the other hand, we did not establish the MTD of MPT0B291-HSA NP formulations administered in a single dose due to the limitation to volume via i.v. administration in mice. The mice showed no painful reactions, and no mice died even after the administration of 200 mg/kg of MPT0B291-HSA NPs during 16 days of observation. Therefore, the MTD of MPT0B291-HSA NP formulations was >200 mg/kg BW (single dose). This demonstrated that mice could tolerate a higher concentration of encapsulated MPT0B291 than of free MPT0B291.

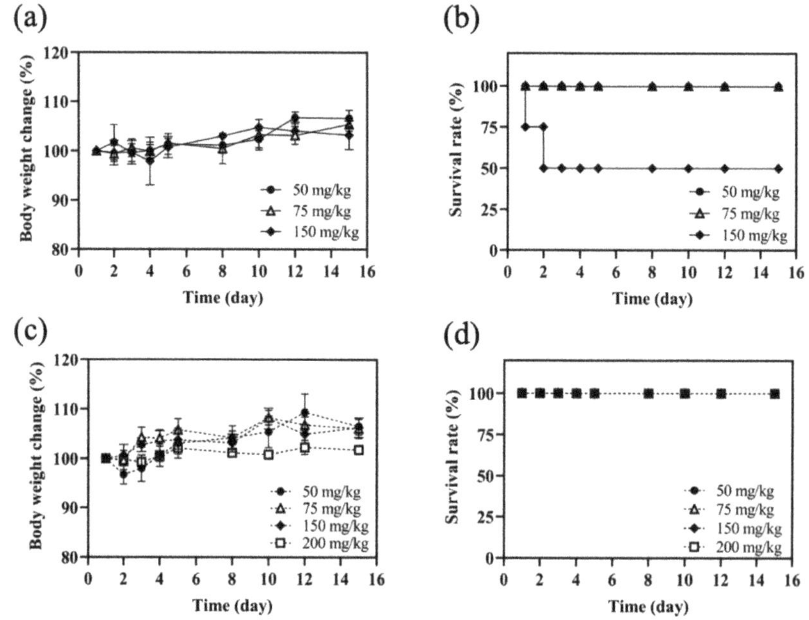

Figure 9. Determination of the maximum tolerated dose (MTD) of MPT0B291 and MPT0B291-human serum albumin (HSA) nanoparticles (NPs) in mice. Body weight changes and survival rates of female BALB/c mice after single-dose intravenous administration with 50, 75 and 150 mg/kg of MPT0B291 solution (**a**,**b**) and with 50, 75, 150 and 200 mg/kg of MPT0B291-HSA NPs (**c**,**d**), respectively. Each point represents the mean ± SD. Error bars represent the standard deviation (n = 4).

3.7. In Vivo PK Study

MPT0B291 concentration-time curves after intravenous administration of different formulations in rats are shown in Figure 10. The PK parameters were calculated and are shown in Table 2. Concentration-time curves of MPT0B291-HSA NPs differed significantly from those of the MPT0B291 solution. The MPT0B291-HSA NPs exhibited much higher AUC0~24h ($p < 0.01$) (2225.09 ± 767.70 vs. 290.98 ± 39.73 h·ng/mL) and slower clearance ($p < 0.0001$) (38.24 ± 10.53 vs. 288.47 ± 36.66 mL/min/kg) as compared to the free MPT0B291 (Table 2). This demonstrates an increased systemic circulation time and enhanced MPT0B291 bioavailability in encapsulated form. A much longer MRT (4.95 ± 1.03 h) was also found after i.v. administration of MPT0B291-HSA NPs, which indicates a prolonged drug duration.

The above results were in agreement with those previously obtained for in vitro drug–release curves, that coating the MPT0B291 with albumin NPs protected the drug from quick diffusion to the system in vivo, yet exhibited sustained release of MPT0B291 (Figure 7). In contrast, the free MPT0B921 induced burst release once injected into the blood which eventually initiated opsonization by the mononuclear phagocyte system (MPS), thus lowering its plasma concentration progressively during the time course (Figure 10). The use of the albumin NPs incorporated in this study seemed to successfully cloak the MPT0B291 from unselective uptake by the MPS, enabling a prolonged circulation time effective drug distribution in the blood and slower elimination [26,50,51]. Furthermore, it was evident that the blood circulation half-life ($t_{1/2}$) of the encapsulated drug was 2.5 times higher than that of the free drug (Table 2), corresponding to the sustained release profile of the MPT0B291 HSA NPs including the influence of absorption and distribution.

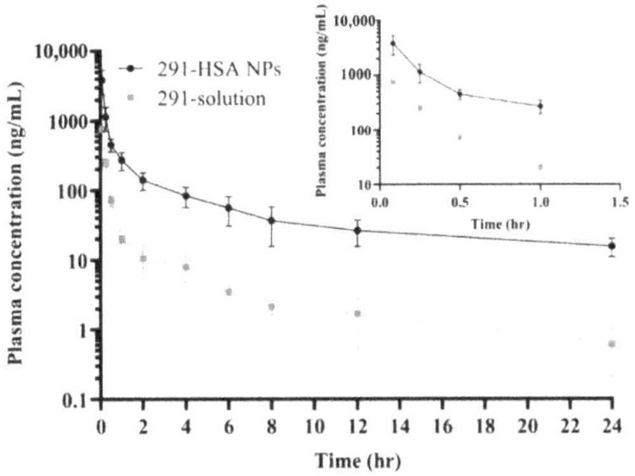

Figure 10. Plasma concentration-time curves of MPT0B291 after intravenous administration with MPT0B291-human serum albumin (HSA) nanoparticles (NPs) and an MPT0B291 solution (at a single dose of 5 mg/kg body weight) to rats. Each point represents the mean ± SD of three determinations (n = 4).

Table 2. Primary pharmacokinetic parameters of MPT0B291 after intravenous administration with MPT0B291-human serum albumin (HSA) nanoparticles (NPs) (at 5 mg/kg body weight) and an MPT0B291 solution (5 mg/kg body weight) to Sprague-Dawley rats. Data shown are the mean ± SD (n = 4).

Parameter	MPT0B291-HSA NPs	MPT0B291 Solution
$AUC_{0\text{–}24h}$ (h·ng/mL)	2225.09 ± 767.70 **	290.98 ± 39.73
$AUC_{0\text{–}\infty}$ (h·ng/mL)	2333.73 ± 764.32 **	292.60 ± 39.17
$t_{1/2}$ (h)	4.71 ± 0.65 **	2.07 ± 0.64
CL (mL/min/kg)	38.24 ± 10.53 ***	288.47 ± 36.66
MRT (h)	4.95 ± 1.03 **	1.86 ± 0.66
V_{ss} (L/kg)	11.49 ± 3.92	32.58 ± 12.26 *

Abbreviations: $AUC_{0\text{–}24h}$, area under the plasma concentration-time curve (AUC) from time 0 to 24 h; $AUC_{0\text{–}\infty}$, AUC extrapolated to infinity; CL, clearance; $t_{1/2}$, elimination half-life; V_{ss}, volume of distribution at steady state; MRT, mean residence time. ** $p < 0.01$, ** $p < 0.001$, *** $p < 0.0001$.

PK parameters showed that MPT0B291-HSA NPs had the advantages of maintaining higher and steadier plasma concentrations than free MPT0B291, which indicated that MPT0B291-HSA NPs could more stably and continuously release MPT0B291. MPT0B291-HSA NPs are likely to have significant potential for in vivo antitumor efficacy in the future.

4. Conclusions

NPs based on albumin have received considerable interest due to their high binding capacity to hydrophobic drugs and biocompatibility with no serious side effects. In this study, HSA was selected as an ideal candidate for drug delivery due to its ready availability, biodegradability, and priority uptake [27,52]. We demonstrated that MPT0B291, a water-insoluble anticancer drug, could be successfully loaded into albumin NPs via a two-stage emulsification method under optimized conditions. These MPT0B291-HSA NPs had a favorable particle size of <200 nm with a high encapsulation efficiency and drug loading, which are desirable for intravenous injections. In vitro studies revealed that the MPT0B291-HSA NPs exhibited sustained release of MPT0B291, which suggested that MPT0B291-HSA NPs are likely to prolong MPT0B291 in the circulation in vivo. Furthermore, in the in vivo experiments, we showed that incorporating MPT0B291 in albumin NPs allowed us to prepare single-dose administration with a higher tolerated dose, resulting in increased biological safety and reduced adverse effects. The PK study also clearly demonstrated that the optimized HSA NPs significantly enhanced the drug bioavailability of MPT0B291. This suggests that MPT0B291-HSA NPs offer promising antitumor activity with low systemic toxicity. In summary, we successfully prepared an injectable, biocompatible, biodegradable, targeted, safe, effective, and controlled-release nanoscale preparation, which may be significant in promoting more nanoscale preparations for hydrophobic drugs to be applied in clinical practice.

Supplementary Materials: The following are available online at https://www.mdpi.com/article/10.3390/pharmaceutics13101728/s1, Table S1: The 50% inhibitory concentration (IC50) of free MPT0B291 and MPT0B291-human serum albumin (HSA) nanoparticles (NPs).

Author Contributions: Experimental investigation and analysis, Y.-L.S. and J.-P.L. (Jia-Pei Lin); supervision and writing—original draft preparation, A.D.P. and P.-S.C.; chemical synthesis and funding acquisition, J.-P.L. (Jing-Ping Liou); writing—review and editing, C.-M.H. All authors have read and agreed to the published version of the manuscript.

Funding: This research was funded by the Ministry of Science and Technology (grant No. MOST 109-2221-E-038-001-MY3).

Institutional Review Board Statement: All animal experiments were carried out in accordance with a protocol approved by the Laboratory Animal Center of Taipei Medical University (approval no: LAC-2016-0287; Approval Date: 26 December 2016) and conducted in compliance with the Taiwanese Animal Welfare Act.

Informed Consent Statement: Not applicable.

Conflicts of Interest: The authors declare no conflict of interest. The funder had no role in the design of the study, in the collection, analyses or interpretation of data, in the writing of the manuscript, or in the decision to publish the results.

References

1. Peserico, A.; Simone, C. Physical and functional hat/hdac interplay regulates protein acetylation balance. *J. Biomed. Biotechnol.* **2011**, *2011*, 371832. [CrossRef] [PubMed]
2. Li, T.; Zhang, C.; Hassan, S.; Liu, X.; Song, F.; Chen, K.; Zhang, W.; Yang, J. Histone deacetylase 6 in cancer. *J. Hematol. Oncol.* **2018**, *11*, 111. [CrossRef]
3. Fraga, M.F.; Ballestar, E.; Villar-Garea, A.; Boix-Chornet, M.; Espada, J.; Schotta, G.; Bonaldi, T.; Haydon, C.; Ropero, S.; Petrie, K. Loss of acetylation at lys16 and trimethylation at lys20 of histone h4 is a common hallmark of human cancer. *Nat. Genet.* **2005**, *37*, 391–400. [CrossRef] [PubMed]
4. Yasui, W.; Oue, N.; Ono, S.; Mitani, Y.; Ito, R.; Nakayama, H. Histone acetylation and gastrointestinal carcinogenesis. *Ann. N. Y. Acad. Sci.* **2003**, *983*, 220–231. [CrossRef] [PubMed]
5. Ropero, S.; Esteller, M. The role of histone deacetylases (hdacs) in human cancer. *Mol. Oncol.* **2007**, *1*, 19–25. [CrossRef]
6. Choudhary, C.; Kumar, C.; Gnad, F.; Nielsen, M.L.; Rehman, M.; Walther, T.C.; Olsen, J.V.; Mann, M. Lysine acetylation targets protein complexes and co-regulates major cellular functions. *Science* **2009**, *325*, 834–840. [CrossRef]
7. Minucci, S.; Pelicci, P.G. Histone deacetylase inhibitors and the promise of epigenetic (and more) treatments for cancer. *Nat. Rev. Cancer* **2006**, *6*, 38–51. [CrossRef]
8. Aldana-Masangkay, G.I.; Sakamoto, K.M. The role of hdac6 in cancer. *J. Biomed. Biotechnol.* **2011**, *2011*, 875824. [CrossRef]
9. Marks, P.A. Discovery and development of saha as an anticancer agent. *Oncogene* **2007**, *26*, 1351–1356. [CrossRef]
10. Grabarska, A.; Łuszczki, J.J.; Nowosadzka, E.; Gumbarewicz, E.; Jeleniewicz, W.; Dmoszyńska-Graniczka, M.; Kowalczuk, K.; Kupisz, K.; Polberg, K.; Stepulak, A. Histone deacetylase inhibitor saha as potential targeted therapy agent for larynx cancer cells. *J. Cancer* **2017**, *8*, 19–28. [CrossRef]
11. Porter, N.J.; Mahendran, A.; Breslow, R.; Christianson, D.W. Unusual zinc-binding mode of hdac6-selective hydroxamate inhibitors. *Proc. Natl. Acad. Sci. USA* **2017**, *114*, 13459–13464. [CrossRef] [PubMed]
12. Ma, Y.; Yue, Y.; Pan, M.; Sun, J.; Chu, J.; Lin, X.; Xu, W.; Feng, L.; Chen, Y.; Chen, D. Histone deacetylase 3 inhibits new tumor suppressor gene dtwd1 in gastric cancer. *Am. J. Cancer Res.* **2015**, *5*, 663.

13. Deng, B.; Luo, Q.; Halim, A.; Liu, Q.; Zhang, B.; Song, G. The Antiangiogenesis Role of Histone Deacetylase Inhibitors: Their Potential Application to Tumor Therapy and Tissue Repair. *DNA Cell Biol.* **2020**, *39*, 167–176. [CrossRef] [PubMed]
14. Buyandelger, B.; Bar, E.E.; Hung, K.S.; Chen, R.M.; Chiang, Y.H.; Liou, J.P.; Huang, H.M.; Wang, J.Y. Histone deacetylase inhibitor mpt0b291 suppresses glioma growth in vitro and in vivo partially through acetylation of p53. *Int. J. Biol. Sci.* **2020**, *16*, 3184–3199. [CrossRef] [PubMed]
15. Lee, H.Y.; Tsai, A.C.; Chen, M.C.; Shen, P.J.; Cheng, Y.C.; Kuo, C.C.; Pan, S.L.; Liu, Y.M.; Liu, J.F.; Yeh, T.K.; et al. Azaindolylsulfonamides, with a more selective inhibitory effect on histone deacetylase 6 activity, exhibit antitumor activity in colorectal cancer hct116 cells. *J. Med. Chem.* **2014**, *57*, 4009–4022. [CrossRef] [PubMed]
16. Din, F.U.; Aman, W.; Ullah, I.; Qureshi, O.S.; Mustapha, O.; Shafique, S.; Zeb, A. Effective use of nanocarriers as drug delivery systems for the treatment of selected tumors. *Int. J. Nanomed.* **2017**, *12*, 7291–7309. [CrossRef] [PubMed]
17. Lahann, J. Protein nanoparticles as multifunctional drug delivery carriers. In *Abstracts of Papers of the American Chemical Society*; American Chemical Society: Washington, DC, USA, 2019; Volume 257.
18. Lohcharoenkal, W.; Wang, L.Y.; Chen, Y.C.; Rojanasakul, Y. Protein nanoparticles as drug delivery carriers for cancer therapy. *Biomed. Res. Int.* **2014**, *2014*, 180549. [CrossRef]
19. Desai, N. Nanoparticle albumin-bound paclitaxel (abraxane®). In *Albumin in Medicine*; Springer: Singapore, 2016; pp. 101–119.
20. Yin, T.J.; Dong, L.H.; Cui, B.; Wang, L.; Yin, L.F.; Zhou, J.P.; Huo, M.R. A toxic organic solvent-free technology for the preparation of pegylated paclitaxel nanosuspension based on human serum albumin for effective cancer therapy. *Int. J. Nanomed.* **2015**, *10*, 7397–7412.
21. Tai, C.J.; Wang, H.; Wang, C.K.; Tai, C.J.; Huang, M.T.; Wu, C.H.; Chen, R.J.; Kuo, L.J.; Wei, P.L.; Chang, Y.J.; et al. Bevacizumab and cetuximab with conventional chemotherapy reduced pancreatic tumor weight in mouse pancreatic cancer xenografts. *Clin. Exp. Med.* **2017**, *17*, 141–150. [CrossRef] [PubMed]
22. Thadakapally, R.; Aafreen, A.; Aukunuru, J.; Habibuddin, M.; Jogala, S. Preparation and characterization of peg-albumin-curcumin nanoparticles intended to treat breast cancer. *Indian J. Pharm. Sci.* **2016**, *78*, 65–72.
23. Shao, H.; Tang, H.; Salavaggione, O.E.; Yu, C.; Hylander, B.; Tan, W.; Repasky, E.; Adjei, A.A.; Dy, G.K. Improved response to nab-paclitaxel compared with cremophor-solubilized paclitaxel is independent of secreted protein acidic and rich in cysteine expression in non-small cell lung cancer. *J. Thorac Oncol.* **2011**, *6*, 998–1005. [CrossRef]
24. Rajeshkumar, N.V.; Yabuuchi, S.; Pai, S.G.; Tong, Z.; Hou, S.; Bateman, S.; Pierce, D.W.; Heise, C.; Von Hoff, D.D.; Maitra, A.; et al. Superior therapeutic efficacy of nab-paclitaxel over cremophor-based paclitaxel in locally advanced and metastatic models of human pancreatic cancer. *Br. J. Cancer* **2016**, *115*, 442–453. [CrossRef]
25. Hoogenboezem, E.N.; Duvall, C.L. Harnessing albumin as a carrier for cancer therapies. *Adv. Drug Deliv. Rev.* **2018**, *130*, 73–89. [CrossRef]
26. Peng, Q.; Mu, H. The potential of protein-nanomaterial interaction for advanced drug delivery. *J. Control. Release* **2016**, *225*, 121–132. [CrossRef]
27. Karimi, M.; Bahrami, S.; Ravari, S.B.; Zangabad, P.S.; Mirshekari, H.; Bozorgomid, M.; Shahreza, S.; Sori, M.; Hamblin, M.R. Albumin nanostructures as advanced drug delivery systems. *Expert Opin. Drug Deliv.* **2016**, *13*, 1609–1623. [CrossRef]
28. Food Drug Administration, U.S. *Bioanalytical Method Validation Guidance for Industry*; US Department of Health Human Services: Washington, DC, USA, 2018; pp. 1–41.
29. Tang, B.; Fang, G.; Gao, Y.; Liu, Y.; Liu, J.; Zou, M.; Cheng, G. Liprosomes loading paclitaxel for brain-targeting delivery by intravenous administration: In vitro characterization and in vivo evaluation. *Int. J. Pharm.* **2014**, *475*, 416–427. [CrossRef] [PubMed]
30. Discher, D.E.; Eisenberg, A. Polymer vesicles. *Science* **2002**, *297*, 967–973. [CrossRef] [PubMed]
31. Lamichhane, S.; Lee, S. Albumin nanoscience: Homing nanotechnology enabling targeted drug delivery and therapy. *Arch. Pharm. Res.* **2020**, *43*, 118–133. [CrossRef]
32. Jun, J.Y.; Nguyen, H.H.; Paik, S.-Y.-R.; Chun, H.S.; Kang, B.-C.; Ko, S. Preparation of size-controlled bovine serum albumin (bsa) nanoparticles by a modified desolvation method. *Food Chem.* **2011**, *127*, 1892–1898. [CrossRef]
33. Lomis, N.; Westfall, S.; Farahdel, L.; Malhotra, M.; Shum-Tim, D.; Prakash, S. Human serum albumin nanoparticles for use in cancer drug delivery: Process optimization and in vitro characterization. *Nanomaterials* **2016**, *6*, 116. [CrossRef] [PubMed]
34. Tazhbayev, Y.; Mukashev, O.; Burkeev, M.; Kreuter, J. Hydroxyurea-loaded albumin nanoparticles: Preparation, characterization, and in vitro studies. *Pharmaceutics* **2019**, *11*, 410. [CrossRef] [PubMed]
35. He, C.; Hu, Y.; Yin, L.; Tang, C.; Yin, C. Effects of particle size and surface charge on cellular uptake and biodistribution of polymeric nanoparticles. *Biomaterials* **2010**, *31*, 3657–3666. [CrossRef] [PubMed]
36. Shen, S.; Wu, Y.; Liu, Y.; Wu, D. High drug-loading nanomedicines: Progress, current status, and prospects. *Int. J. Nanomed.* **2017**, *12*, 4085–4109. [CrossRef] [PubMed]
37. Jain, A.K.; Thareja, S. In vitro and in vivo characterization of pharmaceutical nanocarriers used for drug delivery. *Artif. Cells Nanomed. Biotechnol.* **2019**, *47*, 524–539. [CrossRef] [PubMed]
38. Liu, Y.; Yang, G.; Jin, S.; Xu, L.; Zhao, C.-X. Development of high-drug-loading nanoparticles. *ChemPlusChem* **2020**, *85*, 2143–2157. [CrossRef] [PubMed]
39. Gronroos, A.; Pirkonen, P.; Heikkinen, J.; Ihalainen, J.; Mursunen, H.; Sekki, H. Ultrasonic depolymerization of aqueous polyvinyl alcohol. *Ultrason. Sonochem.* **2001**, *8*, 259–264. [CrossRef]

40. Amini, M.A.; Faramarzi, M.A.; Mohammadyani, D.; Esmaeilzadeh-Gharehdaghi, E.; Amani, A. Modeling the parameters involved in preparation of pla nanoparticles carrying hydrophobic drug molecules using artificial neural networks. *J. Pharm. Innov.* **2013**, *8*, 111–120. [CrossRef]
41. Stinchcombe, T.E. Nanoparticle albumin-bound paclitaxel: A novel cremphor-el-free formulation of paclitaxel. *Nanomedicine* **2007**, *2*, 415–423. [CrossRef]
42. Mohan, S.; Narsimhan, G. Coalescence of protein-stabilized emulsions in a high-pressure homogenizer. *J. Colloid Interface Sci.* **1997**, *192*, 1–15. [CrossRef]
43. Li, Y.; Zhao, X.; Zu, Y.; Zhang, Y. Preparation and characterization of paclitaxel nanosuspension using novel emulsification method by combining high speed homogenizer and high pressure homogenization. *Int. J. Pharm.* **2015**, *490*, 324–333. [CrossRef]
44. Mu, L.; Feng, S.S. A novel controlled release formulation for the anticancer drug paclitaxel (taxol): Plga nanoparticles containing vitamin E TPGS. *J. Control. Release* **2003**, *86*, 33–48. [CrossRef]
45. Jaramillo, D.P.; Roberts, R.F.; Coupland, J.N. Effect of ph on the properties of soy protein–pectin complexes. *Food Res. Int.* **2011**, *44*, 911–916. [CrossRef]
46. De Oliveira, J.K.; Ronik, D.F.; Ascari, J.; Mainardes, R.M.; Khalil, N.M. Nanoencapsulation of apocynin in bovine serum albumin nanoparticles: Physicochemical characterization. *Nanosci. Nanotechnol. Asia* **2018**, *8*, 90–99. [CrossRef]
47. He, X.; Xiang, N.; Zhang, J.; Zhou, J.; Fu, Y.; Gong, T.; Zhang, Z. Encapsulation of teniposide into albumin nanoparticles with greatly lowered toxicity and enhanced antitumor activity. *Int. J. Pharm.* **2015**, *487*, 250–259. [CrossRef] [PubMed]
48. Qu, N.; Sun, Y.; Li, Y.; Hao, F.; Qiu, P.; Teng, L.; Xie, J.; Gao, Y. Docetaxel-loaded human serum albumin (HSA) nanoparticles: Synthesis, characterization, and evaluation. *Biomed. Eng. Online* **2019**, *18*, 11. [CrossRef] [PubMed]
49. Bae, S.; Ma, K.; Kim, T.H.; Lee, E.S.; Oh, K.T.; Park, E.S.; Lee, K.C.; Youn, Y.S. Doxorubicin-loaded human serum albumin nanoparticles surface-modified with tnf-related apoptosis-inducing ligand and transferrin for targeting multiple tumor types. *Biomaterials* **2012**, *33*, 1536–1546. [CrossRef]
50. Ogawara, K.-I.; Furumoto, K.; Nagayama, S.; Minato, K.; Higaki, K.; Kai, T.; Kimura, T. Pre-coating with serum albumin reduces receptor-mediated hepatic disposition of polystyrene nanosphere: Implications for rational design of nanoparticles. *J. Control. Release* **2004**, *100*, 451–455. [CrossRef]
51. Davis, M.E.; Chen, Z.; Shin, D.M. Nanoparticle therapeutics: An emerging treatment modality for cancer. *Nat. Rev. Drug Discov.* **2008**, *7*, 771–782. [CrossRef] [PubMed]
52. Kratz, F. Albumin as a drug carrier: Design of prodrugs, drug conjugates and nanoparticles. *J. Control. Release* **2008**, *132*, 171–183. [CrossRef] [PubMed]

pharmaceutics

MDPI

Article

Leveraging Affinity Interactions to Prolong Drug Delivery of Protein Therapeutics

Alan B. Dogan, **Katherine E. Dabkowski** and **Horst A. von Recum** *

Department of Biomedical Engineering, Case Western Reserve University, Cleveland, OH 44106, USA; abd51@case.edu (A.B.D.); ked87@case.edu (K.E.D.)
* Correspondence: horst.vonrecum@case.edu; Tel.: +1-216-368-5513

Abstract: While peptide and protein therapeutics have made tremendous advances in clinical treatments over the past few decades, they have been largely hindered by their ability to be effectively delivered to patients. While bolus parenteral injections have become standard clinical practice, they are insufficient to treat diseases that require sustained, local release of therapeutics. Cyclodextrin-based polymers (pCD) have been utilized as a platform to extend the local delivery of small-molecule hydrophobic drugs by leveraging hydrophobic-driven thermodynamic interactions between pCD and payload to extend its release, which has seen success both in vitro and in vivo. Herein, we proposed the novel synthesis of protein–polymer conjugates that are capped with a "high affinity" adamantane. Using bovine serum albumin as a model protein, and anti-interleukin 10 monoclonal antibodies as a functional example, we outline the synthesis of novel protein–polymer conjugates that, when coupled with cyclodextrin delivery platforms, can maintain a sustained release of up to 65 days without largely sacrificing protein structure/function which has significant clinical applications in local antibody-based treatments for immune diseases, cancers, and diabetes.

Keywords: antibody; affinity; cyclodextrin; protein therapeutics; sustained drug delivery

Citation: Dogan, A.B.; Dabkowski, K.E.; von Recum, H.A. Leveraging Affinity Interactions to Prolong Drug Delivery of Protein Therapeutics. *Pharmaceutics* **2022**, *14*, 1088. https://doi.org/10.3390/pharmaceutics14051088

Academic Editors: Ana Isabel Fernandes and Angela Faustino Jozala

Received: 22 April 2022
Accepted: 17 May 2022
Published: 19 May 2022

Publisher's Note: MDPI stays neutral with regard to jurisdictional claims in published maps and institutional affiliations.

1. Introduction

Protein and peptide therapeutics have emerged in the past few decades as a major branch of modern pharmacology. Due to their modularity, high specificity, and low off-target activity, protein therapeutics have been utilized to treat diseases including cancers, genetic disorders, autoimmune diseases, and inflammatory diseases by replacing, augmenting, or interfering with cellular pathways or by delivering payloads to achieve a desired outcome. In 2019, protein-based therapeutics contributed to eight out of the top ten drugs by sales globally and encompasses an annual market of around 69.4 billion dollars [1]. A majority of these novel therapeutics, consisting of around 100 FDA-approved therapeutics since their introduction in the 1980s, leverages the high target specificity of monoclonal antibodies (mAbs) and antibody fragments (FABs) [2]. Monoclonal antibody therapeutics have been shown to efficaciously treat autoimmune diseases, cancers, asthma, and have even shown significant potential for treating COVID-19 [3–5].

Despite these advantages, many protein therapeutics suffer from relatively short in vivo half-lives compared with disease prognosis and high accumulation in the liver and spleen [6,7]. This translates to clinical protocols that typically involve parenteral drug administration; however, frequent injections decrease patient compliance, increase risk of infection, and promote nonspecific drug targeting—all of which greatly decrease therapeutic efficacy. Therapeutic efficacy of protein-based drugs with bolus administration is also highly dose dependent, which can also decrease positive patient outcomes. Therefore, there is a need for extending and controlling the delivery of protein and peptide therapeutics.

Polymeric drug delivery systems present a possible solution to extending the delivery of protein and peptide therapeutics. Hydrogels and in situ forming implants, which are composed of polymer matrices such as poly(lactic-co-glycolic acid) (PLGA), have been used to locally deliver small-molecule and protein payloads via diffusion-based mechanisms [8,9]. Nanoparticles and liposomes have also been used to deliver proteins by taking advantage of the enhanced permeation and retention effect and can greatly increase in vivo circulation time [10,11]. However, the mechanism of delivery for a majority of these solutions involves diffusion, degradation, and/or encapsulation, which makes existing protein delivery systems effective for bolus-injection therapeutics but unattractive for sustained, controlled, local delivery.

Affinity-based drug delivery systems have emerged as a popular way to help control and prolong the release of protein therapeutics [12]. Broadly, "affinity-based" delivery encompasses any matrix/guest system that leverages receptor/ligand, electrostatic/ionic, hydrogen bonding, hydrophobic, or van der Waal interactions to increase the thermodynamic interactions between the matrix host and the guest payload [13–15]. A well-established example of this is synthesizing a polymer matrix with exposed streptavidin sites designed to bind with biotinylated protein payloads [16,17]. However, due to the strong interactions between biotin and streptavidin (dissociation constant [K_D] ~ 10^{-15} M), much of the protein payload remains associated with the streptavidin matrix and is never released where it can interact with cells and tissue [17,18].

Polymerized cyclodextrin (pCD) is an alternative affinity-based drug delivery system that utilizes hydrophobic interactions between cyclodextrin's hydrophobic "interior" pocket and hydrophobic payloads [19–21]. Typically, this interaction has been used to enhance loading and extend the release of small-molecule, hydrophobic drugs, as the inclusion pocket of cyclodextrin only ranges from 0.5–0.8 nm in diameter [22]. pCD has been shown to have drug loading and drug release kinetics directly associated with the K_D of its included payload and has the ability to refill in vivo, making it especially useful for long-term therapeutic timelines [23–29]. While many groups have investigated pCD to deliver small molecules such as rifampicin and other smaller therapeutics such as RNA, the delivery of proteins by pCD, to the best of our knowledge, has never been achieved due to their large molecular weights and hydrophilic nature of the therapeutics [30,31].

Recently, our group has shown that conjugating polymer chains capped with "high affinity" groups can increase the overall conjugate's affinity towards pCD polymers [32,33]. Briefly, by taking advantage of the strong interactions between adamantane (Ad) hydrocarbons and beta-cyclodextrin (K_D ~ 5×10^{-4} M), we have shown that the affinity between pCD and the drugs rifampicin and rapamycin can be increased by conjugating polymer tethers end-capped with adamantane groups (referred to as polymer-Ad). The drug–Ad conjugates exhibited a higher loading capacity and an extended window of release in pCD hydrogels [32,33], thereby suggesting that by manipulating the K_D between the payload and pCD matrix, we are able to modulate delivery and loading.

As protein and peptide therapeutics now constitute the current, and possibly future, direction of pharmaceuticals, we proposed to apply the idea of modulating affinity to hydrophilic payloads, such as proteins, so that they can take advantage of the "affinity-driven" loading and release kinetics common to pCD hydrogels. Many current protein delivery systems, such as PLGA hydrogels, are single use and may degrade into unwanted byproducts, many of which can negatively impact the overall therapeutic efficiency of the payload [34]. pCD hydrogels, when prepared with a non-cleavable crosslinker, do not degrade and can be reused and refilled with drugs after initial administration by nearby bolus injection, making it ideal for long-term therapeutic treatments [35,36].

Herein, we use bovine serum albumin (BSA) as a model protein, and monoclonal antibodies (mAb) as a functional example to show that proteins can be delivered from pCD hydrogels by increasing the protein's affinity for the system through the conjugation of polymer–Ad groups (Figure 1). Additionally, we explore the impact that conjugating polymer–Ad groups have on the functionality of mAbs to help assess if pCD can be a viable platform for the clinical delivery of therapeutic proteins and peptides.

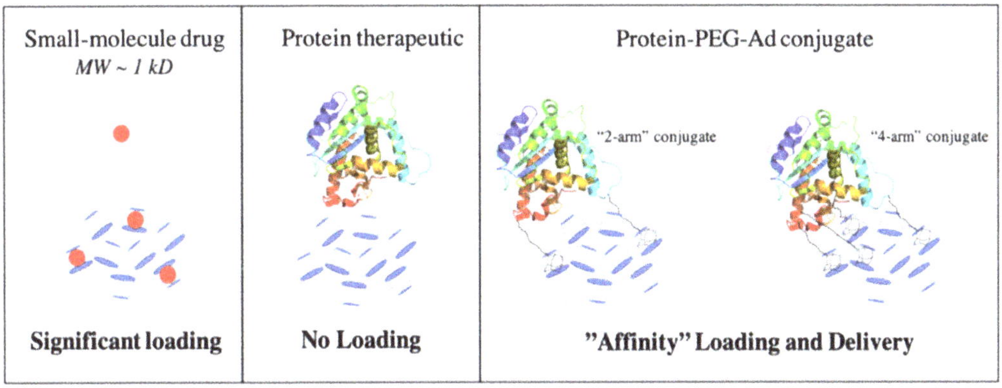

Figure 1. Illustration comparing the loading of small-molecule drugs, protein therapeutics, and protein–PEG–Ad conjugates. Increased conjugation of "PEG-Ad" groups should decrease K_D, increase thermodynamic interactions between payload and pCD matrix, and ultimately increase loading and prolong release.

2. Materials and Methods

2.1. Materials

Bovine Serum Albumin (BSA) heat shock fraction, protease free, fatty acid free, essentially globulin free, pH 7, >98% and QuantiPro BCA Assay Kit were purchased from Sigma-Aldrich (St. Louis, MO, USA). IL-10 ELISA Kit (Interleukin 10) was purchased from Antibodies-online.com accessed on 12 February 2020 (Limerick, PA, USA; MabTag). β-cyclodextrin (β-CD) prepolymer, lightly crosslinked with epichlorohydrin, was purchased from Cyclolab (Budapest, Hungary). Mini-PROTEAN TGX Precast Protein Gels (4–20%) and Precision Plus Protein Dual Color Standards were purchased from Bio-Rad (Hercules, CA, USA). Maleimide PEG Hydroxyl (MW = 5000 g/mol) was ordered from JenKem Technology USA (Plano, TX, USA). All other reagents, solvents, and chemicals were purchased from Fisher Scientific (Hampton, NH, USA) in the highest grade available.

2.2. Protein–PEG–Adamantane Conjugation Synthesis

To synthesize adamantane-capped PEG (Ad–PEG_{5000}–Mal), a 1:1 (w/w) ratio of adamantane carbonyl chloride and maleimide–PEG_{5000}–hydroxyl was dissolved in anhydrous chloroform (5 mL chloroform per 1 g mixture), according to a previous protocol [28,37]. Equal molar amounts of triethylamine to PEG were then added dropwise and the solution was allowed to react for 24 h at room temperature (RT) under agitation (Figure 2a). Once reacted, the product was precipitated with diethyl ether three times (using half of the total volume of chloroform) and solvent was removed in vacuum at 25 °C overnight (ON). As pCD is a covalently bonded polymer network with closely-packed monomer units, PEG_{5000} was selected for adamantane conjugation as its estimated hydrodynamic radius (~2 nm) was predicted to sufficiently "space out" the adamantane groups from the hydrophobic interior of folded proteins (3–14 nm). This was carried out to help ensure adamantane groups were available for complexation within cyclodextrin's interior.

Protein–PEG_{5000}–Ad conjugates were synthesized with sulfhydryl-reactive crosslinker chemistry. Protein samples (Bovine Serum Albumin, BSA, or IL-10 monoclonal antibody, mAb) were incubated with 10x molar excess TCEP (tris(2-carboxyethyl)phosphine) slurry for 1 h at RT on an end-over-end mixer. Once disulfide bonds were reduced, a variable molar excess (2×, 4×, 8×) of Ad–PEG_{5000}–Mal was added to the protein samples and were allowed to react for 4 h at RT (or ON at 4 °C) (Figure 2b). The protein–polymer conjugates were then dialyzed for 48 h (MWCO = 14 kD). In this study, BSA–PEG_{5000}–Ad and mAb–PEG_{5000}–Ad were investigated. The concentration of mAb present in each reaction was according to MabTag kit standards.

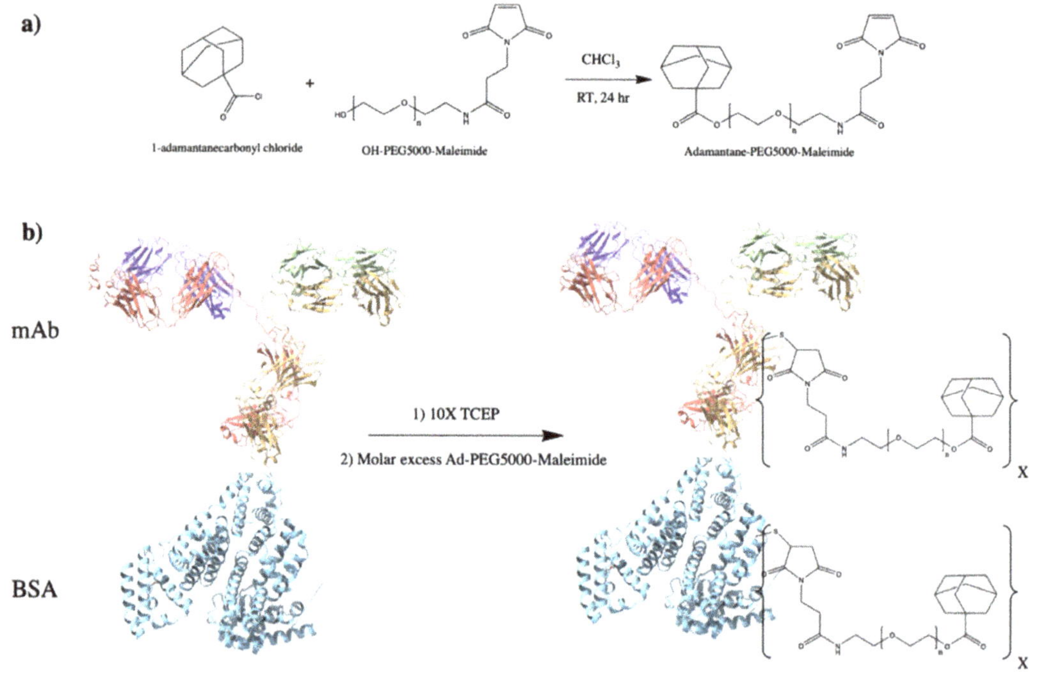

Figure 2. Synthesis overview for protein–PEG–Ad conjugates: (**a**) synthesis of Ad–PEG_{5000}–Mal, a nucleophilic addition/elimination reaction; and (**b**) synthesis of protein–(PEG_{5000}–Ad)$_X$ where X represents the number of PEG_{5000}–Ad "tethers" conjugated to each molecule of protein. BSA (PDB entry 4F5S) is used as a model protein, mAb (PDB entry 1IGT) is used as a "functional example" of an antibody therapeutic. Products for mAb synthesis in (**b**) will also produce two fragmented antibodies (Fabs).

2.3. Nuclear Magnetic Resonance

Nuclear magnetic resonance (NMR) was used to verify successful conjugation during synthesis steps. All spectra of presented chemical species were recorded by Bruker 300 MHz NMR system (Bruker, Germany) in DMSO-d_6 or D_2O solvent, as indicated.

2.4. Rate of Hydrolysis for (Ad–PEG_{5000}–Mal) Species

An amount of 10 mg of Adamantane–PEG_{5000}–Mal was dissolved in 10 mL of D_2O and incubated to 37 °C, agitated at 100 rmp. An amount of 600 µL aliquots were sampled at designated intervals and ^{1}H-NMR spectra were obtained. Percent hydrolysis was determined by comparing the integral of the "hydrolysis alcohol peak" at $\delta = 6.1$ ppm and a fixed peak at $\delta = 4.2$ ppm. Samples were capped with N_2 after obtaining each sample.

2.5. pCD Polymer Synthesis (MPs and SRPL)

pCD polymer microparticles (MPs) and Sustained Release Polymeric Liquid (SRPL), a fluidic pCD formulation, were synthesized to serve as insoluble drug delivery vehicles [38]. As we aimed to investigate the impact of polymer topology on drug loading capabilities for protein payloads, SRPL was used as an example of crosslinked, linear branch topology while MPs were used to represent crosslinked, spherical topology. As polymer macrostructures are widely known to influence drug loading and drug release profiles, we aimed to investigate the differences between a linear, viscous polymer and a compact, dense particle, respectively.

Briefly, microparticles were synthesized from epichlorohydrin-crosslinked β-cyclodextrin prepolymer solubilized in 0.2 M potassium hydroxide (25% w/v) preheated in a 60 °C oil bath for 10 min. Light mineral oil was then added to a beaker with Tween 85/Span 85 (24/76%) and stirred at 500 rpm. Ethylene glycol diglycidyl ether (0.01 M) was added to the prepolymer solution dropwise and then mixed. After vortexing, the prepolymer solution was added to the oil/Span/Tween 85 solution and heated in a 70 °C-oil bath. The stir speed was increased and then the mixture was stirred for 3 h. After incubating, the particles were taken out and centrifuged at 200× g to be separated from the oil mixture and then washed with excess hexanes twice, excess acetone twice, and finally diH_2O twice. The microparticles were then frozen and lyophilized before further use. Based on previous studies, we can estimate that this protocol generates pCD microparticles with a size of 81.88 ± 36.86 µm with a polydispersity index of 0.2 [39].

SRPL was synthesized with β-cyclodextrin crosslinked with epichlorohydrin, dried for 4 h at 70 °C, and then stirred (150 rpm) in a 55 °C-oil bath for 10 min. DMSO (4 mL per gram of dried CD) was then added to the CD and incubated for 10 min. Hexamethylene diisocyanate (HDI) crosslinker (45 µL HDI per gram dried CD) was added to the CD mixture and capped with N_2 gas. The speed of mixing was then increased and after two 15-min intervals, the vial was checked to observe increases in viscosity until the solution appears viscous and glassy (~30 min). Then, diH_2O was added to quench the remaining crosslinker and synthesized polymer was lyophilized overnight (ON).

2.6. *Affinity Testing—Surface Plasmon Resonance*

Experimental "affinity" between β-CD monomers and protein conjugates were measured experimentally through surface plasmon resonance (SPR) with a Biacore X100 system (GE Healthcare Bio-Sciences, Pittsburgh, PA, USA) according to previous protocols [40,41]. The surface of a sensor chip CM-5 was conjugated with EDC (0.4 M) and NHS (0.1 M) followed by 10 mM of 6-amino-6-deoxy-β-cyclodextrin (CycloLab, Budapest, Hungary) suspended in HBS-N buffer (a HEPES balanced salt solution with pH 7.4). The other channel was conjugated similarly with aminodextran (Thermo Fisher Scientific, Waltham, MA, USA) to determine specific versus nonspecific interactions with a chemically similar but non-affinity substrate. The remaining functional groups were capped with ethanolamine. A multi-cycle kinetic experiment was performed with drug dissolved in a MilliQ water solution and was regenerated with 100 mM sodium hydroxide between samples. The differential responses between the channels were fit to steady-state affinity using Biacore evaluation software. Indicated K_D values (*) were within model confidence interval (Chi^2 values below 10% of the maximum SPR response) [20]. A concentration range of 0.125–10 nM was used.

2.7. *Drug Loading and Release*

Affinity and drug loading and release kinetics of protein–$(PEG_{5000}–Ad)_x$ was tested in vitro in both pCD MPs and SRPL. BSA was used as a model protein, as it is relatively inexpensive and easy to detect with BCA assay kits. An amount of 10 mg of dried pCD MPs and SRPL, respectively, were soaked for 48 h in drug solutions (100 µg/mL) of each protein-conjugate species. The loaded pCDs were then washed 3 times with 1 mL of 0.1 sodium phosphate buffer and then incubated in 1 mL of a "physiological release buffer" (phosphate-buffered saline (PBS) and 0.1% Tween$^{8○}$) at 37 °C on a rotary shaker. To simulate "infinite sink" in vivo conditions, aliquots were sampled frequently at recorded time intervals. BSA-conjugate concentrations were measured using a Micro BCA kit that gave a colorimetric readout that was compared with a standard curve for each BSA-conjugate species. Affinity interactions were "maximized" by keeping the number of potential "affinity-groups" under the theoretical maximum "host-groups" (e.g., BSA–$(PEG_{5000}–Ad)_2$ has two potential binding sites). Calculations were based on the following assumptions: β-CD MW = 1135 g/mol, Epichlorohydrin MW = 92 g/mol, BSA MW= 65,000 g/mol, and Mal–PEG_{5000}–Ad at 5330 g/mol.

After the drug release aliquots decreased below detectable concentrations, the polymers were incubated for 96 h in 1 mL of DMSO to extract remaining protein conjugates. DMSO was removed from samples using a SpeedVac concentrator, ON, and reconstituted in 200 µL PBS. "Total loading" values were obtained by combining cumulative drug release results with DMSO-released drug.

2.8. Modified ELISA

To quantify antibody functionality after conjugation of affinity groups, we utilized a modified ELISA protocol to investigate mAb antigen recognition after PEGylation. Briefly, coating-capture antibody and blocking steps were performed according to the MabTag ELISA protocol and 500 pg/mL of rhIL-10 standard was added to each well. Detection-antibody was treated for 1 h with 10× molar excess TCEP and incubated for 4 h at RT with varying molar excess of Mal–PEG–Ad. Upon reaction completion, 100 µL of modified detection-antibody was added to each well, and each group (n = 3) was normalized to unmodified detection antibody. "Antibody functionality" was reported as a percentage of positive controls, which were assumed to have 100% antigen recognition.

2.9. Statistical Analysis

All statistics were calculated in Origin (OriginLab, Northampton, MA, USA). Statistically significance was defined as $p < 0.05$ with further specifications stated in figure captions. Drug release curves were analyzed by one-way ANOVA and Tukey post hoc test ($p < 0.05$).

3. Results

3.1. PEG–Adamantane (PEG–Ad) "Tether" Synthesis

Synthesis of Ad–PEG_{5000}–Mal was confirmed via ^{1}H NMR. Confirmation of Ad conjugation to maleimide–PEG_{5000}–hydroxyl was observed as the coexistence of adamantane's hydrocarbon (-CH_2) peaks at δ = 1.7–1.9 ppm and PEG's repeating backbone (-CH_2-) peak at δ = 3.6 ppm. Reaction yield was determined by comparing the peak integrals of adamantane (δ = 1.7–1.9 ppm; 16 hydrogens) and the last carbon of PEG (δ = 4.2 ppm; 2 hydrogens), and a range of 73–96% conversion (n = 2 batches) was observed (Figure 3).

3.2. PEG–Ad "Tethers" Remain Stable for up to 40 Days

As Ad–PEG_{5000}–Mal contains an ester group prone to hydrolysis, the stability of the chemical species was observed over time via ^{1}H NMR in D_2O. The integral of the terminal hydroxyl peak (-OH) at δ = 6.1 ppm was compared with a constant PEG (-CH_2-) peak at δ = 4.2 ppm, and a percent of species hydrolysis was obtained. Over time, the integral of the terminal hydroxyl peak increased until it equaled half of the integral of the δ = 4.2 ppm, indicating 100% species hydrolysis. We found that at around 40 days, the adamantane is completely dissociated from the PEG linker, which is most likely attributed to the partial solubility of Ad–PEG_{5000}–Mal (Figure 4). Hydrolysis was confirmed to have zero-order kinetics, as the percent of species exhibited a linear relationship relative to time.

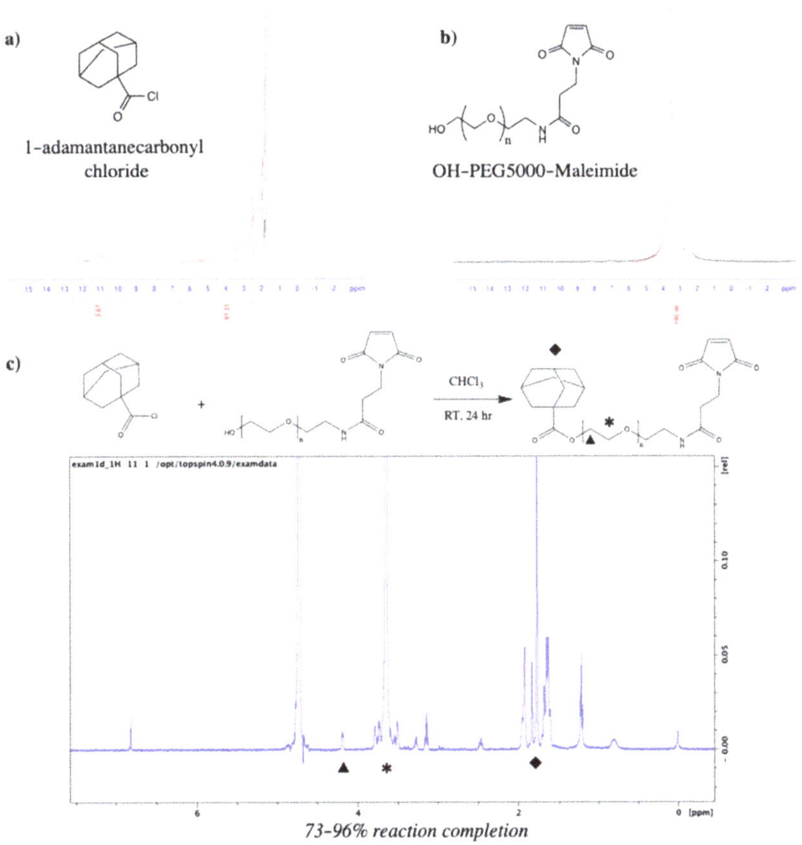

Figure 3. (**a**) ^{1}H NMR (DMSO-d_6) of 1-adamantanecarbonyl chloride which confirmed a 97.33% purity; (**b**) ^{1}H NMR (DMSO-d_6) of maleimide–PEG$_{5000}$–hydroxyl; and (**c**) Ad–PEG$_{5000}$–Mal ^{1}H NMR (DMSO-d_6), with unique peaks at δ = 1.7–1.9 ppm (Ad hydrocarbons, ◆), δ = 4.2 ppm (terminal –CH$_2$– of PEG, ▲), and δ = 3.6 ppm (–CH$_2$– PEG repeat units, *).

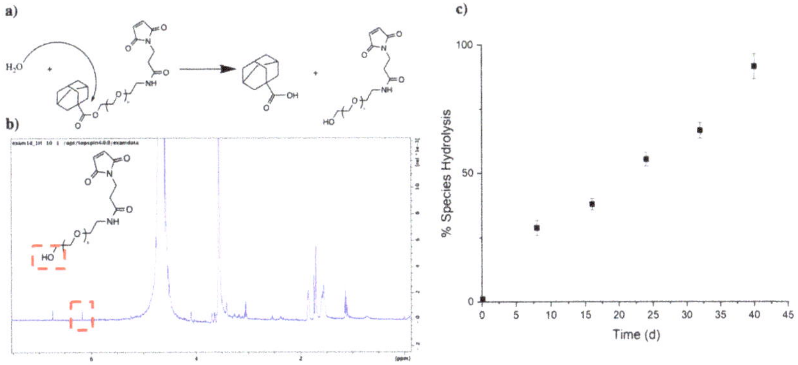

Figure 4. (**a**) Hydrolysis mechanism for PEG–Ad; (**b**) ^{1}H NMR (D_2O) with Bruker 300 MHz, noting a hydrolysis peak at δ = 6.1 ppm and a reference peak at δ = 4.2 ppm (–CH$_2$–); and (**c**) a species percentage was quantitively obtained from hydrolysis peak δ = 6.1 ppm.

3.3. PEG–Ad "Tethers" Successfully Conjugated to Reduced Proteins

To ensure maleimide–sulfhydryl chemistry was successfully taking place, nonreducing SDS-PAGE gels were used to quantify the molecular weight of our BSA and mAb protein–polymer conjugates (Figure 5). An increase in molecular weight was observed for all protein–polymer species, and the estimated conjugation ratio (*ECR*) of each species was obtained by the following equation:

$$ECR = \frac{MW_{conjugate} - MW_{protein}}{MW_{polymer\ 'tether'}} \quad (1)$$

a)

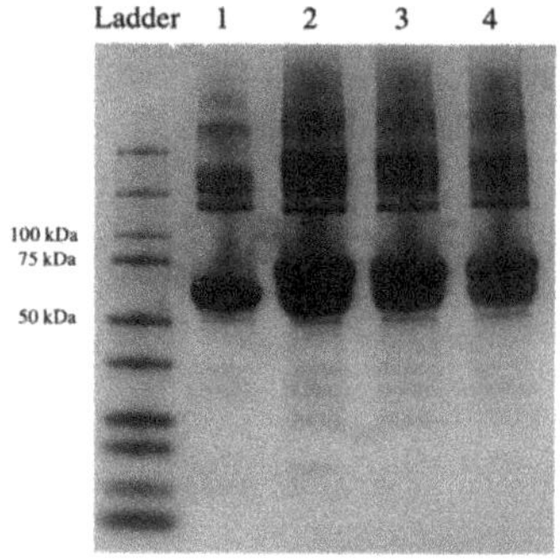

Lane Number	1	2	3	4
	BSA	**BSA-(PEG$_{5000}$-Ad)$_2$**	**BSA-(PEG$_{5000}$-Ad)$_4$**	**BSA-(PEG$_{5000}$-Ad)$_8$**
Average Molecular Weight (kDa)	65.1	79.5	83.9	95.2
Estimated Conjugation Ratio	0	2.8	3.7	5.9

b)

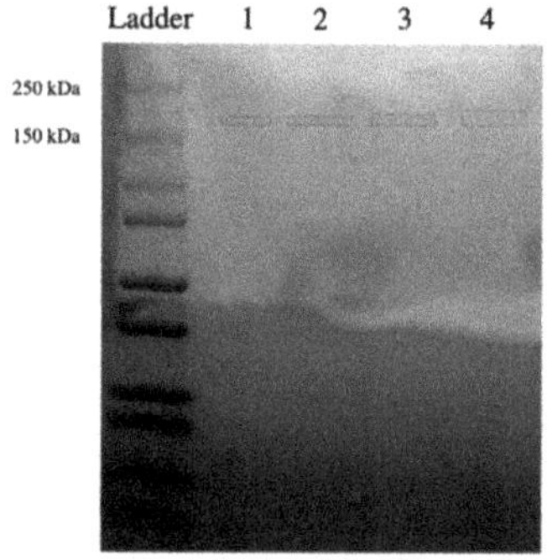

Lane Number	1	2	3	4
	mAb	**mAb-(PEG$_{5000}$-Ad)$_2$**	**mAb-(PEG$_{5000}$-Ad)$_4$**	**mAb-(PEG$_{5000}$-Ad)$_8$**
Average Molecular Weight (kDa)	162.0	175.4	177.4	184.5
Estimated Conjugation Ratio	0	2.5	2.9	4.2

Figure 5. Nonreducing SDS-PAGE gel electrophoresis (12–20% Tris Glycine) of (**a**) BSA conjugates found between 79–95 kDa and (**b**) mAb conjugates found between 175–185 kDa. Average molecular weights were obtained based on ladder band locations in ImageJ. mAb bands were boxed in red to increase visibility, as loaded protein concentration was low.

3.4. PEG–Ad "Tethers" Greatly Increased Protein–Polymer Conjugate Affinity for β-CD

Affinity between our protein–polymer conjugates and β-CD was tested using surface plasmon resonance (SPR). Unmodified protein species had characteristically low affinity for β-CD, while an increase in Ad–PEG_{5000} conjugation corresponded to an increased affinity (decreased K_D). However, we found that as the number of "affinity" groups increased, we were unable to obtain low Chi^2 value curve fittings, as indicated in Table 1. K_D values were determined from steady-state affinity equation curve fitting according to standards set in Biacore's evaluation software.

Table 1. SPR kinetics results for unmodified and modified protein–polymer conjugates against β-CD immobilized CM5 chip, diH_2O running buffer.

Interaction (Host/Ligand)	K_D (M)	Binding Free Energy (KJ/mol)
βCD/BSA	0.001293 [1]	−16.5
βCD/BSA–(PEG_{5000}–Ad)$_2$	7.966×10^{-5} [1]	−23.4
βCD/BSA–(PEG_{5000}–Ad)$_4$	9.090×10^{-9}	−45.9
βCD/BSA–(PEG_{5000}–Ad)$_8$	4.099×10^{-10}	−53.6
βCD/mAb	0.0001443 [1]	−21.9
βCD/mAb–(PEG_{5000}–Ad)$_2$	8.755×10^{-10} [1]	−52.9
βCD/mAb–(PEG_{5000}–Ad)$_4$	3.012×10^{-11}	−54.1
βCD/mAb–(PEG_{5000}–Ad)$_8$	4.515×10^{-13}	−70.4

[1] K_D values were within the model confidence interval with Chi^2 values below 10% of the maximum SPR response.

3.5. PEG–Ad Conjugation to BSA Greatly Increases Loading Capacity into pCD, Regardless of Form

BSA–(PEG_{5000}–Ad)$_2$ was observed to have superior loading over both BSA–(PEG_{5000}–Ad)$_4$ and BSA–(PEG_{5000}–Ad)$_8$ (Figure 6). As BSA–(PEG_{5000}–Ad)$_{4/8}$ had comparable loading, we predict that both species were able to maximize the number of inclusion complexes formed with pCD hydrogels; however, the increase in PEG–Ad groups sterically hindered their ability to diffuse deeply into pCD. While MPs were observed to have slightly higher loading of BSA and BSA–(PEG_{5000}–Ad)$_2$, there were no significant differences in loading between SRPL and MPs in BSA–(PEG_{5000}–Ad)$_{4/8}$.

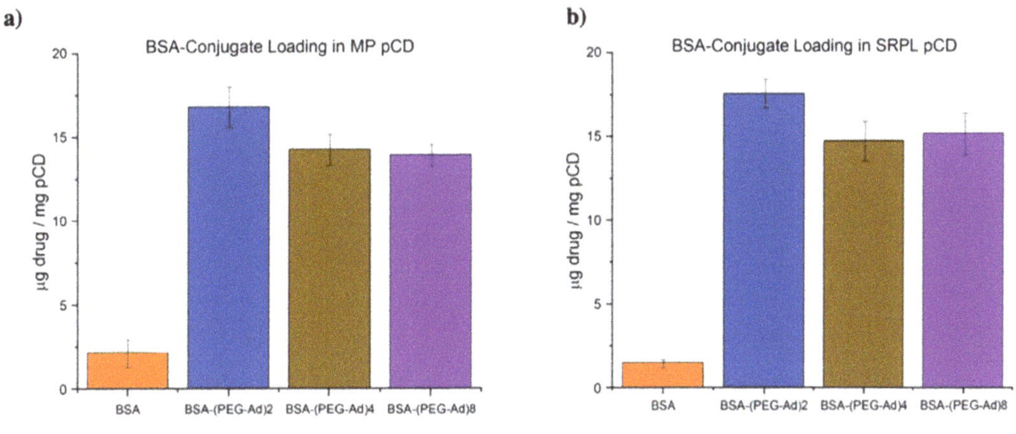

Figure 6. Total loaded drug normalized to pCD weight (10 mg) for BSA–polymer conjugates for (**a**) pCD MPs and (**b**) pCD SRPL.

3.6. Protein–Polymer Conjugates Can Be Delivered for up to 65 Days in pCD Polymers

We observed that all BSA conjugates released for a significantly longer time (45–65 days) than BSA controls (1–2 days). While all groups experienced a "burst" release within days 1–4, a prolonged "affinity" release was observed after day 6 (Figure 7b,d). BSA, which lacks the ability to form inclusion complexes with pCD, was observed to only exhibit a brief, diffusion-based release. However, the extended release observed by BSA conjugates were most likely the combination of diffusion, "affinity" from adamantane groups complexing with pCD, and subsequent hydrolysis of adamantane groups. While MP pCD was found to have more favorable loading capabilities, we found that SRPL was able to sustain release of its payload over a longer period of time. All release curves were found to be statistically significant from one another (one-way ANOVA with Tukey, $p < 0.05$), with the exception of BSA–(PEG_{5000}–Ad)$_4$ and BSA–(PEG_{5000}–Ad)$_8$ in both MP and SRPL pCD. Comparing cumulative release with our total loaded drug values in Figure 6, around 18% of the loaded drug was never released from the pCD MPs while 20% was never released from pCD SRPL.

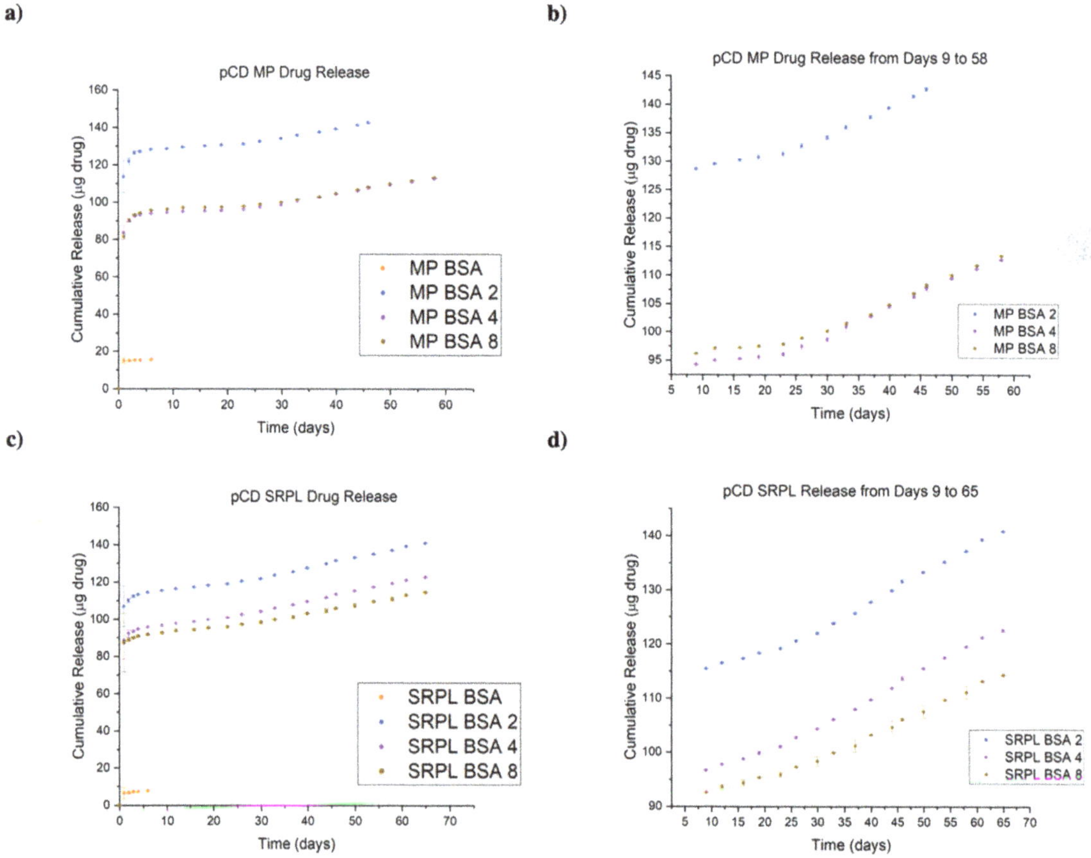

Figure 7. Cumulative drug release curves for BSA–polymer conjugates from (**a**) pCD MPs, (**b**) pCD MPs zoomed in on release days 9–65, and (**c**) pCD SRPL and (**d**) pCD SRPL zoomed in on release days 9–65. All datasets were found to be statistically significant from one another (one-way ANOVA with Tukey, $p < 0.05$), except BSA 4 and BSA 8 curves in both MP and SRPL trials.

3.7. All mAb–Polymer Conjugates Maintained at Least 70% of Antigen-Recognition Ability

As past literature has noted that mAb–polymer conjugates are at risk of losing antigen specificity after alteration, we utilized a modified ELISA to quantify these changes in structure/function. After modifying the detection mAb of an ELISA sandwich assay, we found that given a constant saturation of ligand (human interleukin-10 (hIL-10), 500 pg/mL), a decrease in overall detection occurred, which we attributed to loss of antigen recognition. Normalizing these values to unmodified positive controls, we were able to obtain a quantitative value for the mAb analog's ability to recognize its respective antigen (Figure 8). While all groups were statistically different from the positive controls, one-way ANOVA test revealed that the groups were not statistically different from one another ($p = 0.151$).

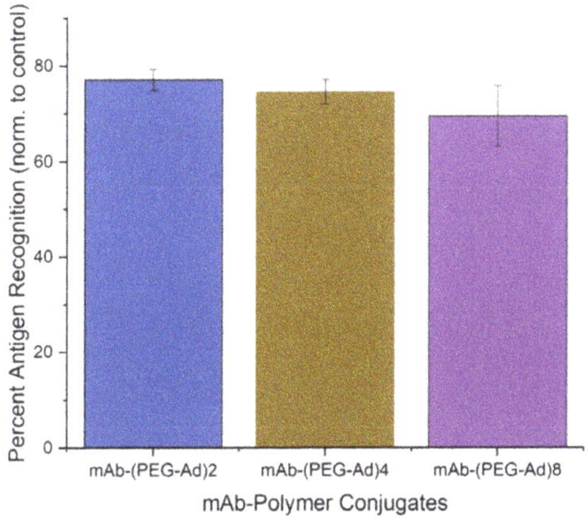

Figure 8. Quantitative estimation of mAb (anti-IL10) structure/function after PEG_{5000}–Ad conjugation. Positive controls (according to MabTag protocol, using unmodified primary antibodies) were assumed to have 100% antigen recognition.

4. Discussion

As pCD has been traditionally used for the prolonged delivery of small-molecule, hydrophobic drugs by complexing with drug ligands in a 1:1 model, this work demonstrates a novel approach for protein-based therapeutic delivery by leveraging the thermodynamic interactions between pCD polymers and protein–polymer conjugates. We successfully synthesized a PEG–Adamantane "tether" group, which was shown to remain unhydrolyzed over the span of 40 days (Figures 3 and 4). We then observed that these high-affinity "tether" groups were able to be successfully conjugated to reduce peptides via maleimide–sulfhydryl chemistry (Figure 5), and that the addition of PEG–Ad groups to peptides significantly increased their affinity for pCD, as shown in decreased K_D values between protein–polymer conjugates and β-CD (Table 1). This increase in affinity, as correlated in previous studies, yielded significant gains in loading capabilities in pCD polymers (Figure 6) and greatly enhanced drug release kinetics (Figure 7). Compared with unmodified BSA, which was delivered at a limited capacity for only 1 day, our BSA conjugates were able to load in pCD polymers at significantly higher amounts and exhibited a profoundly longer window of delivery (Figures 6 and 7).

It is well known that PEGylation and modification of mAbs and other structure-dependent therapeutics decrease their ability to bind to their respective ligand in vitro and in vivo [42]. We sought to investigate the impact PEG_{5000}–Ad conjugation has on mAb antigen recognition in vitro by modifying a sandwich ELISA assay by conjugating the polymer groups to the detection antibody. We found this modified method produced detectable differences in antigen-recognition capabilities between unmodified and modified anti-IL-10 mAbs, and while some mAb function was lost, ~70% specificity was retained between all protein–polymer groups (Figure 8). We recognize this approach to assessing retained receptor recognition is not ideal, and analyzing Fc-mediated binding to Fc gamma receptors or FcRn receptors would provide more accurate insight on retained antibody activity; however, we believe that our simplified, ELISA-derived assay provides an appropriate proxy for antigen recognition for the scope of this study. In addition, due to the low volumes of mAbs we were conjugating, we were not able to complete a molecular weight analysis of the species generated as a result of conjugation. Therefore, future work will need to use a more granular approach to molecular weight analysis, such as mass spectroscopy, to understand the distribution of PEG to antibody ratios.

When measuring affinity, we found that SPR was unable to achieve a statistically significant steady-state curve fitting with chemical species with over two potential complexing domains, namely, BSA–$(PEG_{5000}–Ad)_{4/8}$ and mAb–$(PEG_{5000}–Ad)_{4/8}$ (Table 1). We hypothesize that because SPR measures "affinity" between a monolayered "host" and mobile "ligand", it was unable to accurately detect higher-degree complexation. Nonetheless, based on drug loading and drug release kinetics, we can still conclude that an increase in complexation "high-affinity" groups increased the species' overall affinity for β-CD (Figures 6 and 7). Regardless, it is also important to note that K_D values decreased non-linearly (Table 1), suggesting that as more PEG–Ad groups were added, the molecule was unlikely to maximize interactions with pCD (i.e., not all Ad functional groups were complexed with a CD molecule).

Drug loading and delivery results suggest that there may be an upper limit to how many inclusion complexes a single drug payload can form in pCD. Given the similar performance of BSA–$(PEG_{5000}–Ad)_4$ and BSA–$(PEG_{5000}–Ad)_8$ in both MP and SRPL pCD (Figures 6 and 7), we hypothesize that despite BSA–$(PEG_{5000}–Ad)_8$'s average of 5.9 "affinity groups" per molecule, not all of these groups are being utilized to increase thermodynamic interactions, perhaps due to the limited distancing of Ad from the protein itself. Most likely, only two to four groups are actually available for docking in pCD, while the other PEG–Ad groups only add to molecular steric hindrance, which may explain the decreased overall loading efficiency in BSA–$(PEG_{5000}–Ad)_{4/8}$ (Figure 6). However, we did observe that the increased "affinity" groups decreased the overall "burst" release that occurred both in MP and SRPL pCD (Figure 7). However, the observation of a "burst" release within the first day suggests that the drug payload was only interacting with the outer surface of the pCD structures and not fully encapsulated within the pCD. This superficial interaction would likely only result in weaker thermodynamic interactions, such as van der Waal forces, and not pCD complexation. Future studies will need to focus on how to maximize the entropy of mixing during the loading phase of the protocol or explore other methods for ensuring that larger payloads, such as peptides and proteins, are properly complexed with the delivery vector; doing so would potentially reduce the "burst" phenomenon observed in Figure 7.

pCD structure appeared to not have a large impact on drug loading capabilities; however, SRPL was observed to have an extended window of delivery of up to 65 days, as opposed to 45–58 days in MP pCD (Figure 7). We predict this difference in delivery stems from topology differences between MP spheres and SRPL "branches"—permeable branching architecture allowed for increased interactions between payload and pCD. Furthermore, we observed a notable increase in optical opacity in SRPL samples after BSA-conjugate loading, which may have been a product of PEG–Ad complexation with pCD.

The idea of "multiplexing" interactions between a chemical species and cyclodextrin inclusion complexes has been consistently shown to enhance loading and delivery of small-molecule therapeutics; however, to the best of our knowledge, this study is the first study that showed that multiplexing thermodynamic interactions can help deliver higher molecular weight payloads (>1 kD) [32,33]. While the exact mechanism of loading and release has not been studied, based on previous cyclodextrin kinematic modeling studies, we suspect that our drug release profiles are the integrated result of thermodynamic interactions, diffusion, and aqueous solubility, which are impacted by our "affinity-group" adamantane hydrolysis from PEG [43,44].

While this study specifically examined protein–polymer conjugates synthesized via maleimide–sulfhydryl chemistry, alternative bioconjugation techniques, such as lysine-based conjugation, can be utilized to generate similar species [45]. For example, the ester bond connecting Ad–PEG can be replaced with an amide for more stable tethers or acid/base reactive tethers for controlled and triggered delivery, respectively. In addition, altering PEG-linker lengths may impact the capacity for pCD binding—our attempt to account for this in our experimental design (choosing PEG_{5000} due to its hydrodynamic radius) seems to have sufficiently distanced our adamantane groups from the protein to promote inclusion in cyclodextrins.

BSA was used as a model drug for this study due to its low cost and ease of detection; however, our outlined synthesis and pCD delivery platform can be applied to extend the drug delivery of any peptide or protein therapeutic with modifiable residues. Especially in situations where local, sustained delivery of protein therapeutics is ideal for positive treatment outcomes, such as the delivery of anti-VEGF antibodies to the retina for treating diabetic retinopathy, the local delivery of chemotherapeutics to a tumor, or the local treatment of rheumatoid arthritis. This platform can be utilized to maintain steady local drug concentration over a period of up to 65 days. We recognize that refillable implants are not currently typical in clinical workflows; however, based on the increasing prevalence of lifelong diseases and chronic conditions, we believe in situ, refillable implants may have a place in clinical practice in the future. Furthermore, while extensive in vivo testing is needed before these protein–polymer conjugates can be utilized for patients, we are encouraged that pCD hydrogels have, historically, performed similarly in in vitro versus in vivo models [24,36,46].

5. Conclusions

Herein, we outlined a novel synthesis of protein–polymer conjugates that, when coupled with cyclodextrin delivery platforms, can maintain a sustained release of up to 65 days without largely sacrificing protein structure/function. Antibody and protein-based therapeutics have been increasing in popularity in clinical pharmacology and this study has shown that pCD polymers are suitable for protein drug delivery, not just small-molecule hydrophobic drugs. Compared with traditional administration protocols for peptide therapeutics, many of which involve parenteral injection, pCD hydrogels present a potential effective delivery mechanism. Utilizing a variety of bioconjugation tools, other protein therapeutics can take advantage of pCD's affinity-based release and can potentially be tuned to fit other relevant clinical applications.

Author Contributions: H.A.v.R. devised the project. A.B.D. developed the technical procedures and performed the experiments under the supervision of H.A.v.R., K.E.D. helped perform drug loading and release studies. Under the supervision of H.A.v.R., A.B.D. wrote the manuscript. All authors have read and agreed to the published version of the manuscript.

Funding: This work was funded by the NIH Grant Number: R01 (R01GM121477).

Institutional Review Board Statement: Not applicable.

Informed Consent Statement: Not applicable.

Data Availability Statement: Not applicable.

Acknowledgments: Special thanks to Ashley Djuhadi for helping to brainstorm the early concepts of this project.

Conflicts of Interest: H.v.R. is a co-founder of Affinity Therapeutics but does not receive salary. The other authors have nothing to disclose.

References

1. Urquhart, L. Top companies and drugs by sales in 2019. *Nat. Rev. Drug Discov.* **2020**, *19*, 228. [CrossRef] [PubMed]
2. Lu, R.-M.; Hwang, Y.-C.; Liu, I.-J.; Lee, C.-C.; Tsai, H.-Z.; Li, H.-J.; Wu, H.-C. Development of therapeutic antibodies for the treatment of diseases. *J. Biomed. Sci.* **2020**, *27*, 1. [CrossRef] [PubMed]
3. Shepard, H.M.; Phillips, G.L.; Thanos, C.D.; Feldmann, M. Developments in therapy with monoclonal antibodies and related proteins. *Clin. Med.* **2017**, *17*, 220–232. [CrossRef] [PubMed]
4. Hansen, J.; Baum, A.; Pascal, K.E.; Russo, V.; Giordano, S.; Wloga, E.; Fulton, B.O.; Yan, Y.; Koon, K.; Patel, K.; et al. Studies in humanized mice and convalescent humans yield a SARS-CoV-2 antibody cocktail. *Science* **2020**, *369*, 1010–1014. [CrossRef] [PubMed]
5. Marovich, M.; Mascola, J.R.; Cohen, M.S. Monoclonal antibodies for prevention and treatment of COVID-19. *JAMA* **2020**, *324*, 131. [CrossRef]
6. Patel, A.; Patel, M.; Yang, X.; Mitra, A. Recent advances in protein and peptide drug delivery: A special emphasis on polymeric nanoparticles. *Protein Pept. Lett.* **2014**, *21*, 1102–1120. [CrossRef]
7. Piepenhagen, P.A.; Vanpatten, S.; Hughes, H.; Waire, J.; Murray, J.; Andrews, L.; Edmunds, T.; O'Callaghan, M.; Thurberg, B.L. Use of direct fluorescence labeling and confocal microscopy to determine the biodistribution of two protein therapeutics, Cerezyme®and Ceredase®. *Microsc. Res. Tech.* **2010**, *73*, 694–703.
8. Schaefer, E.; Abbaraju, S.; Walsh, M.; Newman, D.; Salmon, J.; Amin, R.; Weiss, S.; Grau, U.; Velagaleti, P.; Gilger, B. Sustained release of protein therapeutics from subcutaneous thermosensitive biocompatible and biodegradable pentablock copolymers (PTS gels). *J. Drug Deliv.* **2016**, *2016*, 2407459. [CrossRef]
9. Patel, R.B.; Solorio, L.; Wu, H.; Krupka, T.; Exner, A.A. Effect of injection site on in situ implant formation and drug release in vivo. *J. Control. Release* **2010**, *147*, 350–358. [CrossRef]
10. Martins, S.; Sarmento, B.; Ferreira, D.C.; Souto, E.B. Lipid-based colloidal carriers for peptide and protein delivery—Liposomes versus lipid nanoparticles. *Int. J. Nanomed.* **2007**, *2*, 595–607.
11. Villegas, M.R.; Baeza, A.; Vallet-Regí, M. Nanotechnological strategies for protein delivery. *Molecules* **2018**, *23*, 1008. [CrossRef] [PubMed]
12. Infante, J.C. Nanoparticle-based systems for delivery of protein therapeutics to the spinal cord. *Front. Neurosci.* **2018**, *12*, 484. [CrossRef] [PubMed]
13. Zhou, J.; Rao, L.; Yu, G.; Cook, T.R.; Chen, X.; Huang, F. Supramolecular cancer nanotheranostics. *Chem. Soc. Rev.* **2021**, *50*, 2839–2891. [CrossRef]
14. Ding, Y.; Tong, Z.; Jin, L.; Ye, B.; Zhou, J.; Sun, Z.; Yang, H.; Hong, L.; Huang, F.; Wang, W.; et al. An NIR discrete metallacycle constructed from perylene bisimide and tetraphenylethylene fluorophores for imaging-guided cancer radio-chemotherapy. *Adv. Mater.* **2022**, *34*, 2106388. [CrossRef] [PubMed]
15. Nambiar, M.; Schneider, J.P. Peptide hydrogels for affinity-controlled release of therapeutic cargo: Current and potential strategies. *J. Pept. Sci.* **2022**, *28*, e3377. [CrossRef] [PubMed]
16. Shuvaev, V.V.; Dziubla, T.; Wiewrodt, R.; Muzykantov, V.R. Streptavidin–Biotin Crosslinking of Therapeutic Enzymes with Carrier Antibodies: Nanoconjugates for Protection against Endothelial Oxidative Stress. In *Bioconjugation Protocols 003–020*; Humana Press: Totowa, NJ, USA, 2004. [CrossRef]
17. Huynh, V.; Wylie, R.G. Competitive affinity release for long-term delivery of antibodies from hydrogels. *Angew. Chem. Int. Ed.* **2018**, *57*, 3406–3410. [CrossRef] [PubMed]
18. Sano, T.; Cantor, C.R. Cooperative biotin binding by streptavidin. *J. Biol. Chem.* **1990**, *265*, 3369–3373. [CrossRef]
19. Utzeri, G.; Matias, P.M.C.; Murtinho, D.; Valente, A.J.M. Cyclodextrin-based nanosponges: Overview and opportunities. *Front. Chem.* **2022**, *10*, 859406.
20. Shoukat, H.; Pervaiz, F.; Khan, M.; Rehman, S.; Akram, F.; Abid, U.; Noreen, S.; Nadeem, M.; Qaiser, R.; Ahmad, R.; et al. Development of β-cyclodextrin/polyvinypyrrolidone-co-poly (2-acrylamide-2-methylpropane sulphonic acid) hybrid nanogels as nano-drug delivery carriers to enhance the solubility of Rosuvastatin: An in vitro and in vivo evaluation. *PLoS ONE* **2022**, *17*, e0263026. [CrossRef]
21. Xiong, R.; Xu, R.X.; Huang, C.; De Smedt, S.; Braeckmans, K. Stimuli-responsive nanobubbles for biomedical applications. *Chem. Soc. Rev.* **2021**, *50*, 5746–5776. [CrossRef]
22. Cromwell, W.C.; Byström, K.; Eftink, M.R. Cyclodextrin-adamantanecarboxylate inclusion complexes: Studies of the variation in cavity size. *J. Phys. Chem.* **1985**, *89*, 326–332. [CrossRef]
23. Wang, N.X.; von Recum, H.A. Affinity-Based Drug Delivery. *Macromol. Biosci.* **2011**, *11*, 321–332. [CrossRef] [PubMed]
24. Halpern, J.M.; Gormley, C.A.; Keech, M.A.; von Recum, H.A. Thermomechanical properties, antibiotic release, and bioactivity of a sterilized cyclodextrin drug delivery system. *J. Mater. Chem. B* **2014**, *2*, 2764–2772. [CrossRef] [PubMed]
25. Haley, R.M.; von Recum, H.A. Localized and targeted delivery of NSAIDs for treatment of inflammation: A review. *Exp. Biol. Med.* **2019**, *244*, 433–444. [CrossRef] [PubMed]
26. Cyphert, E.L.; von Recum, H.A. Emerging technologies for long-term antimicrobial device coatings: Advantages and limitations. *Exp. Biol. Med.* **2017**, *242*, 788–798. [CrossRef]
27. Rivera-Delgado, E.; von Recum, H.A. Using affinity to provide long-term delivery of antiangiogenic drugs in cancer therapy. *Mol. Pharm.* **2017**, *14*, 899–907. [CrossRef]

28. Singh, R.P.; Hidalgo, T.; Cazade, P.-A.; Darcy, R.; Cronin, M.F.; Dorin, I.; O'Driscoll, C.M.; Thompson, D. Self-assembled cationic β-cyclodextrin nanostructures for siRNA delivery. *Mol. Pharm.* **2019**, *16*, 1358–1366. [CrossRef]
29. He, D.; Deng, P.; Yang, L.; Tan, Q.; Liu, J.; Yang, M.; Zhang, J. Molecular encapsulation of rifampicin as an inclusion complex of hydroxypropyl-β-cyclodextrin: Design; characterization and in vitro dissolution. *Colloids Surfaces B Biointerfaces* **2013**, *103*, 580–585. [CrossRef]
30. Mealy, J.E.; Rodell, C.B.; Burdick, J.A. Sustained small molecule delivery from injectable hyaluronic acid hydrogels through host-guest mediated retention. *J. Mater. Chem. B* **2015**, *3*, 8010–8019. [CrossRef]
31. Wang, Y.; Zhang, R.; Tang, L.; Yang, L. Nonviral delivery systems of mRNA vaccines for cancer gene therapy. *Pharmaceutics* **2022**, *14*, 512. [CrossRef]
32. Thatiparti, T.R.; Averell, N.; Overstreet, D.; Von Recum, H.A. Multiplexing interactions to control antibiotic release from cyclodextrin hydrogels. *Macromol. Biosci.* **2011**, *11*, 1544–1552. [CrossRef] [PubMed]
33. Dogan, A.; von Recum, H. Engineering selective molecular tethers to enhance suboptimal drug properties. *Acta Biomater.* **2020**, *115*, 383–392. [CrossRef] [PubMed]
34. Hoare, T.R.; Kohane, D.S. Hydrogels in drug delivery: Progress and challenges. *Polymer* **2008**, *49*, 1993–2007. [CrossRef]
35. Rohner, N.A.; Dogan, A.B.; Robida, O.A.; von Recum, H.A. Serum biomolecules unable to compete with drug refilling into cyclodextrin polymers regardless of the form. *J. Mater. Chem. B* **2019**, *7*, 5320–5327. [CrossRef] [PubMed]
36. Cyphert, E.L.; Learn, G.D.; Hurley, S.K.; Lu, C.; von Recum, H.A. An additive to pmma bone cement enables postimplantation drug refilling, broadens range of compatible antibiotics, and prolongs antimicrobial therapy. *Adv. Healthc. Mater.* **2018**, *7*, 1800812. [CrossRef]
37. Chen, X.; Dong, C.; Wei, K.; Yao, Y.; Feng, Q.; Zhang, K.; Han, F.; Fuk-Tat Mak, F.; Li, B.; Bian, L. Supramolecular hydrogels cross-linked by preassembled host–guest PEG cross-linkers resist excessive, ultrafast, and non-resting cyclic compression. *NPG Asia Mater.* **2018**, *10*, 788–799. [CrossRef]
38. Rivera-Delgado, E.; Djuhadi, A.; Danda, C.; Kenyon, J.; Maia, J.; Caplan, A.I.; von Recum, H.A. Injectable liquid polymers extend the delivery of corticosteroids for the treatment of osteoarthritis. *J. Control. Release* **2018**, *284*, 112–121. [CrossRef]
39. Rohner, N.A.; Purdue, L.N.; von Recum, H.A. Affinity-Based Polymers Provide Long-Term Immunotherapeutic Drug Delivery Across Particle Size Ranges Optimal for Macrophage Targeting. *J. Pharm. Sci.* **2021**, *110*, 1693–1700. [CrossRef]
40. Rohner, N.A.; Schomisch, S.J.; Marks, J.M.; von Recum, H.A. Cyclodextrin polymer preserves sirolimus activity and local persistence for antifibrotic delivery over the time course of wound healing. *Mol. Pharm.* **2019**, *16*, 1766–1774. [CrossRef]
41. Thatiparti, T.R.; Shoffstall, A.J.; von Recum, H.A. Cyclodextrin-based device coatings for affinity-based release of antibiotics. *Biomaterials* **2010**, *31*, 2335–2347. [CrossRef]
42. Nejadmoghaddam, M.-R.; Minai-Tehrani, A.; Ghahremanzadeh, R.; Mahmoudi, M.; Dinarvand, R.; Zarnani, A.H. Antibody-drug conjugates: Possibilities and challenges. *Avicenna J. Med. Biotechnol.* **2019**, *11*, 3–23. [PubMed]
43. Larrañeta, E.; Martínez-Ohárriz, C.; Vélaz, I.; Zornoza, A.; Machín, R.; Isasi, J.R. In vitro release from reverse poloxamine/α-cyclodextrin matrices: Modelling and comparison of dissolution profiles. *J. Pharm. Sci.* **2014**, *103*, 197–206. [CrossRef] [PubMed]
44. D'Aria, F.; Pagano, B.; Giancola, C. Thermodynamic properties of hydroxypropyl-β-cyclodextrin/guest interaction: A survey of recent studies. *J. Therm. Anal. Calorim.* **2022**, *147*, 4889–4897. [CrossRef]
45. Dennler, P.; Fischer, E.; Schibli, R. Antibody conjugates: From heterogeneous populations to defined reagents. *Antibodies* **2015**, *4*, 197–224. [CrossRef]
46. Rivera-Delgado, E.; Sadeghi, Z.; Wang, N.X.; Kenyon, J.; Satyanarayan, S.; Kavran, M.; Flask, C.; Hijaz, A.Z.; A Von Recum, H. Local release from affinity-based polymers increases urethral concentration of the stem cell chemokine CCL7 in rats. *Biomed. Mater.* **2016**, *11*, 25022. [CrossRef] [PubMed]

pharmaceutics

MDPI

Article

Dual-Acting Zeta-Potential-Changing Micelles for Optimal Mucus Diffusion and Enhanced Cellular Uptake after Oral Delivery

Ahmad Malkawi [1,*], Nasr Alrabadi [2] and Ross Allan Kennedy [3]

[1] Department of Pharmaceutical Sciences, Faculty of Pharmacy, Isra University, Queen Alya Airport Street, Amman 11622, Jordan
[2] Department of Pharmacology, Faculty of Medicine, Jordan University of Science and Technology, Irbid 22110, Jordan; nnalrabadi@just.edu.jo
[3] School of Biomedical Sciences, Charles Sturt University, Wagga Wagga, NSW 2650, Australia; rokennedy@csu.edu.au
* Correspondence: malkawi_ahmad@live.com; Tel.: +43-660-310-5481

Abstract: Context: Overcoming the intestinal mucosal barrier can be a challenge in drug delivery. Nanoemulsions with negative zeta potentials can effectively permeate the mucus layer, but those with positive zeta potentials are better taken up by cells; a nanoemulsion with capricious zeta potential from negative to positive can achieve both good permeation and high uptake. Objective: This study aimed to develop dual-acting zeta-potential-amphoteric micelles enabling optimal muco-permeation and enhancement of cellular uptake. Methods: A micellar pre-concentrate was prepared from 15% Labrasol, 15% Kolliphor EL, 30% Kolliphor RH 40, and 40% dimethylsulfoxide. The micellar pre-concentrate was loaded with anionic stearic acid (SA), forming ionic complexes with cationic polymers at a ratio of 25:1 with Eudragit RS 100 and Eudragit RL 100. Blank micelles and those containing complexes were separately diluted in physiological buffers and examined for their droplet sizes, polydispersity indices (PDIs), zeta potentials, and cytotoxicity. The SA release from the micellar complexes was evaluated in 0.1 mM phosphate buffer (pH 6.8) containing 0.001% fluorescein, thereby enabling an instant decrease in fluorescence. Finally, the micelles were loaded with the model drug fluorescein diacetate (FDA) and evaluated for their muco-permeation behavior and cellular uptake. Results: The micellar dilutions formed micelles at the critical micelle concentration (CMC) of 312 μg/mL and showed a uniform average droplet size of 14.2 nm, with a PDI < 0.1. Micellar dilutions were non-cytotoxic when used at 1:100 in a physiological medium. Micelles loaded with ionic complexes achieved a sustained release of 95.5 ± 3.7% of the SA in 180 min. Moreover, the zeta potential of the complex-loaded micelles shifted from −5.4 to +1.8 mV, whereas the blank micelles showed a stabilized zeta potential of −10 mV. Furthermore, the negatively charged blank and complex-loaded micelles exhibited comparable muco-permeation, with an overall average of 58.2 ± 3.7% diffusion of FDA. The complex-loaded micellar droplets, however, provided a significantly higher cellular uptake of the model drug FDA (2.2-fold, $p \leq 0.01$) Conclusion: Due to undergoing a shift in zeta potential, the modified micelles significantly enhanced cellular uptake while preserving mucus-permeating properties.

Keywords: nanoemulsions; micelles; SEDDS; zeta potential; sustained release

Citation: Malkawi, A.; Alrabadi, N.; Kennedy, R.A. Dual-Acting Zeta-Potential-Changing Micelles for Optimal Mucus Diffusion and Enhanced Cellular Uptake after Oral Delivery. *Pharmaceutics* **2021**, *13*, 974. https://doi.org/10.3390/pharmaceutics13070974

Academic Editors: Ana Isabel Fernandes and Angela Faustino Jozala

Received: 16 June 2021
Accepted: 24 June 2021
Published: 27 June 2021

1. Introduction

Oral delivery is the most common route of drug delivery and offers several advantages for localized and systemic therapeutics [1–3]. However, the intestinal mucosal barriers, which predominantly comprise the mucus gel layer and absorptive mucosa, limit the delivery of many drugs, especially hydrophobic ones [4,5]. Lipid-based nanocarriers allow poorly soluble drugs to penetrate the intestinal mucosa with high stability [6]. Various nanocarrier strategies for overcoming the intestinal mucosal barriers have been proposed in the literature [3]. These primarily rely on modifying the nanocarrier's composition, mucoactive properties, and surface zeta potential. It is well-known that the mobilization of nanocarriers through the intestinal mucus layer is facilitated by a small droplet size, negative surface charge, and slippery PEGylated composition. Conversely, the large cationic droplets formed by less-stabilizing non-PEGylated compositions are prone to entrapment in the intestinal mucus [7,8].

The underlying absorptive epithelial layer presents another challenge for drug absorption. Mucoactive systems such as mucoactive nanocarriers can prolong the contact of a formulation with the mucosal epithelia, allowing more of the drug to be released, but may not actually enhance the cellular uptake of the droplets [2,9]. Consequently, an adaptive nanocarrier system that addresses the different challenges presented by those different barriers is needed.

In this regard, the droplet's surface zeta potential is one of the critical properties in determining a nanodroplet's competency for muco-permeation and cellular internalization through a negatively charged cell membrane. Nanodroplets that have traversed the intestinal mucus layer are taken up by the intestinal cells much more easily when their surface zeta potential changes from negative to positive [8]. The permeation of the mucus by zeta-potential-changing droplets inhibits reverse diffusion, ensuring a sufficient contact time with the underlying absorptive epithelium for cellular uptake [8,10]. The design of effective zeta-potential-changing nanodroplets must preserve the optimized muco-diffusion of the negatively charged droplets to enhance cellular uptake upon the change in zeta potential [11]. To date, zeta-potential-changing systems for overcoming intestinal mucosal barriers, such as self-emulsifying drug-delivery systems (SEDDS), nanoparticles, and micelles, have been based on the cleavage of a covalent bond from negatively charged phosphorylated structures through the action of alkaline phosphatase (AP). The release of the cleaved anionic phosphate substructures provides the desired positive zeta potential changes exhibited by nanodroplets and shows significantly enhanced cellular uptake. However, these nanodroplets need to be pre-incubated with AP, so they can show poor muco-permeation when applied to intestinal mucus [2,5,12].

Therefore, the main focus of this study was to prepare nanoemulsions with increased cellular uptake while preserving mucus penetration without the need for the pre-incubation with materials such as AP. Our approach was based on producing negatively charged nanodroplets that slowly release their negatively charged loads while permeating the mucus. These negatively charged droplets efficiently permeate the mucus and increasingly become positively charged while approaching the intestinal cells. Consequently, the droplets are expected to show significant cellular uptake following this positive shift in charge (zeta potential).

To achieve this aim, this study utilized mixed micelles formed by non-ionic surfactants, including Kolliphor and Labrasol, mixed with the co-solvent dimethylsulfoxide (DMSO) as a method of drug delivery. Micellar droplets with high anionic density were generated by anchoring excess stearic acid (SA) with a hydrophilic carboxylic acid moiety oriented in the hydrophilic shell [13]. To induce a positive shift in micellar zeta potential, excess SA forming hydrophobic ionic complexes with two lipophilic cationic polymers (Eudragit RS 100 and Eudragit RL 100) was formed and incorporated within the micellar hydrophobic core. These polymers were chosen due to their ability to promote the sustained release of their ionically complexed counter-ions from lipid-based nanoemulsions, as reported previously. Additionally, their effective entrapment within nanodroplets predominantly revealed a positive surface charge exhibited by their permanent cationic ammonium-substructures [14]. By the slow release of free and complexed SA from these two micelles, we sought to change their droplet surface zeta potentials gradually via the exhibited charge of the non-releasing cationic polymers. To validate our approach, the hydrophobic model drug fluorescein diacetate (FDA) was loaded in the prepared zeta-potential-changing micellar droplets, and its diffusion and cellular uptake through porcine intestinal mucus were investigated in vitro.

2. Materials and Methods

2.1. Materials

Stearic acid (SA), fluorescein diacetate (FDA), fluorescein, potassium phosphate dibasic, sodium phosphate monobasic, Kolliphor EL (macrogol glycerol ricinoleate), and Kolliphor RH 40 (macrogol glycerol hydroxyl stearate) were purchased from Sigma-Aldrich (Vienna, Austria). The copolymers containing ethyl acrylate, methyl methacrylate and trimethylammonioethyl methacrylate Eudragit RS 100 (1:2:0.1), and Eudragit RL 100 (1:2:0.2) were gifted by Evonik AG (Darmstadt, Germany). Labrasol was provided by Gattefossé (Paramus, NJ, USA). All the other chemicals and solvents used were of analytical grade and obtained from commercial sources.

2.2. Experimental Methods

2.2.1. Preparation of Ionic Complexes

Complexes of SA with Eudragit RS and Eudragit RL according to Table 1 were prepared in DMSO. A 25:1 ratio between the excess carboxylate charge exhibited by SA and Eudragit RS/RL's cationic groups was used. The Eudragit RS (10 mg/mL) and Eudragit RL (5 mg/mL) solutions were prepared in DMSO and added (as 100 µL) thereafter to 100 µL volumes of DMSO containing 2 mg of SA. The mixtures were then frozen at −80 °C and lyophilized. The prepared complexes with excess unbound SA were investigated for the development of novel micelles. Another set of complexes containing the same amount of SA at a 1:1 ratio with the polymer was prepared as above.

Table 1. Hydrophobic ionic complexes of stearic acid with selected cationic polymers.

Stearic Acid	Cationic Polymer	Molar Ratios (Stearic Acid: Polymer)
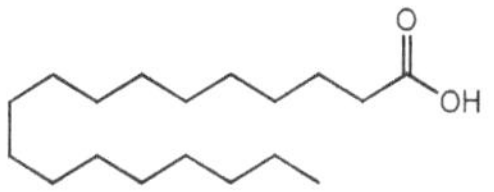 MW = 284.48 g/mol	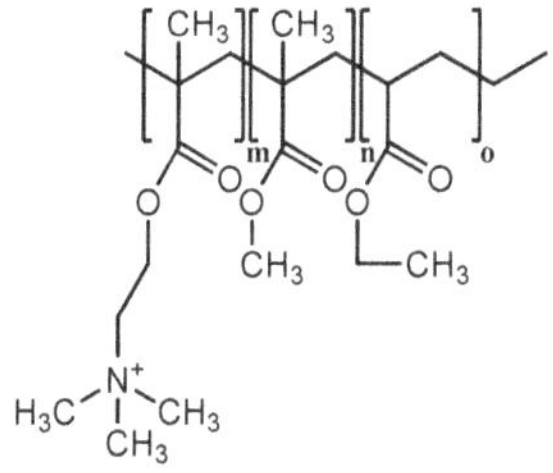 MW = 32 kDa Eudragit RS: m = 0.1, n = 2, o = 1 Eudragit RL: m = 0.2, n = 2, o = 1	25:1 1:1

2.2.2. Characterization of Ionic Complexes Using FT-IR

Using a Bruker ALPHA FT-IR instrument (Billerica, MA, USA) with 22 scans, we recorded the IR spectra of the complex derivatives purified by removing excess SA with n-hexane and their counterparts via platinum attenuated total reflection (ATR). The solids were placed on an ATR tip and scanned at 4000–400 cm^{-1} with a 4 cm^{-1} scanning speed to obtain the FT-IR spectra.

2.2.3. Development of Micellar Complexes

Hydrophobic complexes containing excess SA were dissolved in a mixture of surfactants/co-solvent (% *m*/*v*). The complexes were vortexed at 50 °C in Kolliphor RH 40 (30%), Kolliphor EL (15%), Labrasol (15%), and DMSO (40%) until complete dissolution. Final 0.5 mL micellar solutions containing SA complexed with Eudragit RS and RL were then obtained. Afterward, the micellar complex solutions were mono-dispersed at 1:100 in 0.1 M phosphate buffer (pH 6.8) using a vortex, and the size and polydispersity index (PDI) of the micelles were measured after 0, 2, and 4 h of incubation under shaking at

500 rpm (temperature: 37 °C) using a Malvern Zetasizer device (Malvern Instruments, Worcestershire, UK).

2.2.4. Determination of Critical Micelle Concentration

The critical micelle concentrations (CMCs) of the blank and complex-loaded micellar pre-concentrates were determined using a previously described fluorometric technique [15]. Pyrene—acting as a fluorescent probe partition between the aqueous phase and the micellar hydrophobic core—was dissolved at 6×10^{-7} M in 0.1 M phosphate buffer (pH 6.8.) Next, the micellar pre-concentrates were diluted across a range of 100–1000 µg/mL in pyrene solution, vortexed, thermomixed at 60 °C for 2 h, and cooled under shaking overnight. The fluorescence excitation of the samples at λ_{em} = 390 nm was measured using a Tecan microplate reader (Tecan infinite 200, Tecan Austria GmbH, Salzburg, Austria). A decimal logarithmic concentration-*versus*-I_{338}/I_{333} plot was generated to determine the CMC. Finally, the corresponding dilutions of the micelles and Kolliphor surfactants were analyzed individually for droplet size using 0.0001–0.1 dilutions in the buffer.

2.2.5. Safety Test

We next examined the cytotoxicity of micellar complexes diluted to 0.5:100, 1:100, and 3:100 in 25 mM HEPES-buffered saline (HBS, pH 7.4) toward Caco-2 cells [7]. Caco-2 cells in 24-well plates at a density of 2.5×10^4 cells per well were supplied with fresh red MEM three times per week, and incubated under 5% CO_2 at 37 °C. Following two weeks of incubation, the presence of confluent layers of Caco-2 cells within the plate was verified, and the wells were triple washed with HBS. At this point, 500 µL of micellar complex dilutions were added to each test well, and the plates were incubated for 4, 24, and 48 h at 37 °C. The positive and negative control wells contained blank HBS and 0.5% Triton-X 100 in HBS, respectively. At the end of incubation, the wells were washed twice with HBS again, and a resazurin assay was performed by adding 250 µL of 2.2 mM resazurin in HBS to each well. The resazurin-treated plates were incubated for 3 h, and 100 µL aliquots were then withdrawn from each well and checked for fluorescence at excitation/emission wavelengths of 540/590 nm using a microplate reader (Tecan Infinite 200, Tecan Austria GmbH, Salzburg, Austria). The maximum fluorescence intensity of the positive control based on resazurin's transformation into detectable pink resorufin was used as a reference against which to compare the fluorescence exhibited by the test wells, to calculate the cell viability percentage as per the following equation:

$$Cell\ viability\ (\%) = \frac{Fluorescence\ of\ test\ wells}{Fluorescence\ of\ positive\ control} \times 100. \quad (1)$$

2.2.6. Complex Dissociation and Partition Coefficient

To evaluate the dissociation and partition coefficient, the SA complexes were centrifuged using a MiniSpin device (Eppendorf AG, Hamburg, Germany) in 1 mL of n-hexane until a free SA clear solution was obtained. The supernatants were then removed, and the precipitated complexes were washed with n-hexane. Thereafter, four tubes for each complex labeled with the time points 0.5, 1, 2, and 3 h were shaken at 500 rpm at 37 °C in 1 mL of 1 mM phosphate buffer (pH 6.8), and 10 µL aliquots were added to 980 µL volumes of a fluorescently sensitive quantifying medium: 0.1 mM phosphate buffer (pH 6.8 (containing 0.001% fluorescein)) plus 10 µL of methanol. For the reference, complexes were dissolved in 1 mL of methanol, and 10 µL aliquots were added to 980 µL volumes of quantifying medium plus 10 µL of 1 mM phosphate buffer (pH 6.8). To determine complex dissociation, the values for the test tubes were compared to those for the reference regarding the decrease in fluorescence intensity using excitation/emission wavelengths of 485/515 nm. The complex partition coefficient ($Log\ P_{n\text{-}octanol/water}$) was used to dissolve increasing concentrations of complexes in n-octanol and water until clear solutions were obtained according to the following equation:

$$Log\ P_{n-octanol/water} = log\left(\frac{maximum\ solubility\ in\ n - octanol}{maximum\ solubility\ in\ water}\right). \quad (2)$$

2.2.7. Release of Stearic Acid

The quantification of SA having weak acidic properties (p*K*a = 4.75) in the aqueous medium indicated that SA caused a concentration-dependent decrease in the pH, as detected using a pH electrode, as described previously by Washington and Evans [16]. However, this previous method was modified by transforming the pH changes into instrumentally detectable fluorescent changes. For this purpose, 0.5 mg of pH-sensitive fluorescein were dissolved in a falcon tube containing 50 mL of 0.1 mM phosphate buffer, with the pH adjusted to 6.8, and used as a release medium. The sensitivity of the release medium to decreases in pH was verified by adding gradients of acetic acid and octanoic acid, which caused instant decreases in fluorescent intensity due to fluorescein transformation. Thereafter, 100 µL volumes of 1, 0.5, and 0.25% (m/v) SA solutions in methanol were drawn separately into 15 mL tubes, and, then, the methanol was allowed to evaporate. Different amounts of precipitated SA were reconstituted in 10 mL of the release medium, vortexed, and heated for a few minutes, producing 0.01, 0.005, and 0.0025% (m/v) SA. By measuring the decreases in fluorescence according to different SA concentrations in the release medium, a calibration curve was generated and used as a reference for quantifying the SA released from micellar dispersions. Based on the recommendations by Washington and Evans [16], the domain of colorimetric changes in the release medium was beyond that of the used concentrations of SA and, therefore, permitted the further quenching of fluorescein when needed at higher concentrations. To assess SA's micellar release, 100 µL volumes of the micellar pre-concentrates loaded with different SA complexes were separately mixed with the release medium to 1 mL final volumes and gently vortexed. A dialysis tube (FloatA-Lyzer) was used to dialyze the mixtures against the external phase of a 9 mL release medium in a 50 mL tube at 500 rpm at 37 °C using an Eppendorf ThermoMixer C (Hamburg, Germany). Tubes containing micellar dispersions were tightly closed and incubated for 3 h. We ensured that the release medium's fluorescence intensity was kept constant and considered the effect of blank formulations containing the same polymer ratios as the complexes omitting SA. At predetermined time points every 30 min, an aliquot of 1 mL was drawn from the external phase of each sample and replaced with fresh release medium. The aliquots were centrifuged at 13,400 rpm for 5 min, and the fluorescence of 100 µL sub-aliquots at excitation/emission wavelengths of 485/515 nm was quantified using a microplate reader (Tecan Infinite 200, Tecan Austria GmbH, Salzburg, Austria). The release was determined as a function of the cumulative decline in fluorescence intensity compared to the reference.

2.2.8. Time-Dependent Zeta-Potential Changes

The predicted zeta-potential changes exhibited by micellar droplets after 3 h of SA release were demonstrated via dynamic light scattering utilizing a Zetasizer. Micelles comprising SA-polymer complexes dispersed in an aqueous medium utilizing 1:100 dilutions were vortexed in 10 mM phosphate buffer (pH 6.8) and evaluated for their zeta potentials every 30 min at 37 °C. We assessed the zeta potentials of both blank micelles as pure excipients and those containing the same percentage of polymers used in complexes without SA, which constituted the lower and upper limits of the zeta-potential values, respectively. Furthermore, the tested micellar complex preparations releasing SA that exhibited time-dependent zeta potentials were always within this range. Changes in the zeta potential were continuously evaluated until the zeta-potential values reached a plateau, where they stabilized.

2.2.9. Muco-Permeation Study

The in vitro Transwell diffusion model described previously was used to evaluate the micellar droplets' abilities to penetrate the intestinal porcine mucus [2]. Porcine mucus was collected from fresh pig intestines bought from a local slaughterhouse and stored on ice. The intestines were longitudinally incised, and intraluminal chyme was discarded. Consistent uniform mucus was then scraped and collected in a 200 mL beaker, and bulky debris was removed. Further purification was carried out by gently agitating 200 mg/mL of the mucus in 0.1 M sodium chloride for 1 h. The supernatant was centrifuged in 50 mL tubes for 2 h, and the precipitated pure mucus pellets were stored at −20 °C until further use.

By utilizing the DMSO portions of the micellar pre-concentrates, the FDA model drug was prepared as a stock solution, and 0.2% was used in micelles. FDA-spiked micellar pre-concentrates, either blank or containing micellar complexes, were diluted to 1:100 in 0.1 M phosphate buffer (pH 6.8). To characterize the Transwell model, inserts (as donor chambers) closed with a filtering membrane with a 3.0 μm pore size (ThinCert cell culture insert, Greiner-Bio One, Austria) and evenly distributed mucus (50 mg per insert) were separately immersed in a 24-well plate filled with 500 μL of phosphate buffer as the acceptor chamber. Micellar dilutions in the buffer medium (250 μL) were added to the mucus surface of each insert in the donor chamber. A micellar dilution of the FDA load passing through the insert-filtering membrane in the absence of mucus was used as the positive control, whereas the micellar dilution omitting FDA and diffusing the mucus was used as the negative control. Another positive control utilized a free-FDA-saturated solution in the buffer to account for diffusion. Over 4 h, the plates were incubated with 70 rpm shaking, and 100 μL aliquots of the medium were withdrawn in triplicate each hour from the acceptor chambers and transferred into 96-well black plates, with a fresh buffer replacement in the acceptor chamber. Subsequently, 10 μL of 5 M NaOH were added to each aliquot, and the plate was incubated for 30 min to allow the hydrolysis of FDA into fluorescein quantifiable at excitation/emission wavelengths of 480/520 nm. The micellar droplet permeation through the mucus was quantified as a function of the cumulative amount of permeated FDA.

2.2.10. Cellular Uptake Study

Pre-concentrates of micellar complexes and blank micelles labeled with FDA were evaluated in vitro for cellular uptake in Caco-2 cells following a previously described method [2]. Caco-2 cells seeded at a concentration of 2.5×10^4 cells/well within 24-well plates were grown as described above. After obtaining confluent layers of Caco-2 cells, the cells were washed twice with 25 mM HEPES-buffered saline (HBS) (pH 7.4); then, 500 μL micellar dilutions (1:1000) in HBS were added to the cells, which were then incubated at 37 °C under 5% CO_2 for 4 h. Following incubation, another washing step was performed, and 500 μL of HBS were added to all the wells, excluding those used as positive controls. Subsequent cell lysis was mediated by the addition of 200 μL of 2% Triton-X 100 solution in 5 M NaOH with 30 min incubation to hydrolyze the FDA into detectable sodium fluorescein. The positive control of the FDA reference was represented by cells treated with the lysis solution without removing micellar dilutions, whereas the blank buffer treatment represented the negative control. Aliquots from all the treated wells were transferred to a 96-well plate, and the fluorescence intensity was measured using λ_{ex} = 480 nm and λ_{em} = 520 nm. Cellular uptake was then calculated according to the following equation:

$$Cellular\ uptake\ (\%) = \frac{Fluorescence\ (Sample) - Fluorescence\ (Negative\ control)}{Fluorescence\ (Reference) - Fluorescence\ (Negative\ control)} \times 100. \quad (3)$$

2.2.11. Statistical Analysis

GraphPad Prism V.7 was utilized to assess the significance of the differences between micelles in the release study (two-way ANOVA) and cellular uptake study (column statistics) with 95% confidence intervals ($p \leq 0.05$). * $p \leq 0.05$ was considered significant, ** $p \leq 0.01$ very significant, and *** $p \leq 0.001$ highly significant. The indicated values are expressed as the means ± SD ($n \geq 3$).

3. Results and Discussion

3.1. Hydrophobic Complexes

To ensure the optimum saturation of the polymeric cationic binding sites, excess anionic moiety from the counter ion SA was bound. The organic phase was the co-solvent DMSO used as the ion-pairing medium. Besides its relatively low dielectric constant of 46.7 (encouraging ionic interactions) [17], DMSO has a basic strength comparable to that of water [18] and allows the acidic dissociation of the SA carboxylic moiety (p*K*a = 4.75). Furthermore, the concurrent advantageous presence of permanently charged ammonium groups from Eudragit RS/RL can boost the overall ion-pairing process [19]. The findings of a previous study highlighted a major role for stabilized ionic complexes in producing beneficial zeta-potential changes in nanoemulsions following dispersion in aqueous media within a noticeable timeframe [12]. Inducing slow changes in the zeta potential of nanoemulsions from negative to positive or vice versa—often attributed to a slow release of either counter ion—can significantly improve several aspects of drug delivery.

3.2. Micelle Characterization

The micellar pre-concentrates loading the complexes formed homogenous emulsions when diluted to 1:100 in an aqueous medium. The micellar solutions used as blank or loading complexes were comparable regarding droplet size, exhibiting an average of 14.2 nm, and having a PDI of < 0.1 in an aqueous medium, as illustrated in Figure 1.

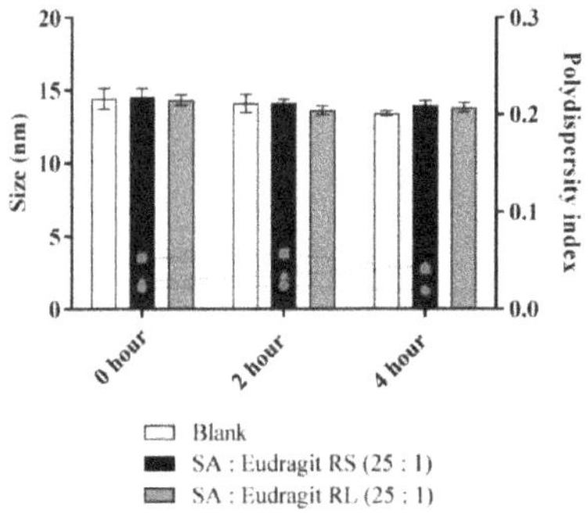

Figure 1. Sizes of micellar droplets used as blank (white bars) or containing SA-polymer complexes with Eudragit RS (black bars) and Eudragit RL (gray bars) and the polydispersity index (red symbols) at 0, 2, and 4 h time points after 1:100 dilution in 0.1 M phosphate buffer (pH 6.8) at 37 °C. Indicated values are the means ± SD ($n \geq 3$).

Micellar dilutions neither showing phase separation nor precipitation preserved the stability of the size when measured over 4 h. It was possible to determine a stabilized micellar size after ≥ 24 h (data not shown). Furthermore, the fluorometry of the fluorescent probe pyrene in the phosphate buffer at pH 6.8 provided information on the CMC of the diluted micelles. Table 2 highlights similar CMC values for the micelles loading SA-polymer complexes, with the blank micelle showing an average CMC (312 µg/mL).

Table 2. Critical micelle concentration (CMC) values of the developed micelles.

Micelle (% *v*/*v*)	Complex	Complex (% *m*/*v*)	CMC (μg/mL)
Labrasol (15%) Kolliphor EL (15%) Kolliphor RH 40 (30%) DMSO (40%)	–	–	314.5 ± 4.8
	SA-Eudragit RS	0.6%	307.8 ± 7.3
	SA-Eudragit RL	0.5%	313.8 ± 4.4

Based on previous observations, altering the hydrophilic-lipophilic balance of the formed surfactant-based micelles towards more lipophilicity reduced their CMC [20]. The concentration of lipophilic complexes from micellar dilutions, however, was too low to alter the self-assembling properties of the diluted surfactants. Moreover, micelles diluted above the CMC before or after the incorporation of complexes exhibited similar stabilized sizes. The corresponding micellar and Kolliphor-based surfactant dilutions in the buffer were examined for droplet size considering the CMC values. As shown in Figure 2, at 0.0001 dilution (<CMC), only the surfactants Kolliphor EL and Kolliphor RH 40 presented an average size of 15.8 ± 1.5 nm, whereas the micellar dilutions showed no measurable size. Above the CMC, dilution at 0.001 showed average sizes of 19.7 ± 3.9 nm and 15.3 ± 0.9 nm for the surfactants and micelles, respectively. Increasing the proportion of polar co-solvents in the micelles interfered with surfactant self-assembly by increasing the CMC [21]. The increased CMC for the present mixture of micellar surfactants compared to that for the individual surfactants in an aqueous medium could be attributed to the use of DMSO as a polar co-solvent. For instance, Anderson et al. noted that the CMC of a cetyltrimethylammonium bromide alkaline solution was shifted from 0.0013 to 0.055 M by using a mixture of water and 60% methanol at 25 °C [22].

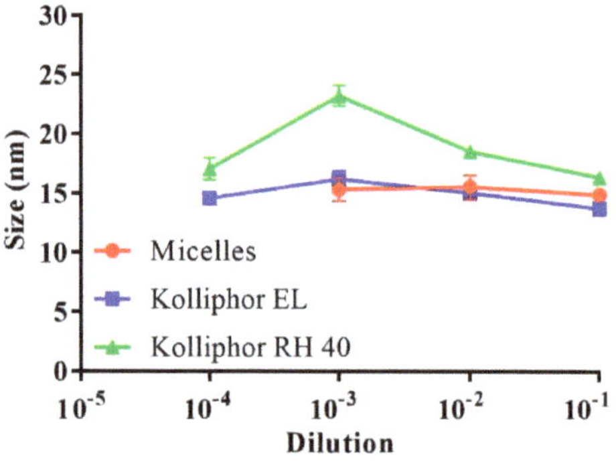

Figure 2. Average droplet size of the micelles and the surfactants Kolliphor EL and Kolliphor RH 40 after 0.1–0.0001 dilutions in 0.1 M phosphate buffer (pH 6.8) at 37 °C. Indicated values are the means ± SD ($n \geq 3$).

Despite the possible impact on the CMC, several advantages were obtained by formulating micellar DMSO. On the one hand, the micellar solubility of the hydrophobic complexes was integrated with the presence of DMSO. On the other hand, DMSO enhanced the miscibility of the relatively small-sized droplets in the surrounding medium. This desired effect facilitated sufficient interactions between the anionic exchange resin anchored within the micellar droplet and the ionic buffer medium to cause dissociation, thereby releasing SA from the micellar complex. Moreover, SA release could be optimized by releasing DMSO while preserving unchanged micellar droplet size, as shown from a previous study [23]. Ultimately, the micellar droplets showed a positive charge in the presence of non-releasing cationic polymers Eudragit.

3.3. Cytotoxicity

The possible cytotoxic effects of micellar solutions bearing different complex loads were tested using a resazurin assay. To evaluate cytotoxicity, we selected Caco-2 cells, bearing the morphological and functional features of intestinal enterocytes, to test for cytotoxicity, intestinal drug delivery, and cellular uptake after the intended oral administration [24]. As shown in Figure 3, the cell viability remained at 100% under significant micellar concentrations of 0.5% and 1% after 4, 24, and 48 h, providing evidence for prolonged high safety. At a 3% micellar concentration, significant cytotoxicity was observed, as indicated by the 40% cut-off safety limit. Therefore, further studies on cells were conducted using a micellar concentration of $\leq$1%.

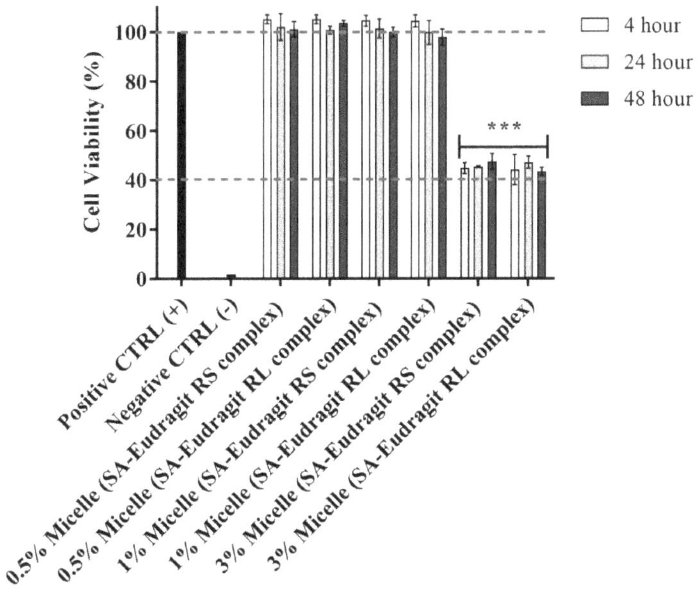

Figure 3. Effects on Caco-2 cell viability of 0.5:100, 1:100, and 3:100 dilutions of micellar preconcentrates containing SA-polymer complexes with Eudragit RS and Eudragit RL in 25 mM HBS (pH 7.4) after 4, 24, and 48 h incubation at 37 °C. A 3:100 versus 1:100 and 0.5:100 micellar dilutions indicated significant decreases in cell viability (*** $p \leq 0.001$). Indicated values are the means ± SD ($n \geq 3$).

In previous observations, the studied non-ionic surfactants incurred no significant cytotoxicity in micellar compositions at relatively high concentrations [25]. However, a significant increase in the concentration of these surfactants in culture medium was reported to reduce cell viability [26,27]. Furthermore, the cationic properties of polymers, commonly associated with the cell membrane and cellular metabolic disturbances, did not show cytotoxic potential [28]. Several previous evaluations concluded that Eudragit methacrylate copolymers have a high safety limit. Zhang et al., for instance, demonstrated no cytotoxic effects on human cornea epithelial cells after utilizing Eudragit RS, at a concentration of 100 µg/mL, for the coating of a structured lipid-based nanocarrier encapsulating genistein [29]. Therefore, the cytotoxicity induced at a 3% micellar concentration may not be related to the high amount of cationic polymers. Among the micellar excipients, however, DMSO was reported to interact with the cellular membrane and metabolic pathways, causing damages at concentrations > 1% (v/v) [30]. This could explain why the 0.2% and 0.4% DMSO concentrations from the 0.5:100 and 1:100 micellar dilutions were not cytotoxic, whereas the DMSO concentration of 1.2% from the 3:100 micellar dilution could have an impact on cell viability. Previous studies also reported that DMSO at relatively low concentrations has no cytotoxic potential on different cell lines following 4–48 h incubation [31–33].

3.4. Dissociation of the Complexes

Despite the indispensable need to form stabilized micellar complexes, the reversible nature of ionic interactions is crucial for releasing the counter ion from its micellar complex. Therefore, we examined the potential of SA-polymer complexes to dissociate in a fluorescently sensitive release medium utilizing thermo-mechanical force. For pre-micellar testing, solid dispersions of the complexes showed continuous dissociation of SA each hour, which reached a plateau within 1 h. Over the 3 h dissociation evaluation, up to 47 ± 8.4% of SA rendered polymers as precipitates that dissociated from all the complexes, as shown in Figure 4. A relatively low complex dissociation rate in an aqueous medium was also expected following lipophilic incorporation in the micellar droplets. Our complexes, characterized by the long hydrocarbon SA with insoluble lipophilic Eudragit polymers featuring a tested $Log\ P_{n\text{-}octanol/water} > 5$, were found to be sufficiently lipophilic. Moreover, this enhanced lipophilicity ensured the ability to anchor lipophilic complexes within the micellar hydrophobic core, resembling the lipophilicity of the n-octanol phase. Therefore, micelles preserving stabilized complexes over a relatively long period of time were responsible for significant time-dependent changes in the zeta potential throughout the study.

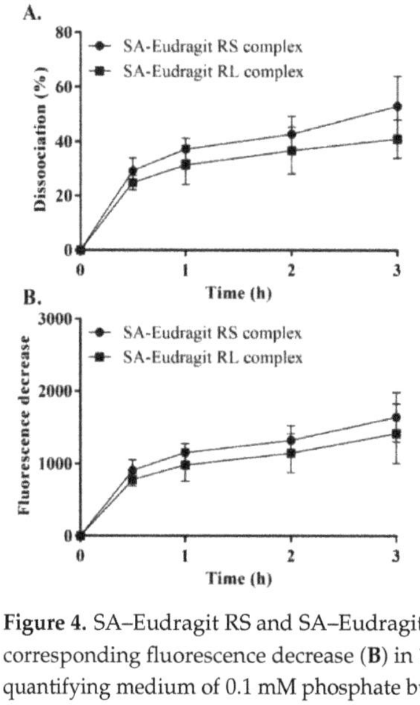

Figure 4. SA–Eudragit RS and SA–Eudragit RL: pure complex dissociation percentage (**A**) and the corresponding fluorescence decrease (**B**) in 1 mM phosphate buffer (pH 6.8) following dilution in a quantifying medium of 0.1 mM phosphate buffer (pH 6.8) containing 0.001% fluorescein at a 1 h time interval for a duration of 3 h. Indicated values are the means ± SD ($n \geq 3$).

3.5. Release Study

The micellar release profiles according to Figure 5 are presented as the released SA percentages corresponding to a fluorescence intensity decrease against time in a fluorescently sensitive aqueous phase at 37 °C. As shown in Figure 5a,b, when SA presented a 25-fold-higher molar equivalence than the micellar Eudragit RS/RL, up to 77.1 ± 5.6% of the released SA (assessed at 30 min) exhibited a rapid release kinetics. As a function of decreasing the pH, Washington and Evans reported a few minutes for the release of >90% free arachidic acid describing a relatively long hydrocarbon fatty acid from submicron emulsion in an aqueous medium [16].

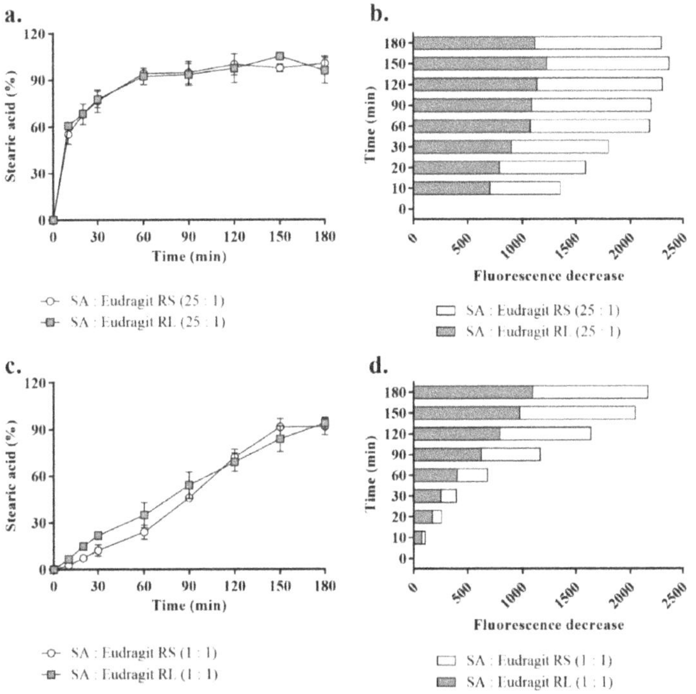

Figure 5. The profiles of SA release from SA-polymer complexes featuring SA-to-polymer ratios of 25:1 with Eudragit RS/RL as a percentage (**a**) and the corresponding fluorescence decrease (**b**) and those of complexes with a SA-to-polymer ratio of 1:1 as a percentage (**c**) and the corresponding fluorescence decrease (**d**) after 1:100 dilution in a release medium of 0.1 mM phosphate buffer (pH 6.8) containing 0.001% fluorescein, taken at 30 min time intervals for 180 min at 37 °C. A 1:1 versus 25:1 SA-to-Eudragit RS/RL ratio led to a significantly greater sustained release of SA ($p \leq 0.001$). Indicated values are the means ± SD ($n \geq 3$).

In another study, Torotta et al. also observed the immediate release of the free acidic species indomethacin (log P = 4.27) from micro-emulsions as a function of decreasing pH (monitored with a conventional pH electrode) [34]. Data obtained from these two studies proved that acidic dissociation of poorly soluble acidic species in aqueous media to a large extent enhanced their solubility by showing optimum release. Similarly, as the aim of the present study was to recover a polymeric cationic charge of the micellar droplet by releasing SA, acidic dissociation of free SA was ensured through micellar droplet direct contact with the ionic strength of the aqueous medium. In parallel, the complexed portion of SA showed slower release. The permanently charged ammonium substructures from these two polymers independent of pH formed a sufficiently strong ionic interaction with SA [19,35]. In the subsequent time points, more of the complexed SA released from micelles at a slow rate with > 95% free and complex micellar SA released at 180 min. However, the complexed portion of micellar SA in a ratio of 25:1 to the polymer between time points highlighted insignificant increases in the released SA percentages according to Figure 5a,b. To highlight significant changes in fluorescence decreases (released SA) between the time points, equal amounts of micellar SA were introduced through micellar complexes with the polymers at a 1:1 ratio. Based on this used ratio, the lower portion of Figure 5c,d compared the most consistent SA release profiles representing a significantly sustained release ($p \leq 0.001$). The release behavior, showing a slow dissociation of the SA complex portion, was crucial for observing a positive shift in the micellar droplet zeta potential caused by the cationic moiety of the complex polymer in a controlled manner. The use of excess SA ensured the longer-term stability of the complexes and favored slower dissociation from the permanently charged non-releasing Eudrgit. Lu et al. described a reciprocal relationship between counter ions in a way that increases the ratio of the model drug to the polymer or vice versa, encouraging longer stability of the other counterpart within nanoemulsions dispersed in a release medium [36].

Furthermore, in this study, the ionic strength of the release medium at pH 6.8 with the dissolved fluorescein (0.001%) was reduced in the magnitude of 10^{-1} multiplication. After observing a change in the pH to around ~6.2 at 0.1 mM ionic strength, it was adjusted to 6.8 using sodium hydroxide. This change ensured that the phosphate buffer medium at 0.1 mM would not mask pH changes reflecting the release of SA [16]. Figure 6 shows the calibration curve of the used SA concentrations, indicating linearity with an r^2 of 0.99 ± 0.002.

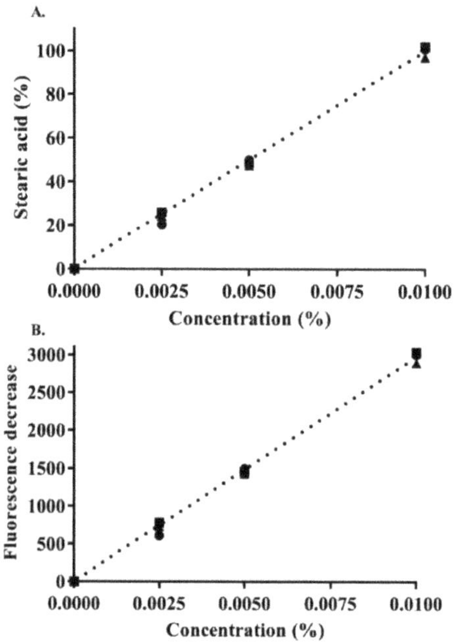

Figure 6. Concentration-dependent SA calibration curve: SA percentage (**A**) as a function of the decrease in fluorescence (**B**) in 0.1 mM phosphate buffer (pH 6.8) containing 0.001% fluorescein. Indicated values are the means ± SD ($n \geq 3$).

At the point that releasing SA stabilized, the release medium verifying > 5 pH indicated further quenching of ionically transformed fluorescein as dianion (phenolic p*K*a ~ 6.5) or monoanion (carboxylic p*K*a ~4) was still feasible with increasing SA (carboxylic p*K*a = 4.75) concentrations [37,38]. To accomplish this, up to 20% acetic acid in a fresh release medium completely vanished any fluorescent properties checked physically and instrumentally after measuring fluorescence. Provided that the p*K*a of releasing SA was not approached in the release medium, quantifying a larger concentration of SA was possible, as it depends on quenching fluorescein demonstrating lower p*K*a. Moreover, SA concentration from the used micellar dilutions having predictable quantification in the release medium in referral to its calibration curve did not form micellar structures and was significantly below its previously reported CMC [13]. Therefore, it can be concluded that the unreached saturation, predictable acid dissociation, and the concentration-dependence of fluorescence sensitivity to SA justified the choice of the release medium [16].

3.6. Zeta-Potential Changes

The average zeta potential of SA-polymer complex-loaded micellar droplets at time zero was determined to be −5.4 mV, as shown in Figure 7. Within a 3 h follow-up time, the first positive change in the zeta potential of +0.72 mV was observed for micellar complexes at 150 min, and a further zeta-potential increase to +1.8 mV was minimally observed at 180 min, after which the micellar droplets' zeta potential stabilized. These zeta-potential values were in the range of −10 to +2 mV, with the lower limit characteristic of a blank micellar dispersion and the upper limit attributed solely to the micellar load of the polymers excluding SA by assuming its full release. The zeta-potential values exhibited by the micelles separately loading these polymers without SA were similar, as both of the polymers were used in charge-equimolar concentrations. Moreover, the use of non-ionic surfactants was necessary. However, further analyses were necessary to refine the surfactant choice to a PEGylated type, such as the Kolliphor type reported to show a negative droplet surface charge [39,40]. Additionally, we observed well-adapted zeta-potential changes corresponding to the added concentrations of cationic polymers dissolved in these micellar surfactants. Therefore, the polymers were adjusted to the lowest possible concentration in the micelles able to provide a positive read and remain masked from excess SA for a considerable duration in the buffer medium. Conversely, the use of SA equivalent from the polymers demanded significantly larger concentrations of the related cationic property that cannot be sufficiently neutralized by the equivalent SA carboxylate. Therefore, micelles loading complexes of equivalent polymeric charge to SA showed significant positive charge transformations in the aqueous medium shortly after dispersion.

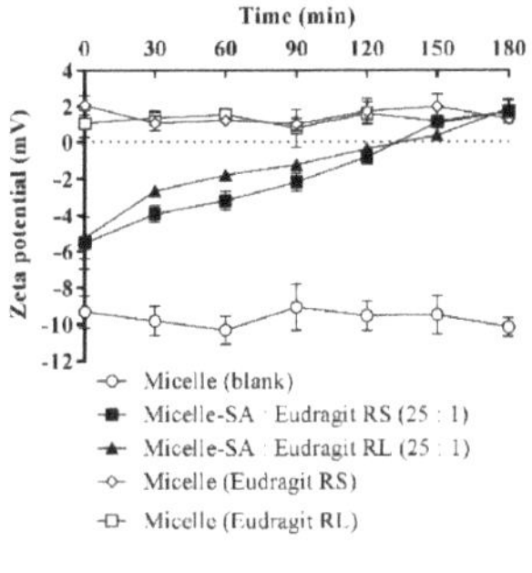

Figure 7. Time-dependent zeta-potential changes of micellar droplets containing SA-polymer complexes featuring a SA-to-polymer ratio of 25:1 with Eudragit RS/RL after 1:100 dilution in 10 mM phosphate buffer (pH 6.8), at 30 min time intervals for 180 min at 37 °C. Zeta-potential values of the blank micelle and micelles containing the same polymer amount used in micellar complexes without SA were also assessed after 1:100 dilution in the buffer. Indicated values are the means ± SD ($n \geq 3$).

3.7. Mucus Permeation

The zeta-potential-changing micellar droplets were evaluated in vitro for their diffusion capacity through the intestinal mucus using Transwell diffusion. Figure 8 illustrates dilutions from different micellar complexes and the blank micelle in a 0.1 M buffer (pH 6.80) at 37 °C having an average of 58.2 ± 3.7% of the model drug FDA diffused in the mucus over 4 h.

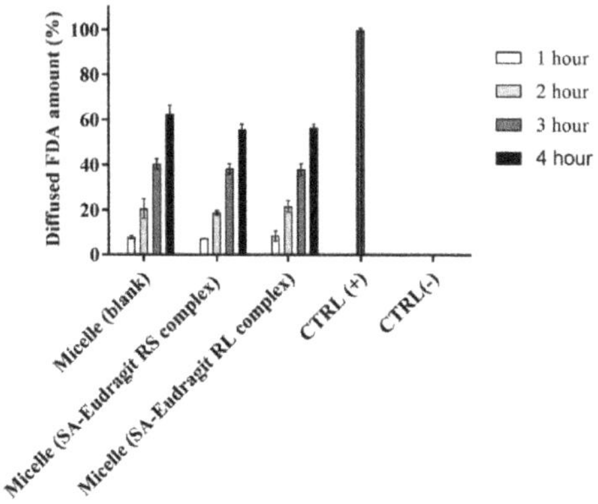

Figure 8. Diffusion behavior of micellar droplets loaded with 0.2% FDA through the intestinal porcine mucus as a blank or containing SA-polymer complexes after 1:100 dilution in 0.1 M phosphate buffer (pH 6.8) for 4 h at 37 °C. Indicated values are the means ± SD ($n \geq 3$).

Generally, several factors must be considered for the efficient muco-permeation of the dispersed nanoemulsion in an aqueous medium, including the droplet size, the droplet surface charge or zeta potential, and the type of excipients forming the nanodroplets [3,41]. The relatively small micellar droplet size was exploited in significantly high muco-permeation of the model drug FDA. The inverse relation between nanoemulsion droplet size and muco-permeation has been described by Friedl et al. In their study, nanoemulsions showing droplet size of 12 nm diffused up to 70% of the model drug through the mucus which was significantly larger than the diffused model drug amount of 8% from relatively large droplets bearing a 455 nm droplet size. They further showed that increasing the proportion of specific excipients such as Kolliphor forming PEGylated corona in aqueous media provides the ultimate flexible and deforming shape of the droplets diffusing the mucus gel layer [42]. Our evaluation utilizing 45% micellar excipients from the Kolliphor source led to efficient muco-permeation. Other research also provided conclusive evidence regarding the aforementioned study [2,43]. Because of droplet size spotting an average below the reported average mucus pore size of 20–200 nm, other factors hindering micellar droplets traversing the mucus could be overcome [41]. On the other hand, the zeta potential exhibited by nanodroplets strongly influences their muco-permeation. The composition of mucin fibers from negatively charged proteoglycans forming the mucus displays selectivity towards the positively charged droplets electrostatically interacting with the mucus, causing major entrapment and poor permeation [8,39]. On the contrary, the diffusion of neutral or particularly negatively charged droplets repelling electrostatic interactions with the mucus is favorable [8]. The amount of zeta-potential-changing micelles penetrating the mucus compared to blank micelle highlighted the insignificant differences. The exhibited negative charge by the zeta-potential-changing micellar droplets lasting sufficiently long helps mitigating interactions with negatively charged mucus components [5]. Therefore, changing the negative zeta potential of studied permeating micellar droplets taking considerable time could explain their similar muco-permeation profiles to that of negatively charged blank micellar droplets not changing the zeta potential. Moreover, shifting the zeta potential of the droplets having already penetrated the mucus to a positive value desirably prolongs their contact time with the underlying absorptive mucosal epithelium for efficient cellular uptake by the means of preventing back-diffusion [10]. It can be concluded that micellar droplets achieved the desired zeta-potential changes while effectively permeating the mucus in a time-dependent manner.

3.8. Cellular Uptake

Intestinal absorption by mucosal epithelium accounts for another barrier hindering the mucosal drug delivery of nanoemulsions, especially those exhibiting a negative charge at the droplet surface [44]. As the time for human intestinal mucosal turnover is 4–6 h, nanodroplets shifting the zeta potential to a positive value within this time are desired for cellular uptake [2,45]. Therefore, the achieved positive zeta-potential changes from the studied micellar droplets in 150–180 min (Section 3.6) allowed sufficient time for cellular uptake.

Figure 9 illustrates significantly higher Caco-2 cellular uptake of the zeta-potential-changing micelles by ~2.2-fold ($p \leq 0.01$) from micellar droplets loading SA-Eudragit RS/RL hydrophobic complexes as compared to the blank micelle after 4 h. The permanently negative zeta potential of -10 mV for the blank micelle shifted to a less negative value following SA-polymer complex incorporation and showed further transformation to a positive value upon SA release. This dramatic shift in the zeta potential enhanced micellar droplets' cellular uptake from 31.7 ± 3% to 68.9 ± 4.9%.

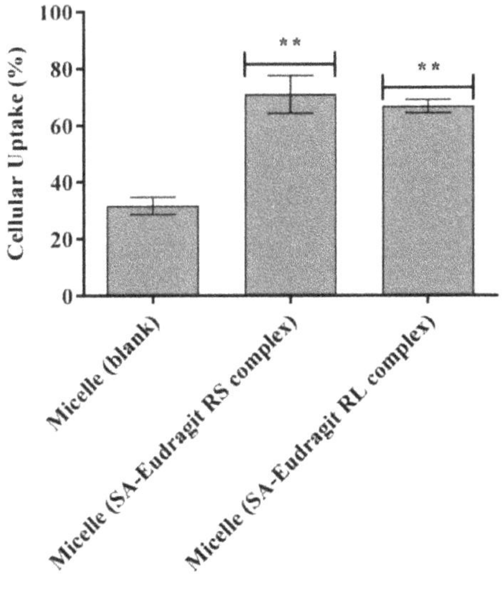

Figure 9. Cellular uptake of FDA-labeled micelles as blank or loaded with SA-polymer complexes after 4 h at 37 °C. ** $p \leq 0.01$ indicates significant differences regarding SA–Eudragit RS and SA–Eudragit RL complex-loaded micelles versus the blank micelle. Indicated values are the means of at least three experiments ± SD.

The enhanced cellular uptake of the zeta-potential-changing system has been proven in the literature. The majority of these systems employed cleavable anionic phosphate sub-structures from a backbone lipophilic domain, spiking the zeta-potential-changing nanodroplet by the action of alkaline phosphatase (AP). Applying these nanodroplets having phosphate groups already cleaved in aqueous media, however, was strongly linked to poor permeation of the mucus [2,12,40]. A previous evaluation incorporating 1% of a phosphorylated product of the structure N,N′-Bis (polyoxyethylene) oleylamine in SEDDS showed potent zeta potential change from -15.1 mV to +6.5 mV by the mean of phosphate cleavage following incubation with the AP release medium. This change in zeta potential was desired for enhancing cellular uptake of the AP-pretreated SEDDS but significantly lowered the amount of AP-non-pretreated SEDDS, permeating the mucus to one-third [40]. Moreover, the stringent need of these systems nevertheless to in vitro pretreatment with AP may pose to in vivo variability induced by fluctuations in intestinal enzymatic secretions.

Within the study, the zeta-potential-changing micelles releasing SA from regenerated anionic-exchange resins offered a dual action in terms of enhancing cellular uptake after efficient permeation of the mucus. Our approach changing the zeta potential independent of enzymatic activity therefore could be of practical relevance for in vivo applications.

4. Conclusions

The blank micelle and the zeta-potential-changing micelles loading anionic SA as hydrophobic ionic complexes with the cationic polymers Eudragit RS and Eudragit RL showed an average CMC of 312 μg/mL, a uniform droplet size of 14.2 nm, and a stability of < 0.1 PDI. Micelles diluted up to 1:100 in physiological medium proved no cytotoxicity on Caco-2 cells. Micellar release combined excess free SA relatively quickly, and SA from the complex was released in an adequately sustained manner. This release pattern caused a significant time-dependent change in the micellar droplet zeta potential, shifting from −5.4 to +1.8 mV. Conversely, blank micellar droplets showed a permanently negative zeta potential of −10 mV. Zeta-potential-changing micellar droplets were shown to be significant, with comparable diffusion behavior between the intestinal porcine mucus and blank micellar droplets. However, they also presented up to a 2.2-fold significantly higher cellular uptake ($p \leq 0.01$) compared to the blank micelles. Due to the slow and time-dependent changes in zeta potential, micellar droplets, therefore, offer dual benefits in drug delivery by achieving both optimal mucus-permeating properties and significant cellular uptake.

Author Contributions: Conceptualization, A.M.; Data curation, N.A. and R.A.K. Formal analysis, N.A. and R.A.K.; Methodology, A.M.; Resources, N.A.; Writing—original draft, A.M.; Writing—review & editing, N.A. and R.A.K. All authors have read and agreed to the published version of the manuscript.

Funding: Isra University (Amman, Jordan) under grant number: I.u-27-2441.

Institutional Review Board Statement: Not applicable.

Informed Consent Statement: Not applicable.

Data Availability Statement: Not applicable.

Acknowledgments: The authors are thankful and would like to extend their Acknowledgments to Isra University (Amman, Jordan) for providing fund to support this work.

Conflicts of Interest: The authors declare that they have no conflict of interest.

References

1. Zhang, H.; Zhang, J.; Streisand, J.B. Oral mucosal drug delivery: Clinical pharmacokinetics and therapeutic applications. *Clin. Pharm.* **2002**, *41*, 661–680. [CrossRef] [PubMed]
2. Nazir, I.; Fürst, A.; Lupo, N.; Hupfauf, A.; Gust, R.; Bernkop-Schnürch, A. Zeta potential changing self-emulsifying drug delivery systems: A promising strategy to sequentially overcome mucus and epithelial barrier. *Eur. J. Pharm. Biopharm.* **2019**, *144*, 40–49. [CrossRef] [PubMed]
3. Dünnhaupt, S.; Kammona, O.; Waldner, C.; Kiparissides, C.; Bernkop-Schnürch, A. Nano-carrier systems: Strategies to overcome the mucus gel barrier. *Eur. J. Pharm. Biopharm.* **2015**, *96*, 447–453. [CrossRef]
4. Prüfert, F.; Fischer, F.; Leichner, C.; Zaichik, S.; Bernkop-Schnürch, A. Development and in vitro evaluation of stearic acid phosphotyrosine amide as new excipient for zeta potential changing self-emulsifying drug delivery systems. *Pharm. Res.* **2020**, *37*, 79. [CrossRef] [PubMed]
5. Le-Vinh, B.; Le, N.N.; Nazir, I.; Matuszczak, B.; Bernkop-Schnürch, A. Chitosan based micelle with zeta potential changing property for effective mucosal drug delivery. *Int. J. Biol. Macromol.* **2019**, *133*, 647–655. [CrossRef]
6. Mohsin, K.; Alamri, R.; Ahmad, A.; Raish, M.; Alanazi, F.K.; Hussain, M.D. Development of self-nanoemulsifying drug delivery systems for the enhancement of solubility and oral bioavailability of fenofibrate, a poorly water-soluble drug. *Int. J. Nanomed.* **2016**, *11*, 2829–2838.
7. Nazir, I.; Leichner, C.; Le-Vinh, B.; Bernkop-Schnürch, A. Surface phosphorylation of nanoparticles by hexokinase: A powerful tool for cellular uptake improvement. *J. Colloid Interface Sci.* **2018**, *516*, 384–391. [CrossRef]

8. Suchaoin, W.; Pereira de Sousa, I.; Netsomboon, K.; Lam, H.T.; Laffleur, F.; Bernkop-Schnürch, A. Development and in vitro evaluation of zeta potential changing self-emulsifying drug delivery systems for enhanced mucus permeation. *Int. J. Pharm.* **2016**, *510*, 255–262. [CrossRef]
9. Köllner, S.; Dünnhaupt, S.; Waldner, C.; Hauptstein, S.; Pereira de Sousa, I.; Bernkop-Schnürch, A. Mucus permeating thiomer nanoparticles. *Eur. J. Pharm. Biopharm.* **2015**, *97*, 265–272. [CrossRef]
10. Griesser, J.; Burtscher, S.; Köllner, S.; Nardin, I.; Prüfert, F.; Bernkop-Schnürch, A. Zeta potential changing self-emulsifying drug delivery systems containing phosphorylated polysaccharides. *Eur. J. Pharm. Biopharm.* **2017**, *119*, 264–270. [CrossRef] [PubMed]
11. Salimi, E.; Le-Vinh, B.; Zahir-Jouzdani, F.; Matuszczak, B.; Ghaee, A.; Bernkop-Schnürch, A. Self-emulsifying drug delivery systems changing their zeta potential via a flip-flop mechanism. *Int. J. Pharm.* **2018**, *550*, 200–206. [CrossRef]
12. Akkus, Z.B.; Nazir, I.; Jalil, A.; Tribus, M.; Bernkop-Schnürch, A. Zeta potential changing polyphosphate nanoparticles: A promising approach to overcome the mucus and epithelial barrier. *Mol. Pharm.* **2019**, *16*, 2817–2825. [CrossRef] [PubMed]
13. Fameau, A.-L.; Ventureira, J.; Novales, B.; Douliez, J.-P. Foaming and emulsifying properties of fatty acids neutralized by tetrabutylammonium hydroxide. *Colloids Surf. A Physicochem. Eng. Asp.* **2012**, *403*, 87–95. [CrossRef]
14. Malkawi, A.; Jalil, A.; Nazir, I.; Matuszczak, B.; Kennedy, R.; Bernkop-Schnürch, A. Self-emulsifying drug delivery systems: Hydrophobic drug polymer complexes provide a sustained release in vitro. *Mol. Pharm.* **2020**, *17*, 3709–3719. [CrossRef]
15. Astafieva, I.; Zhong, X.F.; Eisenberg, A. Critical micellization phenomena in block polyelectrolyte solutions. *Macromolecules* **1993**, *26*, 7339–7352. [CrossRef]
16. Washington, C.; Evans, K. Release rate measurements of model hydrophobic solutes from submicron triglyceride emulsions. *J. Control. Release* **1995**, *33*, 383–390. [CrossRef]
17. Jones, J.W.; Gibson, H.W. Ion pairing and host−guest complexation in low dielectric constant solvents. *J. Am. Chem. Soc.* **2003**, *125*, 7001–7004. [CrossRef]
18. Kolthoff, I.M.; Reddy, T.B. Acid-base strength in dimethyl sulfoxide. *Inorg. Chem.* **1962**, *1*, 189–194. [CrossRef]
19. Kunin, R.; Winger, A.G. Liquid ion-exchange technology. *Angew. Chem. Int. Ed.* **1962**, *1*, 149–155. [CrossRef]
20. Zana, R. Ionization of cationic micelles: Effect of the detergent structure. *J. Colloid Interface Sci.* **1980**, *78*, 330–337. [CrossRef]
21. Jiang, H.; Beaucage, G.; Vogtt, K.; Weaver, M. The effect of solvent polarity on wormlike micelles using dipropylene glycol (DPG) as a cosolvent in an anionic/zwitterionic mixed surfactant system. *J. Colloid Interface Sci.* **2018**, *509*, 25–31. [CrossRef] [PubMed]
22. Anderson, M.T.; Martin, J.E.; Odinek, J.G.; Newcomer, P.P. Effect of methanol concentration on CTAB micellization and on the formation of surfactant-templated silica (STS). *Chem. Mater.* **1998**, *10*, 1490–1500. [CrossRef]
23. Jörgensen, A.M.; Friedl, J.D.; Wibel, R.; Chamieh, J.; Cottet, H.; Bernkop-Schnürch, A. Cosolvents in Self-emulsifying drug delivery systems (SEDDS): Do they really solve our solubility problems? *Mol. Pharm.* **2020**, *17*, 3236–3245. [CrossRef] [PubMed]
24. Kauffman, A.L.; Gyurdieva, A.V.; Mabus, J.R.; Eferguson, C.; Eyan, Z.; Hornby, P.J. Alternative functional in vitro models of human intestinal epithelia. *Front. Pharmacol.* **2013**, *4*, 79. [CrossRef] [PubMed]
25. Desai, H.H.; Bu, P.; Shah, A.V.; Cheng, X.; Serajuddin, A.T.M. Evaluation of cytotoxicity of self-emulsifying formulations containing long-chain lipids using Caco-2 cell model: Superior safety profile compared to medium-chain lipids. *J. Pharm. Sci.* **2020**, *109*, 1752–1764. [CrossRef]
26. Sha, X.; Yan, G.; Wu, Y.; Li, J.; Fang, X. Effect of self-microemulsifying drug delivery systems containing Labrasol on tight junctions in Caco-2 cells. *Eur. J. Pharm. Sci.* **2005**, *24*, 477–486. [CrossRef] [PubMed]
27. Kiss, L.; Walter, F.R.; Bocsik, A.; Veszelka, S.; Ózsvári, B.; Puskás, L.G.; Szabó-Révész, P.; Deli, M.A. Kinetic analysis of the toxicity of pharmaceutical excipients cremophor EL and RH40 on endothelial and epithelial cells. *J. Pharm. Sci.* **2013**, *102*, 1173–1181. [CrossRef]
28. Loh, J.W.; Saunders, M.; Lim, L.-Y. Cytotoxicity of monodispersed chitosan nanoparticles against the Caco-2 cells. *Toxicol. Appl. Pharmacol.* **2012**, *262*, 273–282. [CrossRef]
29. Pan, W.; Zhang, W.; Li, X.; Ye, T.; Chen, F.; Yu, S.; Chen, J.; Yang, X.; Yang, N.; Zhang, J.; et al. Nanostructured lipid carrier surface modified with Eudragit RS 100 and its potential ophthalmic functions. *Int. J. Nanomed.* **2014**, *9*, 4305–4315. [CrossRef]
30. Da Violante, G.; Zerrouk, N.; Richard, I.; Provot, G.; Chaumeil, J.C.; Arnaud, P. Evaluation of the cytotoxicity effect of dimethyl sulfoxide (DMSO) on Caco2/TC7 colon tumor cell cultures. *Biol. Pharm. Bull.* **2002**, *25*, 1600–1603. [CrossRef]
31. Yue, G.G.L.; Cheng, S.-W.; Yu, H.; Xu, Z.-S.; Lee, J.K.M.; Hon, P.-M.; Lee, M.Y.H.; Kennelly, E.J.; Deng, G.; Yeung, S.K.; et al. The role of turmerones on curcumin transportation and P-glycoprotein activities in intestinal Caco-2 cells. *J. Med. Food* **2012**, *15*, 242–252. [CrossRef]
32. Rajan, R.; Jain, M.; Matsumura, K. Cryoprotective properties of completely synthetic polyampholytes via reversible addition-fragmentation chain transfer (RAFT) polymerization and the effects of hydrophobicity. *J. Biomater. Sci. Polym. Ed.* **2013**, *24*, 1767–1780. [CrossRef]
33. Aguilar, J.; Roy, D.; Ghazal, P.; Wagner, E. Dimethyl sulfoxide blocks herpes simplex virus-1 productive infection in vitro acting at different stages with positive cooperativity. Application of micro-array analysis. *BMC Infect. Dis.* **2002**, *2*, 9. [CrossRef] [PubMed]
34. Trotta, M. Influence of phase transformation on indomethacin release from microemulsions. *J. Control. Release* **1999**, *60*, 399–405. [CrossRef]
35. Hauptstein, S.; Prüfert, F.; Bernkop-Schnürch, A. Self-nanoemulsifying drug delivery systems as novel approach for pDNA drug delivery. *Int. J. Pharm.* **2015**, *487*, 25–31. [CrossRef] [PubMed]

36. Lu, H.D.; Rummaneethorn, P.; Ristroph, K.; Prud'Homme, R.K. Hydrophobic ion pairing of peptide antibiotics for processing into controlled release nanocarrier formulations. *Mol. Pharm.* **2018**, *15*, 216–225. [CrossRef] [PubMed]
37. Panchompoo, J.; Aldous, L.; Baker, M.; Wallace, M.; Compton, R.G. One-step synthesis of fluorescein modified nano-carbon for Pd(ii) detection via fluorescence quenching. *Analyst* **2012**, *137*, 2054–2062. [CrossRef]
38. Stearic Acid. National Library of Medicine, National Center for Biotechnology Information. Available online: https://pubchem.ncbi.nlm.nih.gov/compound/Stearic-acid. (accessed on 15 March 2019.).
39. Efiana, N.A.; Phan, T.N.Q.; Wicaksono, A.J.; Schnürch, A.B. Mucus permeating self-emulsifying drug delivery systems (SEDDS): About the impact of mucolytic enzymes. *Colloids Surf. B Biointerfaces* **2018**, *161*, 228–235. [CrossRef] [PubMed]
40. Wolf, J.D.; Kurpiers, M.; Götz, R.X.; Zaichik, S.; Hupfauf, A.; Baecker, D.; Gust, R.; Bernkop-Schnürch, A. Phosphorylated PEG-emulsifier: Powerful tool for development of zeta potential changing self-emulsifying drug delivery systems (SEDDS). *Eur. J. Pharm. Biopharm.* **2020**, *150*, 77–86. [CrossRef]
41. Rohrer, J.; Partenhauser, A.; Hauptstein, S.; Gallati, C.M.; Matuszczak, B.; Abdulkarim, M.; Gumbleton, M.; Bernkop-Schnürch, A. Mucus permeating thiolated self-emulsifying drug delivery systems. *Eur. J. Pharm. Biopharm.* **2016**, *98*, 90–97. [CrossRef]
42. Friedl, H.; Dunnhaupt, S.; Hintzen, F.; Waldner, C.; Parikh, S.; Pearson, J.P.; Wilcox, M.D.; Bernkop-Schnurch, A. Development and evaluation of a novel mucus diffusion test system approved by self-nanoemulsifying drug delivery systems. *J. Pharm. Sci.* **2013**, *102*, 4406–4413. [CrossRef] [PubMed]
43. Netsomboon, K.; Bernkop-Schnürch, A. Mucoadhesive vs. mucopenetrating particulate drug delivery. *Eur. J. Pharm. Biopharm.* **2016**, *98*, 76–89. [CrossRef] [PubMed]
44. Bonengel, S.; Prüfert, F.; Jelkmann, M.; Bernkop-Schnürch, A. Zeta potential changing phosphorylated nanocomplexes for pDNA delivery. *Int. J. Pharm.* **2016**, *504*, 117–124. [CrossRef] [PubMed]
45. Leichner, C.; Menzel, C.; Laffleur, F.; Bernkop-Schnürch, A. Development and in vitro characterization of a papain loaded mucolytic self-emulsifying drug delivery system (SEDDS). *Int. J. Pharm.* **2017**, *530*, 346–353. [CrossRef] [PubMed]

pharmaceutics

MDPI

Article

Synthesis and Evaluation of Thiol-Conjugated Poloxamer and Its Pharmaceutical Applications

Muhammad Zaman [1,*], Sadaf Saeed [2], Rabia Imtiaz Bajwa [2], Muhammad Shafeeq Ur Rahman [1], Saeed Ur Rahman [3], Muhammad Jamshaid [1], Muhammad F. Rasool [4], Abdul Majeed [4], Imran Imran [5], Faleh Alqahtani [6,*], Sultan Alshehri [7], Abdullah F. AlAsmari [6], Nemat Ali [6] and Mohammed Alasmari [6]

1 Faculty of Pharmacy, University of Central Punjab, Lahore 54000, Pakistan; shafeeq.rahman@ucp.edu.pk (M.S.U.R.); dr.jamshaid@ucp.edu.pk (M.J.)
2 Department of Pharmaceutics, Faculty of Pharmacy, The University of Lahore, Lahore 54000, Pakistan; sadafsaeed14@gmail.com (S.S.); rabiabajwa370@gmail.com (R.I.B.)
3 Oral Biology, Institute of Basic Medical Sciences, Khyber Medical University, Peshawar 59000, Pakistan; saeed.ibms@kmu.edu.pk
4 Department of Pharmacy Practice, Faculty of Pharmacy, Bahauddin Zakariya University, Multan 60800, Pakistan; fawadrasool@bzu.edu.pk (M.F.R.); abdulmajeed@bzu.edu.pk (A.M.)
5 Department of Pharmacology, Faculty of Pharmacy, Bahauddin Zakariya University, Multan 60800, Pakistan; imran.ch@bzu.edu.pk
6 Department of Pharmacology and Toxicology, College of Pharmacy, King Saud University, Riyadh 11451, Saudi Arabia; afalasmari@ksu.edu.sa (A.F.A.); nali1@ksu.edu.sa (N.A.); 442106674@student.ksu.edu.sa (M.A.)
7 Department of Pharmaceutics, College of Pharmacy, King Saud University, Riyadh 11451, Saudi Arabia; salshehri1@ksu.edu.sa
* Correspondence: m.zaman2157@gmail.com (M.Z.); Afaleh@ksu.edu.sa (F.A.)

Citation: Zaman, M.; Saeed, S.; Imtiaz Bajwa, R.; Shafeeq Ur Rahman, M.; Rahman, S.U.; Jamshaid, M.; Rasool, M.F.; Majeed, A.; Imran, I.; Alqahtani, F.; et al. Synthesis and Evaluation of Thiol-Conjugated Poloxamer and Its Pharmaceutical Applications. *Pharmaceutics* **2021**, *13*, 693. https://doi.org/10.3390/pharmaceutics13050693

Academic Editors: Ana Isabel Fernandes and Angela Faustino Jozala

Received: 15 March 2021
Accepted: 6 May 2021
Published: 11 May 2021

Abstract: The current study was designed to convert the poloxamer (PLX) into thiolated poloxamer (TPLX), followed by its physicochemical, biocompatibilities studies, and applications as a pharmaceutical excipient in the development of tacrolimus (TCM)-containing compressed tablets. Thiolation was accomplished by using thiourea as a thiol donor and hydrochloric acid (HCl) as a catalyst in the reaction. Both PLX and TPLX were evaluated for surface morphology based on SEM, the crystalline or amorphous nature of the particles, thiol contents, micromeritics, FTIR, and biocompatibility studies in albino rats. Furthermore, the polymers were used in the development of compressed tablets. Later, they were also characterized for thickness, diameter, hardness, weight variation, swelling index, disintegration time, mucoadhesion, and in vitro drug release. The outcomes of the study showed that the thiolation process was accomplished successfully, which was confirmed by FTIR, where a characteristic peak was noticed at 2695.9968 cm^{-1} in the FTIR scan of TPLX. Furthermore, the considerable concentration of the thiol constituents (20.625 μg/g of the polymer), which was present on the polymeric backbone, also strengthened the claim of successful thiolation. A mucoadhesion test illustrated the comparatively better mucoadhesion strength of TPLX compared to PLX. The in vitro drug release study exhibited that the TPLX-based formulation showed a more rapid ($p < 0.05$) release of the drug in 1 h compared to the PLX-based formulation. The in vivo toxicity studies confirmed that both PLX and TPLX were safe when they were administered to the albino rats. Conclusively, the thiolation of PLX made not only the polymer more mucoadhesive but also capable of improving the dissolution profile of TCM.

Keywords: poloxamer; thiourea; thiolation; mucoadhesion; drug release; in vivo analysis; in vitro dissolution studies

1. Introduction

The development and evaluation of novel polymers have become the topic of interest for many years. Different polymeric excipients have been introduced to the pharmaceutical industry for the delivery of various active pharmaceutical ingredients (APIs).

Such polymers, which can enhance the efficacy, pharmacodynamics, and pharmacokinetic characteristics of different APIs, are being widely investigated as novel drug carriers in pharmaceutical research. Successful biomedical applications of pharmaceutical materials encourage scientists and researchers to explore and discover more advanced ingredients with modifiable characteristics under certain conditions. The synthetic polymeric material can be premeditated in various structures to fulfill biomedical objectives. For that reason, the acquirement of comprehensive knowledge regarding biocompatible materials is of great importance. In this respect, the applied polymers, either from natural or synthetic sources, can be modified by considering their ultimate use, like the delivery of the drug and protein and peptide and chemotherapy. Among synthetic polymers, poloxamer has found a wide range of applications because of its triblock structure. Both water-soluble and lipid-soluble constituents are present in its structure, which grants exclusive properties, including thermos-sensitivity and micellar formation [1].

One of the most promising techniques is thiolation, which is used to impart enhanced mucoadhesive properties to the polymers. The mucoadhesive drug delivery system usually intermingles with the mucin components, which are present in the mucus of the mucosal membrane. The interaction of the mucoadhesive drug delivery system with the mucus membrane prolongs the residence time at the specific site and hence provides the drug with an opportunity to get entered into the systemic circulation, ultimately enhancing the drug's bioavailability and therapeutic effect [2]. Thiolated polymers entitled "thiomers" are produced by the covalent interaction of thiol moieties to the backbone of polymers. The incorporation of such a thiol group is the main reason for the increased mucoadhesion of the polymers. Thiolated polymers are intrinsically employed as drugs [3,4]. The efficiency of thiomers largely depends on the nature and structure of the parent polymer. Usually, the mucoadhesive polymers are used for thiolation [5]. Different drugs are compounded with thiomers to increase their absorption across the mucus membrane, as there is an increase in the residence time of the drug in a specific part of the body due to prolonged adhesion. It has been found that upon thiolation, the mucoadhesive property of the polymer increases by 2–140 times [6]. Mucoadhesive drug delivery systems are important because they exhibit many advantages over other drug delivery systems, such as increased contact time with the site of absorption, improved drug permeability, and enhanced drug concentration in plasma circulation [7]. Another additional benefit of thiol-conjugated polymeric material is its ability to protect against the enzymatic degradation of certain drugs, like peptides and proteins [8]. Moreover, the thiomers have the potential to be utilized in the development of various drug delivery systems that are aimed at different routes of administration [9,10].

Tacrolimus (TCM) is an immunosuppressant that belongs to BCS class II and has a low solubility, a high permeability, and a poor bioavailability of 24% [11]. The purpose of the study was to achieve the successful thiolation of PLX, the evaluation of its physicochemical properties, the confirmation of its biocompatibility, and its application as a suitable pharmaceutical excipient in the development of a modified release compressed tablet of TCM.

2. Materials and Methods

2.1. Material

PLX and Ellman's reagent (5,5dithio-bis-(2-nitrobenzoic acid) were purchased from Sigma-Aldrich GmbH Chemie, Germany. Thiourea, methanol, potassium chloride, acetic acid, hydrochloric acid (Merck, Darmstadt, Germany), and distilled water were obtained from the research laboratory of The University of Lahore. All the chemicals and reagents used were of analytical grade.

2.2. Thiolation of PLX

The thiolation of PLX was done by using the method explained by Bernkop-Schnürch and co-worker in 2019 [3]. Briefly, the reaction was carried out in the presence of HCl as a catalyst. A 1% aqueous solution of PLX was prepared in a 100 mL glass beaker using distilled water under continuous stirring with hot plate magnetic stirrer at 500 rpm. Afterwards, 2 g of thiourea were mixed in the polymeric solution, followed by the addition of a catalytic amount of HCl (4–5 drops) to carry out the reaction. Initially, the thiourea, being a good nucleophile, and its nucleophilic reaction with HCl led to the production of an intermediate product. In the next step, the mixture was treated with alkali, which ultimately brought about the synthesis of TPLX (Figure 1). During the process, the reaction mixture was subjected to mixing for several minutes using a hot plate magnetic stirrer in order to get a homogenized mixture. Afterwards, it was kept in a water bath at 70 °C for 90 min. After the completion of the specified reaction time, the methanol was added into the mixture to cool it down. The resultant was filtered and washed again and again with HCl and distilled water to remove untreated thiourea. The final product was cooled at −80 °C and lyophilized at −47 °C and at 0.013 millibars of pressure to get a dried polymer. The freeze-dried polymer was kept in a closed container for further analysis. Both PLX and TPLX were used to prepare the modified-release tablets of TCM. A schematic representation of the synthesis of TPLX is given in Figure 1.

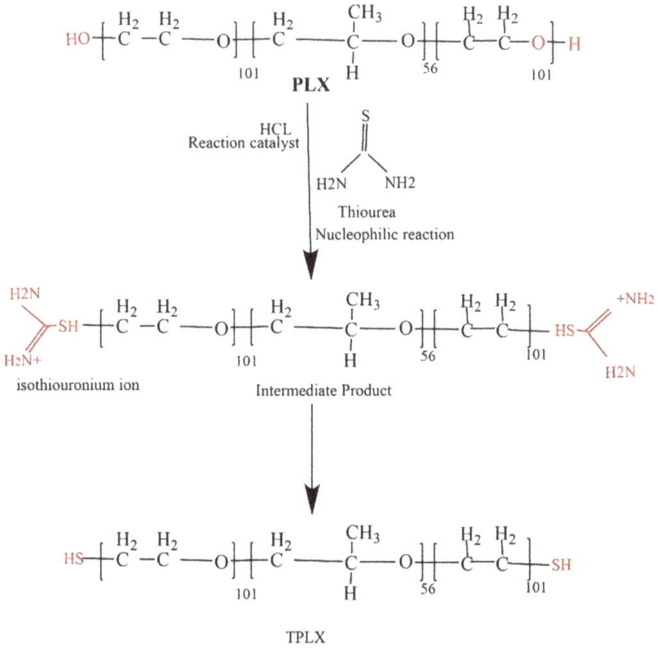

Figure 1. Schematic representation for the synthesis of TPLX using thiourea as the thiol donor.

2.3. *Physicochemical Properties of PLX and Thiolated PLX*

2.3.1. Solubility Studies and Swelling Index (SI)

PLX and TPLX were also checked for their aqueous solubility. Ten milligrams of TPLX and PLX were separately dissolved in 10 mL of water and checked for their aqueous solubility. To observe the residual insoluble material, the prepared solutions were filtered through No. 2 Whatman filter paper (Schleicher Schuell) with a pore size of 8 µm and a weight of 21 mg. After filtration, the filter paper was dried and weighed again to observe the weight gain due to the presence of any residue of the polymer on the paper's surface. One gram each of thiolated and non-thiolated polymer was taken individually in the cylinders, and the initial volume was noted. Then, water was added to make the final volume 50 mL in both cylinders. It was covered with aluminum foil and left to stand overnight. After that, the final volume was recorded, and the swelling index of the polymers was calculated using the following formula:

$$\text{Swelling index} = (\text{Final volume} - \text{Initial volume})/(\text{Initial volume}) \times 100 \quad (1)$$

2.3.2. pH of Aqueous Dispersion

The pH of thiolated and non-thiolated polymers was measured by preparing a 1% (*w*/*v*) aqueous dispersion. The probe of a pH meter (A120-Benchtop pH meter, BANTE instruments, China) was dipped in the aqueous dispersion until a constant pH was observed.

2.3.3. Loss on Drying

One gram of both thiolated and non-TPLX was taken and allowed to dry separately in a digital moisture analyzer (MOC63U Unibloc Moisture Analyzer, Shimadzu, Quezon, Japan). The drying was continued until a constant weight was achieved and the LOD was recorded.

2.3.4. Micromeritic Studies

Micromeritic parameters including bulk density, tapped density, Carr's index, Hausner's ratio, and the angle of repose were calculated for the analysis of the flow properties of the polymers [12]. The bulk density was calculated using the cylinder method. The weighed amount of polymer was poured in a graduated cylinder, and the volume was noted as the bulk volume to calculate the bulk density by comparing the mass and volume of the polymer. Similarly, the tapped density was determined by employing the tapping method, where a graduated cylinder with a known amount of polymer was tapped until a constant volume was achieved, which was noted as the tapped volume. This tapped volume was used to calculate the tapped density. The Carr's index and Hausner's ratio were calculated by using the values of bulk and tapped densities. Additionally, the angle of repose was determined by the fixed funnel method.

2.3.5. Determination of Thiol Content by Ellman's Reagent Method

The standard linearity graph of the thiourea was plotted against the concentration on the x-axis and the corresponding absorbance on the y-axis. For this purpose, 2 mg of thiourea were accurately weighed and added in a test tube to prepare a 1 mL solution using a 0.5 M phosphate buffer of pH 8.0 as the solvent. Furthermore, the serial dilutions were prepared from this solution in the concentration range of 10–100 µg/mL. The absorbance of the prepared dilutions was determined by using a UV–visible spectrophotometer (PG Instruments T80, Leicestershire, United Kingdom) at 280 nm.

The thiol contents of TPLX were determined by using Ellman's reagent technique [13]. In the 1st step, a 2% *w*/*v* solution of the polymer conjugate was prepared by dissolving it in a sufficient volume of deionized water. After that, 1350 µL of 0.1 M PBS at pH 7.4 were prepared. Then 150 µL of Ellman's reagent were prepared by dissolving 3.96 mg of reagent in 10 µL of PBS, and 150 µL of polymer conjugate were added to 1350 µL of deionized water. The mixture was incubated at room temperature for 90 min, and then its absorbance was measured at a wavelength of 412 nm with a UV spectrophotometer [14]. The amount of the thiol group attached to the polymer was determined by a thiourea calibration curve.

2.3.6. Fourier Transformed Infrared Spectroscopy (FT-IR)

FT-IR studies were performed to confirm the thiol modification of PLX. Both PLX and TPLX were taken, and the samples were scanned by using FTIR (Agilent Carry 360 FTIR, United States) in the range of 500–4000 cm^{-1} [15].

2.3.7. Surface Morphology Studies

The surface appearances of the prepared solid dispersion of thiolated and non-thiolated polymers were done by SEM. A small amount of powder was placed on the stage of SEM (JSM-6490A, Tokyo, Japan), and photographs were taken using a lens at a 1000X magnification power [16].

2.3.8. X-Ray Diffractometry (XRD)

An X-ray diffractometer (JDX-3532 JEOL Japan) was used to observe the impact of thiolation on the crystalline nature of PLX. An XRD diffractogram was plotted between the angle of diffraction (2θ) and the counts, and scanning was performed between 5 and 50° under a tube voltage of 45 kV and a tube current 40 mA [17].

2.3.9. Acute Toxicity Studies of PLX and TPLX

Acute toxicity studies of PLX and TPLX were carried out according to OECD guidelines by administering a single dose of the individual polymers to the animals as 50, 300, and 2000 mg/kg body weight of each animal [18]. Fifteen albino rats of an average weight of 150–200 g were selected from the animal house of the University of Lahore and kept in clean cages with food and water supply. The animal study was approved by the Institutional Research Ethics Committee of The University of Lahore under project file no. IREC-2019-101, dated: September, 5, 2019.

2.3.10. Preparation of Test Animal

Fifteen (15) rats were kept in clean cages in the laboratory for one week to acclimatized to the environment. These rats were then divided into 3 groups. Each group had 5 rats. Groups I and II were titled for the administration of doses of PLX and TPLX, while Group III was used as a control group and was only administered food and water. Afterwards, the animals were subjected to acute oral and dermal toxicity studies.

2.3.11. Preparation of Dose

According to OECD guidelines, the dose was prepared according to the weight of each rat and moistened with water before administration. According to the guidelines, the volume of dose should not be greater than 1 mL/100 g. The single dose given for acute toxicity was up to 2000 mg/kg of the animal. Rats were observed for the first 4 h and then after the 3rd, 7th, and 14th days of the study, and the number of rats that survived after 14 days of study was noted. On the 15th day, the animals were sacrificed for further analysis.

2.3.12. Physical Examination

Rats were examined once daily for health and any response to treatment, like changes in skin, hair, eyes, mucus membranes, and behavior, as well as convulsion, saliva production, diarrhea, sleep disorder, and coma, for 14 days.

2.3.13. Skin Irritation and Dermal Toxicities

The animals were tested for skin irritation; for this purpose, hair was removed with a razor from the skin, and 500 mg of thiolated and non-thiolated polymers were individually applied to the naked skin. Then, rats were observed on a daily basis for skin irritation and any other sort of dermal incompatibility [19]. Animals were arranged into 3 groups. One group served as a control group, while the other 2 groups were treated with thiolated and non-thiolated polymers. Three percent solutions of PLX and TPLX were individually applied to the skin of the respective animals. After the application of a 3% solution, the skin was taped with gauze and observed for different time intervals. After 24 h, the gauze was removed and hair growth was observed until the 15th day.

2.3.14. Bodyweight, Food, and Water Consumption

The body weight of rats of all the groups was recorded before and after the administration of the dose. After dosing, the weight was measured on the 7th and 14th days of the study.

2.3.15. Hematological and Biochemical Examination

Hematological and biochemical examinations were done on all the animals used in the study. Blood was taken from the posterior vena cava of the rat under anesthesia, and the samples were examined for hematological observations, including Hb, WBCs, RBCs, and platelet count. Serum was analyzed via liver function tests (LFTs), renal function tests (RFTs), and lipid profiling.

2.3.16. Relative Organ Weight (ROW)

On the 15th day, all albino rats were sacrificed. Three vital organs—the kidney, liver, and heart—were examined for the presence of any abnormality and lesion. These organs were then removed and weighed, and the relative organ weight was calculated by using the following formula [20].

$$\text{ROW} = (\text{Absolute organ weight (g)})/(\text{Body weight of mice on sacrifice day (g)}) \times 100 \quad (2)$$

Then, organs were preserved in a 10% formalin solution for histopathological investigation.

2.4. Preparation of Modified-Released Tablet of TCM

The direct compression method was used to prepare the tablets of TCM while using PLX and TPLX as polymers. The other excipients that were used in the study were talc (lubricant), magnesium stearate (glidant), lactose (diluent), polyvinyl pyrrolidone (binder), avicel at pH 102 (flow modulator), and aspartame (sweetener). All the ingredients were accurately weighed and passed through a No. 40 sieve. After that, all the excipients were added one by one into the mortar and pestle and mixed for 30 min to confirm uniform mixing. Finally, the powder blend was directly compressed by using a single punch compression machine (Table 1).

Table 1. Composition of modified-release tablets of TCM.

Ingredients	F1 (PLX) (mg)	F2 (TPLX) (mg)
TCM	4	4
Polymer	45	45
PVP k-30	7.5	7.5
Mg-Stearate	1.5	1.5
Talc	1.5	1.5
Aspartame	3	3
Avicel pH 102	87	87

2.5. Calibration Curve of TCM

A stock solution of TCM was prepared by dissolving 2 mg of TCM in 1 mL of a 7.4 pH PBS solution in a volumetric flask with a capacity of 50 mL. The standard solution was prepared by diluting 0.5 mL of stock solution in 9.5 of the solution. Then, serial dilutions were prepared in the concentration range of 10–100 μg/mL. The absorbance of all the dilutions was taken at 253 nm using a UV spectrophotometer, and a calibration curve of TCM was drawn.

2.6. Post-Compression Studies of PLX- and TPLX-Based Tablets of TCM

The following post-compression tests were performed on TCM modified-release tablets.

2.6.1. Thickness and Diameter

The diameter and thickness of tablets of F1 and F2 were measured using a vernier caliper. Twenty tablets of each formulation were selected, and then the average thickness and diameter of these 20 tablets were calculated [21].

2.6.2. Tablet Hardness and Friability Test

The ability of tablets to resist any breakage during storage, transportation, and handling is called hardness. A Monsanto hardness tester was used to measure the hardness of all formulations, and it was calculated as kilogram per centimeter square [22]. On the other hand, for the determination of friability, 10 tablets of each formulation after weighing and dusting were placed in a Friabilator at 100 rpm for 4 min (25 rpm/min). Tablets were taken out, and the total weight of the tablets was recorded. Friability was calculated by using the following equation [23].

$$\text{Friability} = (\text{Initial weight} - \text{Final weight})/(\text{Initial weight}) \times 100 \quad (3)$$

2.6.3. Weight Variation Test

The weight variation test was performed by individually weighing 20 tablets of each formulation of F1 and F2 on an analytical balance and then taking the average weight of these 20 tablets. The final values were compared to the USP pharmacopeia limits [24].

$$\text{W.V} = (\text{IW} - \text{AW})/\text{AW} \times 100 \quad (4)$$

2.6.4. Disintegration Test

A disintegration test was carried out in the disintegration apparatus (Microprocessor Disintegration Test Apparatus, JL-DTA-2213). Six tablets from each formulation (F1 and F2) were placed in the basket, which was filled with distilled water and maintained at temperature 37 ± 2 °C. In the end, the basket was lifted and checked for disintegration. The disintegration time of 6 individual tablets was determined, and the average time was recorded [25].

2.6.5. Swelling Index

The swelling index was calculated to determine the ability of the tablet to absorb and retain the liquid. The weight of each tablet was measured (W1) and then separately placed on slides. The weight of the slide was tarred and placed in a petri dish. Five milliliters of PBS at 7.4 pH was added, and swelling studies were performed. The glass slides containing tablets were removed from the petri dish, the excess of the solution was removed with the help of filter paper, and then the weight was measured after different time intervals (15 min, 30 min, 45 min, 1 h, 2 h, 4 h, 6 h, 8 h, and 24 h) until a constant weight was achieved. The swelling index was measured by using the following equation.

$$\text{SI} = (\text{W2} - \text{W1})/\text{W1} \times 100 \quad (5)$$

where W1 is the initial weight and W2 is the final weight [26].

2.6.6. In Vitro Dissolution

The paddle method was used to determine the release rate of the drug from thiolated and non-thiolated polymer-based tablets of TCM. A 900 mL 7.4 pH buffer solution was used as the dissolution media. Tablets were transferred and continuously stirred at 50 rpm under the maintained temperature condition of 37 ± 5 °C. Next, 5 mL samples were withdrawn after specified time intervals of 2 min, 5 min, 10 min, 15 min, 20 min, 30 min, 1 h, 2 h, 4 h, 6 h, and 8 h. The solution was replaced with fresh dissolution media to maintain the sink condition. The absorption of these samples was recorded at 253 nm using a UV–visible spectrophotometer. A curve of the percentage of drug release against time was drawn to observe the drug release pattern [27].

2.6.7. Drug Content

A standard solution of TCM was prepared by dissolving 4 mg of the pure drug in a phosphate-buffered solution (PBS) of pH 7.4 in 100 mL volumetric flasks. On the other hand, ten (10) tablets of each formulation of TCM were taken and crushed individually, and the mass of the crushed powder equivalent to 4 mg of the drug was taken and dissolved in a 100 mL volumetric flask containing PBS of pH 7.4. These solutions were analyzed on a UV spectrophotometer at a wavelength of 253 nm, and then the dissolution factor was applied and drug contents were calculated by the following formula.

$$\% \text{ Drug content} = (\text{Absorbance of sample})/(\text{Absorbance of standard}) \times (\text{Concentration of standard})/(\text{Concentration of sample}) \quad (6)$$

2.6.8. Mucoadhesion Strength

Prepared tablets were subjected to the determination of mucoadhesion strength by using a modified physical balance that consisted of two pans. Three glass slides were taken and attached to the pan in such a way that one slide was stuck to the bottom of the pan and the second one was right beneath that pan. The third slide was placed on the other pan to tare the balance (Figure 2). Mucosa pieces of rabbit were taken and cut into pieces. Mucosa pieces were then placed on the glass slides. A compressed tablet was taken and individually placed between the pieces of the mucosa that was attached to slides 1 and 2. The tablet was gently pressed between the pieces of the mucosa to properly attach. A force of 50 gm was applied to the second pan, and this was gradually increased until slides 1 and 2 were separated from each other. The mucoadhesion strength was calculated for each formulation and reported [28].

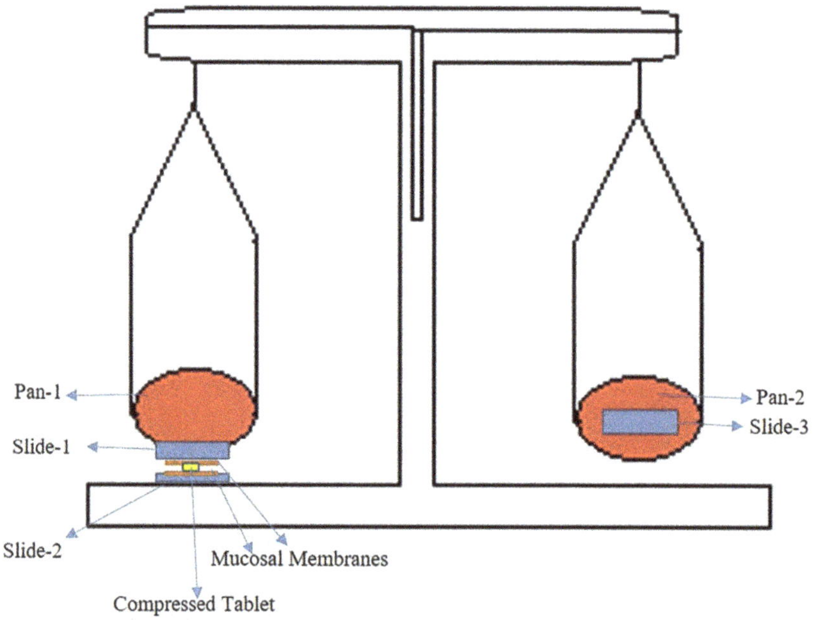

Figure 2. Graphical representation for the determination of mucoadhesion strength of tablets by sandwiching them between glass slides mounted with pieces of mucosal membranes.

2.7. Statistical Analysis

Statistical analysis was conducted to evaluate the drug release profiles of F1, F2, and marketed products. For this purpose, an ANOVA was applied followed by Tukey's multiple comparison test at a level of significance of 95%.

3. Results

3.1. Physicochemical Evaluation of PLX and TPLX

The physicochemical properties of PLX and TPLX were evaluated, and a comparison was made between thiolated and non-thiolated polymers.

The solubility of thiolated and non-TPLX was checked in water. Both PLX and TPLX are soluble in water. The weight of the filter paper after drying was approximately the same (21.003 mg) as observed before filtration (21 mg).

The swelling index of both PLX and TPLX was checked, and it was observed that they did not show considerable swelling abilities. When the polymers were exposed to water for the swelling study, they initially showed swelling (≈3.03%) to some extent but later dissolved, making it difficult to further measure the swelling index.

Similarly, for the determination of pH, 1% *w*/*v* solutions of PLX and TPLX were separately prepared. The outcomes of the study showed that the pH values of PLX and TPLX were 7.85 and 6.68, respectively. On the other hand, the loss on drying for PLX and TPLX were calculated to be 1.4% and 11.2%, respectively (Table 2).

Table 2. Physicochemical properties of PLX and thiolated PLX.

Parameters	PLX ± S.D	TPLX ± S.D
Solubility	Soluble	Soluble
pH (1% Solution)	7.85 ± 0.04	6.68 ± 0.02
Loss on drying (%)	1.4 ± 0.03	11.2 ± 0.04

3.2. Micromeritics

The micromeritic properties of PLX and TPLX were observed and compared to check the flowability of the polymers. The bulk density and tapped density of PLX were calculated to be 0.466 and 0.523 cm^3/mL, respectively. On the other hand, the Hausner's ratio and Carr's index were found to be 1.16 and 10.9, respectively. The value of the angle of repose for PLX was found to be 25.78. These results confirmed that the flow properties of PLX were good, whereas the bulk density and tapped density of TPLX were found to be 0.505 and 0.566 cm^3/mL. The Hausner's ratio, Carr's index, and angle of repose were calculated to be 1.15, 10.7, and 21.80, respectively, exhibiting excellent flow properties (Table 3).

Table 3. Micromeritics analysis of PLX and TPLX.

Parameters	PLX ± S.D (n = 5)	TPLX ± S.D (n = 5)
Bulk Density (g/cm^3)	0.466 ± 0.002	0.505 ± 0.003
Tapped Density (g/cm^3)	0.523 ± 0.002	0.566 ± 0.001
Hausner's Ratio	1.16 ± 0.017	1.15 ± 0.013
Carr's Index (%)	10.9 ± 0.0215	10.7 ± 0.020
Angle of Repose (°)	25.78 ± 0.09	21.80 ± 0.201

3.3. Thiol Contents

The thiolation of the polymers was done by reacting PLX with thiourea. A thiol group attached to the polymeric backbone was confirmed by Ellman's reagent method, as analyzed on a spectrophotometer. Ellman's reagent was used to determine the thiol content present in the polymers. The thiol content of TPLX was found to be 20.625 µg/g of the polymer. The presence of the thiol group confirmed the successful thiolation.

3.4. Calibration Curve of Thiourea

Different dilutions of thiourea, ranging from 10 to 100 µg using a 2 mg/mL stock solution, were prepared. These dilutions were analyzed on a UV–visible spectrophotometer at a wavelength of 280 nm. A linear calibration curve was obtained by plotting concentration µg/mL along the x-axis and absorbance along the y-axis (Supplementary Figure S1).

3.5. FTIR Studies

Thiolated and non-thiolated polymers were subjected to FTIR analysis, which revealed the successful thiolation of polymers. In comparison to PLX, TPLX showed a characteristic peak at 2695.9968 cm^{-1} that confirmed the attachment of a thiol moiety to the polymer. A C–O stretch was seen at 1079.9415 cm^{-1}, and an N–H bend was observed at a wavenumber of 1610.2699 cm^{-1}, which was due to the amine group of thiourea (Figure 3).

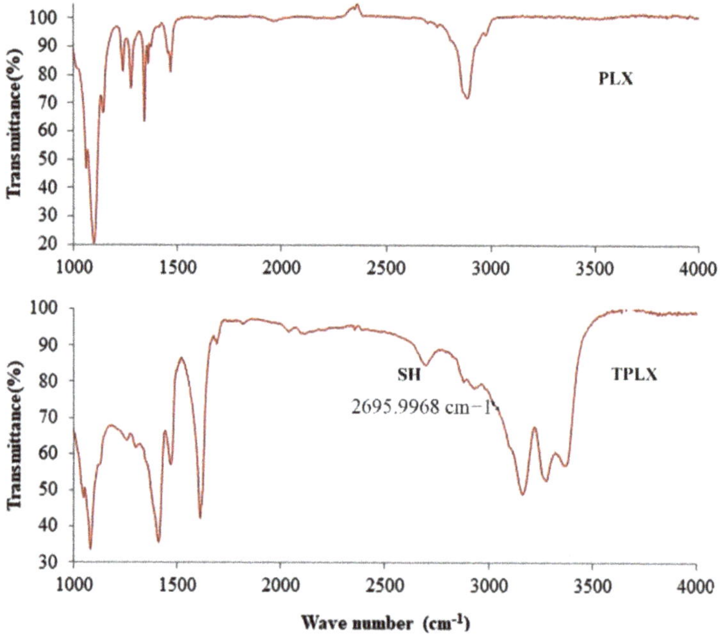

Figure 3. Comparative illustration through FTIR scans of both LX and TPLX, confirming the occurrence of chemical changes in the structure of PLX. The appearance of the characteristic peak in the scan of TPLX at 2695.9968 cm^{-1} indicated the successful modification of the polymer.

3.6. Scanning Electron Microscope (SEM)

SEM images of PLX illustrated a crystalline and shiny surface, whereas when the thiol group was attached to the polymer, distinct changes in the surface were noticed. Apparently, they seem to be more compact but irregular in shape. Figure 4 confirms the observed changes in the surface morphology of PLX.

3.7. XRD Studies

The effect of thiolation on the crystalline structure was observed using an XRD diffractogram. The XRD diffraction spectra of PLX exhibited sharp peaks at diffraction angles (2θ) 180 and 220 and a less intense peak at 260. However, peaks were also observed in the diffractogram of TPLX, but their intensity was reduced to a greater extent (Figure 5).

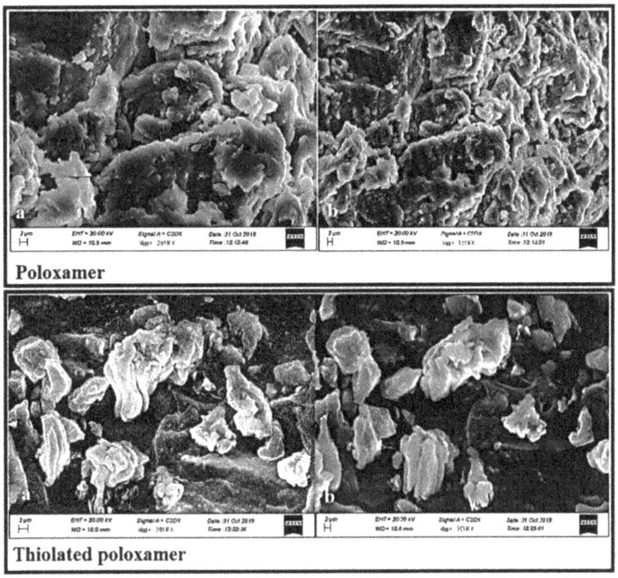

Figure 4. SEM images describing the surface morphology of PLX and TPLX at different magnifications (**a**) 1000X and (**b**) 500X. A change in the apparent surface morphology of TPLX can be observed, thus indicating the chemical modification of PLX.

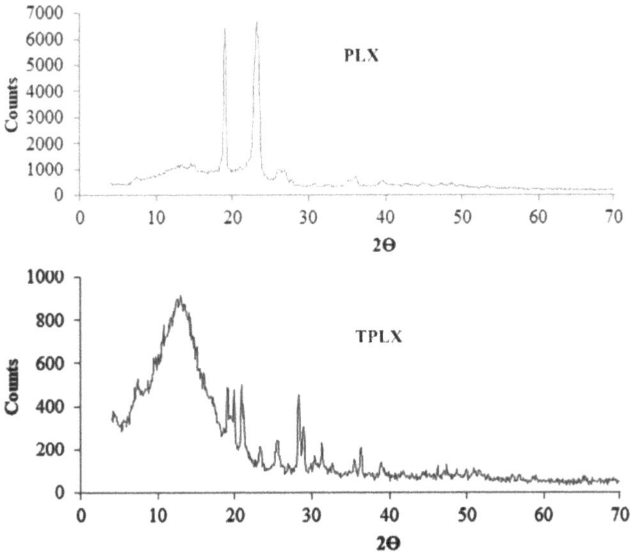

Figure 5. XRD diffractogram of PLX and TPLX exhibiting various peaks between 20 and 40. Sharp peaks present in the structure of PLX was found to be diminished in the graph of TPLX, indicating a noticeable change in its structure upon thiolation.

3.8. Acute Toxicity Studies of PLX and Thiolated PLX

3.8.1. Physical Examination

After treatment, the physical examination showed that the animals were found to be normal. The skin was intact, and normal hair growth and eye color were noted. After the oral administration of the contents, no abnormal behavior was observed during the study because normal gate, food intake, and water drinking were witnessed. Moreover, neither diarrheal conditions (as normal stools have been observed) nor any other abdominal discomfort was observed.

3.8.2. Skin Irritation and Dermal Toxicity

The albino rats did not show any toxic effects—not even skin irritation or signs of dermal toxicities were observed. The outcomes revealed that both the treated and normal groups exhibited similar findings, as no skin irritation or any sort of dermal toxicities from the 1st hour to the 14th day of the study were found.

3.8.3. Body Weight, Food, and Water Consumption

All the groups except for the control group were orally administered with a 2 mL solution of modified and unmodified polymers to perform a single-dose toxicity study.

Bodyweight of control and tested rats were observed before dosing, and then after 1, 3, 7, and 14 days right before their necropsy procedure. A gradual weight change was observed for tested animals in the first seven days. Later on, the weight continued to improve until the last day (Table 4).

Table 4. Bodyweight, hematology, and blood chemistry of albino rats.

Sr. No	Animals Group Test	Group 1	Group 2	Group 3
	Clinical observations	Nil	Nil	Nil
1	Body weight (g)			
	1st day	152	153	175
	3rd day	14	145	174
	7th day	149	148	174
	14th day	150	151	175
2	Hematology (Hb (g/dL) (10–15 g/dL)	12.6	13.4	14.2
	Total WBCs ($\times 10^3$ µL)	8.7	7.8	9.6
	RBC's ($\times 10^6$ µL)	7.11	6.56	6.7
	Platelets ($\times 10^3$ µL)	691	740	934
3	Blood chemistry			
	Liver profile			
	AST (U/L)	111	134	148
	ALT (U/L)	35	39	40
	ALP2S (U/L)	128.2	127.1	129
	Bilirubin(mg/dL)	0.05	0.05	0.04
	Total protein (g/dL)	6.2	5.4	6.4
	Renal profile			
	Urea (mg/dL)	25	28	25
	Creatinine (mg/dL)	0.4	0.3	0.3

footer Content.(All values are expressed as mean; $n = 3$).

3.8.4. Hematological and Biochemical Examination

All the data obtained from blood chemistry and hematology indicated no abnormal values, hence proving that no toxic effect was observed during the acute toxicity study arranged for 14 days. Blood profiles observed during the study included complete blood count, renal profile, and kidney profile. The results disclosed that both PLX and TPLX were safe for in vivo use.

3.8.5. Necropsy

Necropsy was done on the 15th day on all rats. To check any kind of abnormal effects, three organs, i.e., kidney, heart, and liver, were observed. The necropsy showed that all the organs were normal in appearance.

3.8.6. Relative Organ Weight

After dissection, the relative organ weight of animals was calculated. All the weights noted were in the normal range and expressed as the mean of n = 3 (Table 5).

Table 5. Relative organ weight.

Organ(s)	Control (g)	PLX (g)	TPLX (g)
Heart	0.411	0.417	0.413
Liver	3.690	3.751	3.735
Kidney	0.406	0.399	0.393

3.8.7. Histopathological Evaluation

The three vital organs were selected as the heart, liver, and kidney from all groups. After washing with normal saline preserved in a 10% formalin solution for further histopathological investigation, vital organ tissues were stained with hematoxylin and eosin for evaluation purposes (Figure 6). Images of vital organs of control and treated animals were taken at a magnification power of 400X. Histopathological evaluation showed that the observed vital organs (heart, liver, and kidney) of all the animals, placed in different groups, were found to be unaffected. The cardio-myocytes, hepatic cells, and renal tissues of both treated groups were comparable to those of the control group. No signs of toxicity, swelling, inflammation, or damaged cells were noticed during histopathological observation. Hence, the findings confirmed that both modified and unmodified polymers might be employed in the development of oral dosage forms for the delivery of TCM.

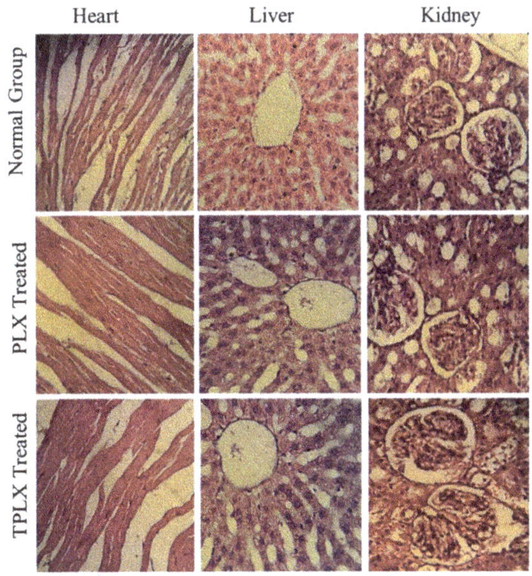

Figure 6. Histopathological evaluation of control group, PLX-treated group, and TPLX-treated group, illustrating the safety profile of modified and unmodified polymers. All the vital organs had normal physiological and anatomical features.

3.9. Preparation of Modified-Release Tablets of TCM

Modified release tablets of TCM using PLX were prepared by the direct compression method. A net weight of 150 mg, amounting to 4 mg of the drug, were kept for the formulation. The other included excipients were polyvinyl pyrrolidone as a binder, magnesium stearate as a glidant, aspartame as a sweetener, avicel at a pH of 102 as a diluent, and talc as a lubricant.

3.10. Calibration Curve of TCM

Different dilutions of TCM, ranging in concentration from 10 to 100 µg/mL using a 2 mg/mL stock solution. These dilutions were analyzed on a UV–visible spectrophotometer at a wavelength of 253 nm. A linear calibration curve was obtained by plotting concentration (µg/mL) along the x-axis and absorbance along the y-axis. The coefficient of correlation (R^2) was 0.9922, describing the good linearity of the standard graph (Supplementary Figure S2).

3.11. Post-Compression Tests

TCM tablets of the F1 and F2 formulations were tested for thickness, diameter, hardness, friability, weight variation, disintegration, in vitro drug release, swelling index, and drug content.

3.11.1. Diameter and Thickness

Thickness and diameter were measured using a Vernier caliper. The mean diameters for the F1 and F2 formulations were found to be 1.1 ± 0.08 and 1.1 ± 0.073 mm, respectively. Thickness was found to be 0.5 ± 0.009 mm for F1 and 0.6 ± 0.147 mm for F2. The negligible value of standard deviation showed that the tablets of both the formulations were uniform in thickness and diameter.

3.11.2. Hardness and Friability Test

A Monsanto hardness tester was used to determine the mechanical strength of the PLX- and TPLX-based tablets. The hardness was found to be 4.1–4.25 ± 0.234 kg/cm^3 for F1 and 4.1–4.2 ± 0.132 for F2. Similarly, the tablets were found to be of good mechanical strength, as the friability was found to be less than 1% for both formulations.

3.11.3. Weight Variation Test

Twenty (20) tablets from each formulation (F1 and F2) were used to report variation among the weight of the tablets. The average weights of the PLX and TPLX-based tablets were found to be 148–160 and 145–162 mg, respectively. The average weight was calculated and compared to the individual weight of the tablets. The results satisfied the USP specification of ±10%.

3.11.4. Disintegration

Six (6) tablets of formulations F1 and F2 were allowed to disintegrate in the disintegration apparatus. The time taken by the tablets to completely disintegrate was noted and compared. The F1 and F2 formulations took 9 ± 0.07 and 10 ± 0.08 min, respectively, to disintegrate.

3.11.5. Swelling Studies

The potential of the polymer to absorb and retain moisture was found via swelling studies. Tablets based on PLX and TPLX showed gradual increases in swelling. Swelling was observed until the constant weight was achieved. It was observed that after an hour, the tablets were dispersed. The maximum swelling values of the PLX- and TPLX-based tablets were found to be 5.9% and 7.6%, respectively. Figure 7 illustrates the significant difference between the swelling behavior between the two different formulations, where F2 was swelling more rapidly. It might be the reason that TPLX has a greater ability to retain moisture contents and a faster rate of hydration, thus allowing for comparatively greater swelling [29].

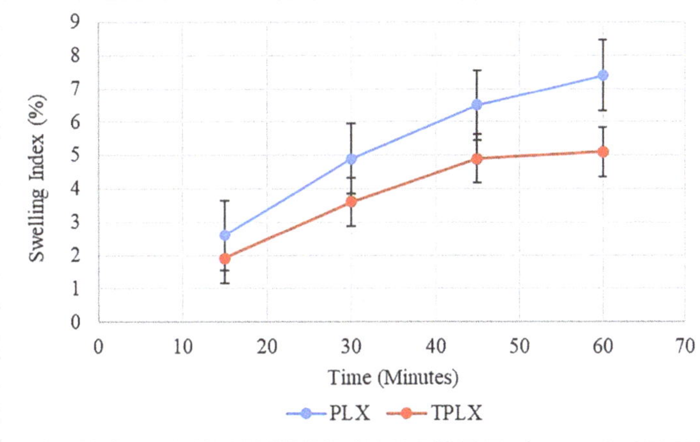

Figure 7. Swelling index of PLX- and TPLX-based tablets of TCM.

3.11.6. In Vitro Drug Release

PLX is considered to be an effective solubilizer and dissolution profile enhancer, and the literature has shown evidence of its properties [30,31]. Here, it was observed that the PLX-based formulation (F1) released more than 60% of the drug in the initial 15 min of the study. On the other hand, TPLX exhibited a more rapid response and a significantly improved dissolution output. As illustrated in Figure 8, F2 released more than 70% of incorporated drugs in a similar period. Furthermore, the prepared formulation was compared with that of the marketed product, and similar types of outcomes were observed. The findings of the study advocated that, by incorporating the thiol group, the dissolution-enhancing abilities of PLX could be further improved to a significant extent. ANOVA statistically proved ($p < 0.05$) that TPLX had a better dissolution enhancement impact than PLX.

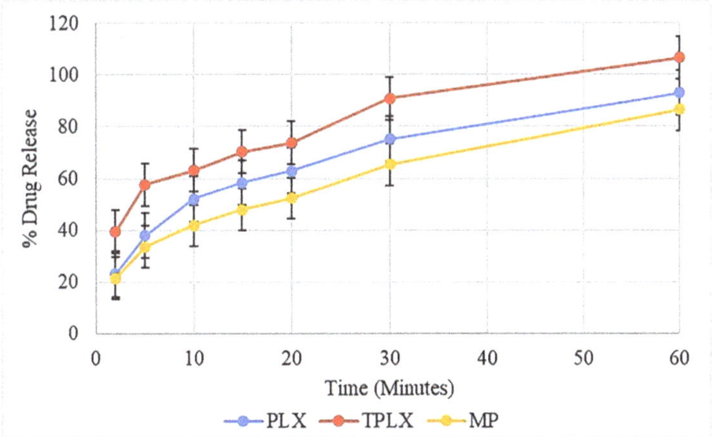

Figure 8. Describing the significant difference ($p < 0.05$) in release of the drug from PLX- and TPLX-based formulations.

3.11.7. Drug Content (DC%)

Formulations F1 and F2 were checked for their % drug content. The results showed that the % drug content for F1 and F2 were 95.89% ± 1.2 and 97.46% ± 1.85%, respectively, which were under the USP specification range (85–115%) (Table 6).

Table 6. Outcomes of post-compression studies of both PLX- and TPLX-based modified-release compressed tablets of TCM

Post-Compression Studies	F1	F2
Diameter (mm)	1.1 ± 0.086	1.1 ± 0.073
Thickness (mm)	0.5 ± 0.009	0.6 ± 0.147
Weight Variation (%)	Within Limit (±10%)	Within Limit (±10%)
Hardness (N)	4.1–4.25 ± 0.234	4.1–4.26 ± 0.132
Friability (%)	0.34 ± 0.006	0.35 ± 0.005
Disintegration Test (min)	9 ± 0.07	10 ± 0.08
Drug Content (%)	95.89 ± 1.22	97.46 ± 1.85

3.11.8. Kinetic Modeling

Different kinetic models like zero order, first order, Higuchi, and Korsmeyer Peppas were applied to find the release kinetics of formulations F1 and F2. In the F1 and F2 formulations, the release kinetics were not dependent on the initial concentration of the drug, as the R^2 of the zero-order model (0.9157) was greater than that of the first order model (0.760) for F2 and F1. Hence, it can be considered that TPLX could also help to control the release of the drug. The best fit model was found to be the Korsmeyer Peppas model, as it got the highest R^2 value of the other applied models. Higher values of R^2 for the Higuchi model (F1: 0.8037; F2: 0.6878) confirmed the diffusion-type release pattern of the drug from the prepared tablets. The correspondent values of 'n' suggested that the release of the drug did not follow Fick's law of diffusion (Table 7).

Table 7. Kinetic modeling of release data obtained from dissolution studies of F1 and F2.

Kinetic Models	F1 (PLX)	F2 (TPLX)
Zero Order (R^2)	0.8935	0.9157
First Order (R^2)	0.7904	0.760
Higuchi Model (R^2)	0.8037	0.6878
Korsmeyer Peppas Model (R^2)	0.9723	0.9816
(n)	$n = 0.61$	$n = 0.65$

Mucoadhesion Strength of Formulations (F1 and F2)

The results of the study indicated that the mucoadhesive strength of TPLX-based tablets was greater than that of PLX-based tablets. The incorporation of an –SH moiety in PLX led to an increase in mucoadhesion strength from 0.99 to 2.95 N (Table 8).

Table 8. Mucoadhesion strength of PLX- (F1) and TPLX- (F2) based compressed tablets.

Formulations	F1	F2
Mucoadhesion Strength (N)	0.99 ± 0.39	2.95 ± 0.35

Statistical Analysis

Statistical analysis showed that the effect of TPLX on drug release was significantly different from that of PLX and the marketed product on the release of TCM from compressed tablets (Table 9).

Table 9. The output of the statistical analysis.

Tukey's Multiple Comparison Test	Mean Diff.	Significant	Summary	*p*-Value
TPLX vs. PLX	11.97	Yes	***	<0.0001
TPLX vs. MP	14.97	Yes	***	<0.0001

*** highly significant values.

4. Discussion

Thiolation is considered to be an approach that can modify the characteristics of the polymer. Here, thiol modification was confirmed by the presence of the considerable amount of the thiol contents (20.625 μg/g of the polymer) in the modified polymer. The claim of successful thiolation was further strengthened by the emergence of a characteristic peak at 2695.9968 cm^{-1} in an FTIR scan of TPLX. Different characteristic changes were observed after the incorporation of thiol moieties in the structure of PLX, as detected in SEM, where intensive peaks confirming the crystalline structure were found to be converted into comparatively broader peaks. The decrease in the intensity of the crystallinity were predicted by the x-ray diffractogram. Poor swelling properties were displayed by PLX and its modified form, which might have been due to the presence of linear chain monomeric units in the structure of PLX.

These findings were comparable to those of various reported studies, where researchers have disclosed that thiolation might not significantly improve the swelling index of certain polymers. Bernkop-Schnürch and his co-worker observed the swelling index of tablets prepared with thiolated and non-thiolated carboxymethyl cellulose, and they revealed that there were no considerable differences in the characteristics of the tablets [32]. Furthermore, in another study that was based upon the modified and unmodified chitosan, the author statistically evaluated the swelling index by using a Student's t-test. He observed that there was no noticeable difference in the swelling profile of both of the polymers [33]. The conversion of PLX into TPLX markedly changed the behavior of the polymer, as well as its impact on the release of the drug. The formulation based on TPLX showed a more rapid drug release than PLX, as confirmed by the statistical analysis ($p < 0.05$), where a significant difference was observed in the amount of the drug released (Table 9). Similarly, the tablets were found to be rapidly disintegrating, and this might have been the reason that the maximum amount of the drug was released in 1 h. This short period might not have been sufficient for the tablets to get attached to the mucus membrane, allowing the mucoadhesive properties of the thiolated polymer to get in and play their role. However, by adjusting the suitable concentrations of the polymer, a better sustained effect could be produced, which may have allowed the tablets to get attached to the mucosal surface. This interaction of the dosage form may have provided the drug an opportunity to get permeated across the mucus membrane in a greater concentration from a specific site, hence benefiting an increased permeation and leading to an enhanced bioavailability and therapeutic effects.

The mechanism of drug release was predicted to be independent of the initial concentration of the drug in tablets, which was the indication that PLX might be used for the development of a controlled release drug delivery system. Another important point that was noticed was the diffusion-type drug release pattern. Though the pattern was non-Fickian, it could be helpful to control the release of the drug by controlling the thickness of the diffusive layer, which is dependent on the concentration of the polymer. In the same way, the tablet assay showed that each dosage form contained a sufficient amount of the drug to satisfy the official limits of the drug contents. It proved that PLX and TPLX have satisfactory drug loading capacities. The property of good drug loading capacity was might be due to the fact that PLX is an amphiphilic polymer [34], and it can therefore also hold poorly water-soluble drugs, such as TCM. After toxicity study evaluation, the findings established the fact that the addition of a thiol group might not cause any sort of toxic effects in the body. It was an important outcome that could help to suggest the initiation of in vivo studies of the prepared formulation. Similarly, another study also found that the thiomer could be safe for in vivo use [35]. PLX has also been widely studied by other researchers to confirm its biocompatibilities, and several studies have confirmed that it is one of those excipients that can be safely used as a carrier for drug administration [36,37].

The oral and dermal compatibilities of the polymers have opened a gateway for their diverse applications. Such modified polymers can be effectively used for both the oral and topical administration of the drug, as thiolation can enhance adhesion strength from 2 to 140 folds, providing a better contact time for the formulation on the skin [38].

5. Conclusions

The objectives of the study were productively achieved, as PLX was invariably converted into TPLX and proved to be a key potential carrier of TCM. These results showed the polymers' reliable compatibility and sufficient loading capacity of the drug. The polymer was found to be non-toxic in the studied concentrations, confirming its suitability for oral use. The polymers were found to be suitable for the development of compressed tablets loaded with TCM, and their evaluation advocated their appropriateness for the oral delivery of the said drug.

Supplementary Materials: The following are available online at https://www.mdpi.com/article/10.3390/pharmaceutics13050693/s1. Supplementary Figure S1: Calibration curve of thiourea, exhibiting good linearity in the selected range of concentration. Supplementary Figure S2: Calibration curve of TCM, showing linearity in the selected concentration range of the drug.

Author Contributions: Conceptualization, M.Z., M.S.U.R., and M.J.; formal analysis, M.Z., M.F.R., A.M., and A.F.A.; funding acquisition, F.A.; Investigation, M.Z., S.S., R.I.B., S.U.R., A.M., I.I., S.A., A.F.A., N.A., and M.A.; methodology, M.Z., S.S., R.I.B., M.S.U.R., S.U.R., M.J., I.I., F.A., and S.A.; project administration, N.A. and M.A.; validation, M.F.R.; writing—original draft, M.Z., S.S., R.I.B., M.S.U.R., S.U.R., M.J., M.F.R., A.M., I.I., A.F.A., N.A., and M.A.; writing—review and editing, M.F.R., F.A., and S.A. All authors have read and agreed to the published version of the manuscript.

Funding: This research was funded by the Deanship of Scientific Research at King Saud University for funding this work through the Research Group No. RG-1441-451.

Institutional Review Board Statement: The animal study was approved by the Institutional Research Ethics Committee of The University of Lahore under project file no. IREC-2019-101.

Informed Consent Statement: Not applicable.

Data Availability Statement: Data is contained within the article or supplementary material.

Acknowledgments: Authors are grateful to CCL Pharmaceuticals Lahore, Pakistan for providing tacrolimus to accomplish the project. The authors extend their appreciation to the Deanship of Scientific Research at King Saud University for funding this work through the Research Group No. RG-1441-451.

Conflicts of Interest: The authors declare no conflict of interest.

References

1. Zarrintaj, P.; Ramsey, J.D.; Samadi, A.; Atoufi, Z.; Yazdi, M.K.; Ganjali, M.R.; Amirabad, L.M.; Zangene, E.; Farokhi, M.; Formela, K. Poloxamer: A versatile tri-block copolymer for biomedical applications. *Acta Biomater.* **2020**, *110*, 37–67. [CrossRef]
2. Alawdi, S.; Solanki, A.B. Mucoadhesive Drug Delivery Systems: A Review of Recent Developments. *J. Sci. Res. Med. Biol. Sci.* **2021**, *2*, 50–64.
3. Leichner, C.; Jelkmann, M.; Bernkop-Schnürch, A. Thiolated polymers: Bioinspired polymers utilizing one of the most important bridging structures in nature. *Adv. Drug Deliv. Rev.* **2019**, *151*, 191–221. [CrossRef] [PubMed]
4. Bonengel, S.; Bernkop-Schnürch, A. Thiomers—From bench to market. *J. Control. Release* **2014**, *195*, 120–129. [CrossRef] [PubMed]
5. Prüfert, F.; Bonengel, S.; Menzel, C.; Bernkop-Schnürch, A. Enhancing the efficiency of thiomers: Utilizing a highly mucoadhesive polymer as backbone for thiolation and preactivation. *Eur. J. Pharm. Sci.* **2017**, *96*, 309–315. [CrossRef]
6. Hanif, M.; Zaman, M.; Qureshi, S. Thiomers: A blessing to evaluating era of pharmaceuticals. *Int. J. Polym. Sci.* **2015**, *2015*. [CrossRef]

7. Davidovich-Pinhas, M.; Harari, O.; Bianco-Peled, H. Evaluating the mucoadhesive properties of drug delivery systems based on hydrated thiolated alginate. *J. Control. Release* **2009**, *136*, 38–44. [CrossRef]
8. Iqbal, J.; Shahnaz, G.; Dünnhaupt, S.; Müller, C.; Hintzen, F.; Bernkop-Schnürch, A. Preactivated thiomers as mucoadhesive polymers for drug delivery. *Biomaterials* **2012**, *33*, 1528–1535. [CrossRef]
9. Carvalho, F.C.; Bruschi, M.L.; Evangelista, R.C.; Gremião, M.P.D. Mucoadhesive drug delivery systems. *Braz. J. Pharm. Sci.* **2010**, *46*, 1–17. [CrossRef]
10. Prüfert, F.; Hering, U.; Zaichik, S.; Le, N.-M.N.; Bernkop-Schnürch, A. Synthesis and in vitro characterization of a preactivated thiolated acrylic acid/acrylamide-methylpropane sulfonic acid copolymer as a mucoadhesive sprayable polymer. *Int. J. Pharm.* **2020**, *583*, 119371. [CrossRef]
11. Patel, P.; Patel, H.; Panchal, S.; Mehta, T. Formulation strategies for drug delivery of tacrolimus: An overview. *Int. J. Pharm. Investig.* **2012**, *2*, 169. [CrossRef]
12. Bhatia, M.; Ahuja, M. Thiol modification of psyllium husk mucilage and evaluation of its mucoadhesive applications. *Sci. World J.* **2013**, *2013*. [CrossRef]
13. Zaman, M.; Adnan, S.; Saeed, M.A.; Farooq, M.; Masood, Z.; Chishti, S.A.; Qureshi, J.; Khan, R. Formulation and in-vitro evaluation of sustained release matrix tablets of cellulose based hydrophilic and hydrophobic polymers loaded with loxoprofen sodium. *Indo Am. J. Pharma Res.* **2013**, *3*, 7389–7398.
14. Bhatia, M.; Ahuja, M.; Mehta, H. Thiol derivatization of Xanthan gum and its evaluation as a mucoadhesive polymer. *Carbohydr. Polym.* **2015**, *131*, 119–124. [CrossRef]
15. Bravo-Osuna, I.; Teutonico, D.; Arpicco, S.; Vauthier, C.; Ponchel, G. Characterization of chitosan thiolation and application to thiol quantification onto nanoparticle surface. *Int. J. Pharm.* **2007**, *340*, 173–181. [CrossRef]
16. Abdelbary, A.; Bendas, E.R.; Ramadan, A.A.; Mostafa, D.A. Pharmaceutical and pharmacokinetic evaluation of a novel fast dissolving film formulation of flupentixol dihydrochloride. *AAPS Pharmscitech* **2014**, *15*, 1603–1610. [CrossRef]
17. Mahajan, H.S.; Tyagi, V.K.; Patil, R.R.; Dusunge, S.B. Thiolated xyloglucan: Synthesis, characterization and evaluation as mucoadhesive in situ gelling agent. *Carbohydr. Polym.* **2013**, *91*, 618–625. [CrossRef]
18. Yu, H.; Feng, Z.-g.; Zhang, A.-y.; Hou, D.; Sun, L.-g. Novel triblock copolymers synthesized via radical telomerization of N-isopropylacrylamide in the presence of polypseudorotaxanes made from thiolated PEG and α-CDs. *Polymer* **2006**, *47*, 6066–6071. [CrossRef]
19. Botham, P.A. Acute systemic toxicity—Prospects for tiered testing strategies. *Toxicol. Vitr.* **2004**, *18*, 227–230. [CrossRef]
20. Erum, A.; Bashir, S.; Saghir, S.; Tulain, U.R.; Saleem, U.; Nasir, M.; Kanwal, F.; Hayat Malik, M.N. Acute toxicity studies of a novel excipient arabinoxylan isolated from Ispaghula (*Plantago ovata*) husk. *Drug Chem. Toxicol.* **2015**, *38*, 300–305. [CrossRef]
21. Halim, S.; Abdullah, N.; Afzan, A.; Rashid, B.A.; Jantan, I.; Ismail, Z. Acute toxicity study of Carica papaya leaf extract in Sprague Dawley rats. *J. Med. Plants Res.* **2011**, *5*, 1867–1872.
22. Corti, G.; Cirri, M.; Maestrelli, F.; Mennini, N.; Mura, P. Sustained-release matrix tablets of metformin hydrochloride in combination with triacetyl-β-cyclodextrin. *Eur. J. Pharm. Biopharm.* **2008**, *68*, 303–309. [CrossRef] [PubMed]
23. Pahade, M.A.A.; Jadhav, V.M.; Kadam, V. Formulation and development of a bilayer sustained released tablets of isosorbide mononitrate. *Stud. Int. J. Pharm. Bio Sci.* **2010**, *8*, 9.
24. Ray, D.; Prusty, A.K. Designing and in-vitro studies of gastric floating tablets of tramadol hydrochloride. *Int. J. Appl. Pharm.* **2010**, *2*, 12–16.
25. Erum, S.; Hassan, F.; Hasan, S.M.F.; Jabeen, S. Formulation of aspirin tablets using fewer excipients by direct compression. *Pak. J. Pharm.* **2011**, *28*, 31–37.
26. Zhao, N.; Augsburger, L.L. Functionality comparison of 3 classes of superdisintegrants in promoting aspirin tablet disintegration and dissolution. *AAPS PharmSciTech* **2005**, *6*, E634–E640. [CrossRef] [PubMed]
27. El-Kamel, A.; Sokar, M.; Naggar, V.; Al Gamal, S. Chitosan and sodium alginate—Based bioadhesive vaginal tablets. *AAPS PharmSci* **2002**, *4*, 224–230. [CrossRef]
28. Kumari, S.D.C.; Tharani, C.; Narayanan, N.; Kumar, C.S. Formulation and characterization of Methotrexate loaded sodium alginate chitosan Nanoparticles. *Indian J. Res. Pharm. Biotechnol.* **2013**, *1*, 915.
29. Saxena, A.; Tewari, G.; Saraf, S.A. Formulation and evaluation of mucoadhesive buccal patch of acyclovir utilizing inclusion phenomenon. *Braz. J. Pharm. Sci.* **2011**, *47*, 887–897. [CrossRef]
30. Hanif, M.; Zaman, M. Thiolation of arabinoxylan and its application in the fabrication of controlled release mucoadhesive oral films. *Daru J. Pharm. Sci.* **2017**, *25*, 6. [CrossRef]
31. Kajdič, S.; Vrečer, F.; Kocbek, P. Preparation of poloxamer-based nanofibers for enhanced dissolution of carvedilol. *Eur. J. Pharm. Sci.* **2018**, *117*, 331–340. [CrossRef]
32. Han, H.; Li, Y.; Peng, Z.; Long, K.; Zheng, C.; Wang, W.; Webster, T.J.; Ge, L. A Soluplus/Poloxamer 407-based self-nanoemulsifying drug delivery system for the weakly basic drug carvedilol to improve its bioavailability. *Nanomed. Nanotechnol. Biol. Med.* **2020**, *27*, 102199. [CrossRef]
33. Bernkop-Schnürch, A.; Scholler, S.; Biebel, R.G. Development of controlled drug release systems based on thiolated polymers. *J. Control. Release* **2000**, *66*, 39–48. [CrossRef]
34. Bernkop-Schnürch, A.; Egger, C.; Imam, M.E.; Krauland, A.H. Preparation and in vitro characterization of poly (acrylic acid)–cysteine microparticles. *J. Control. Release* **2003**, *93*, 29–38. [CrossRef]

35. Giuliano, E.; Paolino, D.; Cristiano, M.C.; Fresta, M.; Cosco, D. Rutin-Loaded Poloxamer 407-Based Hydrogels for In Situ Administration: Stability Profiles and Rheological Properties. *Nanomedicine* **2020**, *10*, 1069.
36. Zaman, M.; Hanif, M.; Sultana, K. Synthesis of thiolated arabinoxylan and its application as sustained release mucoadhesive film former. *Biomed. Mater.* **2018**, *13*, 025019. [CrossRef]
37. Giuliano, E.; Paolino, D.; Fresta, M.; Cosco, D. Drug-loaded biocompatible nanocarriers embedded in poloxamer 407 hydrogels as therapeutic formulations. *Medicines* **2019**, *6*, 7. [CrossRef]
38. Zaman, M.; Bajwa, R.I.; Saeed, S.; Hussain, M.A.; Hanif, M. Synthesis and characterization of thiol modified beta cyclodextrin, its biocompatible analysis and application as a modified release carrier of ticagrelor. *Biomed. Mater.* **2020**, *16*, 015023. [CrossRef]

pharmaceutics

MDPI

Article

Enhancement of the Bioavailability and Anti-Inflammatory Activity of Glycyrrhetinic Acid via Novel Soluplus®—A Glycyrrhetinic Acid Solid Dispersion

Hao Wang [1,†], Runwei Li [1,†], Yuan Rao [1], Saixing Liu [1], Chunhui Hu [2], Yong Zhang [3], Linchao Meng [4], Qilin Wu [4], Qiuhong Ouyang [1], Hao Liang [1,*] and Meng Qin [1,*]

1 Beijing Advanced Innovation Centre for Soft Matter Science and Engineering, State Key Laboratory of Chemical Resource Engineering, College of Life Science and Technology, Beijing University of Chemical Technology, Beijing 100029, China
2 Medical College, Qinghai University, Xining 810001, China
3 Technology Corporation, Beijing 100029, China
4 Star Health Botanical Technology Corporation, Beijing 100029, China
* Correspondence: lianghao@mail.buct.edu.cn (H.L.); qinmeng212@mail.buct.edu.cn (M.Q.)
† These authors contributed equally to this work.

Citation: Wang, H.; Li, R.; Rao, Y.; Liu, S.; Hu, C.; Zhang, Y.; Meng, L.; Wu, Q.; Ouyang, Q.; Liang, H.; et al. Enhancement of the Bioavailability and Anti-Inflammatory Activity of Glycyrrhetinic Acid via Novel Soluplus®—A Glycyrrhetinic Acid Solid Dispersion. *Pharmaceutics* **2022**, *14*, 1797. https://doi.org/10.3390/pharmaceutics14091797

Academic Editor: Bruno Sarmento

Received: 12 June 2022
Accepted: 8 August 2022
Published: 26 August 2022

Abstract: Glycyrrhetinic acid (GA) is an anti-inflammatory drug with potential for development. However, the poor solubility of GA in water leads to extremely low bioavailability, which limits its clinical applications. Solid dispersions have become some of the most effective strategies for improving the solubility of poorly soluble drugs. Soluplus®, a non-cytotoxic amphiphilic solubilizer, significantly improves the solubility of BCS II drugs and improves the bioavailability of insoluble drugs. l-arginine (L-Arg) can be used as a small molecular weight excipient to assist in improving the solubility of insoluble drugs. In this study, we developed a new formulation for oral administration by reacting GA and L-Arg to form salts by co-solvent evaporation and then adding the polymer-solvent Soluplus® with an amphiphilic chemical structure to prepare a solid dispersion GA-SD. The chemical and physical properties of GA-SD were characterized by DLS, TEM, XRD, FT-IR and TG. The anti-inflammatory activity of GA-SD was verified by LPS stimulation of RAW 267.5 cells simulating a cellular inflammation model, TPA-induced ear edema model in mice, and ethanol-induced gastric ulcer model. The results showed that the amide bond and salt formation of GA-SD greatly improved GA solubility. GA-SD effectively improved the anti-inflammatory effect of free GA in vivo and in vitro, and GA-SD had no significant effect on liver and kidney function, no significant tissue toxicity, and good biosafety. In conclusion, GA-SD with L-Arg and Soluplus® is an effective method to improve the solubility and bioavailability of GA. As a safe and effective solid dispersion, it is a promising anti-inflammatory oral formulation and provides some references for other oral drug candidates with low bioavailability.

Keywords: glycyrrhetinic acid; Soluplus®; solid dispersions; anti-inflammatory; biosafety; bioavailability

1. Introduction

Inflammation is the first protective response in biological systems and can protect against injury caused by harmful stimuli, such as physical insults, chemical insults, or infection [1,2]. However, an excessive inflammatory response can damage normal tissues [3]. Due to low or no toxicity, characteristics of natural biologically active substances can greatly reduce the risk of complications in treating excessive inflammation [4]. Therefore, the public is increasingly interested in the use of traditional plant-based medicines to prevent and treat inflammatory diseases. This trend has prompted the further development of natural products with anti-inflammatory properties. A variety of plant extracts have been scientifically shown to exhibit anti-inflammatory activity by modulating the expression levels of inflammation-related genes [5,6].

Glycyrrhetinic acid (GA) is a triterpene saponin generated by the hydrolysis of glycyrrhizic acid to remove the sugar and acid chains and is the main active ingredient in licorice. According to the Biopharmaceutical Classification System, GA is a type II drug [7]. GA has shown a variety of pharmacological actions, such as antiallergic, antimicrobial, antiviral, antihepatotoxic and antitumor activities [8]. Many studies have further confirmed the good immunomodulatory effects of GA. Peng et al. [9] found that GA could modulate the innate immune response by binding to the TLR4 receptor to induce the expression of its downstream signaling molecules. Wang et al., demonstrated that GA can exert anti-inflammatory effects by inhibiting the activity of PI3Kp110δ and p110γ in the PI3K/Akt/GSK3β signaling pathway, blocking Ser phosphorylation of the p65 subunit, a key subunit required for NF-kB activation, indirectly inhibiting NF-kB activation and reducing the release of downstream inflammatory cytokines. GA also promotes dissociation of a glucocorticoid receptor-heat shock protein 90 (GR-HSP90) complex and inhibits excessive inflammatory responses [2,5]. GA is an anti-inflammatory drug with developmental potential. However, it is composed of two hydrophilic glucuronic acid residues and one hydrophobic glycogen, granting it high hydrophobicity and low solubility in aqueous solutions and pH-dependent solubility [10]. Its lower solubility makes it less bioavailable, limiting its clinical applications [11]. Therefore, the use of appropriate strategies to increase the solubility of GA will greatly improve the bioavailability of GA and enhance the clinical efficacy of GA for the treatment of inflammatory diseases.

Solid dispersions have become some of the most effective strategies for improving the solubility of poorly soluble drugs [12,13]. The drug can be dispersed in the polymer, which may have a higher porosity, reduced particle size and improved wettability [13]. The choice of polymer in a solid dispersion can help prevent the recrystallization of the drug [14]. Sui and Chu et al., investigated the effect of polyvinylpyrrolidone (PVP) as a GA solid dispersions carrier at different molecular weights, investigating the dissolution behavior and physicochemical properties. PVP-GA-SDs displayed a good enhancement of dissolution rate and equilibrium solubility compared with pure drugs and corresponding physical mixtures [15]. Dong et al., prepared ternary solid dispersion (TSD) systems containing alkalizers to increase the dissolution of GA; GA-TSD significantly improved the solubility and dissolution of GA [16]. These studies confirmed that the preparation of solid dispersion is one of the important ways to improve the solubility of GA. However, there are few studies on the preparation of GA solid dispersion, and discussions on drug loading, entrapment efficiency, and anti-inflammatory effect of solid dispersion are incomplete. Polyethylene caprolactam-polyvinyl acetate-polyethylene glycol graft copolymer (Soluplus®) is a noncytotoxic amphiphilic solubilizer, absorbent, and penetrant that can be used as a carrier in the formulation of solid dispersions [17]. The bifunctional character of Soluplus® allows it to act as a matrix polymer for solid solutions and to increase the solubility of insoluble drugs [18]. The low critical micelle concentration of Soluplus® is 6.63×10^{-3} mg/mL [19]. When the concentration of Soluplus® exceeds the low critical micelle concentration, Soluplus® encapsulates the hydrophobic drug in a hydrophobic core where the carbonyl group in the molecular structure binds to the hydroxyl group of the drug. At the same time, Soluplus® prevents crystal formation by reducing the energy of the particle surface, further improving the stability of the micelles [20,21]. Studies have shown that Soluplus® can significantly increase the dissolution of BCS II drugs and improve the bioavailability of insoluble drugs [22]. L-arginine (L-Arg) can be used as a small molecular weight excipient and undergo specific molecular interactions with drugs to produce an amorphous material, thus, assisting in improving the solubility of insoluble drugs [23]. These interactions include salt formation between L-arginine and the drug, which changes the pH, improves the solubility of pH-dependent drugs, and controls the aggregation of drug crystals [24]. It has been demonstrated that L-Arg can act as an alkalizer to form salts with glycyrrhetinic acid through strong electrostatic attraction, which can significantly improve the solubility of pH-dependent drugs [16].

This study aimed to prepare solid dispersions with L-Arg as an excipient and Soluplus® as a polymer to improve the solubility and bioavailability of free GA and provide a new scheme for the preparation of GA-SD. The effects of GA-SD on the anti-inflammatory activity of free GA were analyzed in an LPS-stimulated cellular inflammation model, a mouse ear edema model and an alcohol-induced gastric ulcer model. The biosafety of GA-SD was also demonstrated. The results showed that the GA-SD solid dispersion system developed in this study is promising for improving the bioavailability and anti-inflammatory effects of free GA. With the improvement of the solubility and utilization of GA, the application scope of GA in the treatment of many inflammatory diseases will be expanded.

2. Materials and Methods

2.1. Materials

GA was purchased from Beijing Mairuida Technology Co., Ltd., Soluplus® was purchased from BASF (Ludwigshafen, Germany), and L-Arg was purchased from Beijing Aibifan Biotechnology Co. 12-O-tetradecanoylphorbol-13-acetate (TPA) (p1585, Sigma-Aldrich, Munich, Germany). All other related chemicals and reagents were analytically pure.

2.2. Animals and Cell Line

The mouse macrophage RAW264.7 cell line was purchased from the Cell Resource Center of Peking Union Medical College Hospital. RAW264.7 cells were cultured in DMEM complete medium (Gibco™, Grand Island, NY, USA) containing 10% fetal bovine serum (Gibco™, Sydney, Australia) at 37 °C in a 5% CO_2 incubator and passaged by gently scraping the adherent cells with a cell scraper at a ratio of 1:6–1:8.

Experimental animals: KM mice (18~22 g, male) were purchased from Beijing Huafukang Biotechnology Co. All animals were kept under stable temperature conditions (20–26 °C) and 12 h light/dark cycles for three days. All experiments were conducted by the regulations of the National Institutes of Health (NIH) and the Beijing Laboratory Animal Ethics Committee.

2.3. Fabrication of GA-SD

To prepare GA-SD, the co-solvent evaporation method was used [25,26]. Briefly, solutions of GA, L-Arg and Soluplus® were prepared in the proportions shown in Table S1. GA was dissolved in 50 mL of anhydrous ethanol, L-Arg was dissolved in 50 mL of deionized water, and both were ultrasonicated to dissolve them completely. The GA and L-Arg solutions were stirred on a magnetic stirrer at room temperature until thoroughly mixed and then left to stand for 30 min to allow GA to salt with L-Arg. The mixture was spin-dried at 40 °C and 100 rpm. The Soluplus® solution was prepared with 50 mL of deionized water, and the sample was redissolved by adding the prepared Soluplus® solution to the rotary dried sample. The hydrophilic L-Arg fraction allowed the GA-L-Arg complex to disperse in water and the hydrophobic GA fraction combined with the hydrophobic structure of Solulplus® to form the GA-L-Arg-Solulplus® ternary complex. The resulting solution was a GA solid dispersion. The samples were freeze-dried to obtain a solid dispersion powder.

2.4. Drug Loading Analysis

In this study, the drug loading capacity of the prepared GA-SD was tested to screen for the optimal reagent ratio for the preparation of solid dispersions. GA solid dispersions prepared under different mass ratios of substances were first taken and dissolved in deionized water, and then the drug loading was detected by HPLC under the following conditions: phase A methanol, phase B 0.2% phosphoric acid, A:B = 90:10, flow rate

1 mL/min; wavelength 250 nm, column temperature 35 °C; each injection volume was 20 μL.

2.5. Characterizations of GA-SD

2.5.1. Particle Size and Zeta Potentials

A Nano-ZS 2000 (Malvern Instruments Ltd., Malvern, UK) was used to determine the particle size and Zeta potential. Before measurement, an appropriate amount of Soluplus® and GA-SD were weighed respectively and configured into a 2 mg/mL solution. All the samples were diluted 3 times with deionized water at a ratio of 1:3 (v/v), and then the average particle size and Zeta Potentials were measured by a nanoparticle size potential analyzer.

2.5.2. Transmission Electron Microscopy

Morphological observation of GA-SD was performed using a Hitachi-HT7700 (120 kV) transmission electron microscope. Double distilled water was used to dilute the GA-SD powder and ultrasonically disperse it for 30 min. A drop of diluent (approximately 5 μL) was loaded onto a copper mesh (200 mesh, EMS) coated with formaldehyde/carbon, and the sample was air-dried before observation.

2.5.3. Fourier Transform Infrared Spectroscopy

Infrared analysis was performed to identify the formation of complexes by evaluating deviations in peak shape, position, and intensity. A certain amount of GA, Soluplus®, L-Arg, a physical mixture of the three, and GA-SD powder were scanned in the range of 4000–400 cm^{-1} by FT-IR (Thermo Scientific Nicolet iS20).

2.5.4. X-ray Diffraction

To observe the state of the GA before and after wrapping, the GA-SD powder was characterized by X-ray crystal diffraction (XRD) (Pert3 Powder). Certain amounts of GA, Soluplus®, L-Arg, their physical mixture and GA-SD powder were taken and laid flat on a sample table and then analyzed by XRD. The scanning speed was 5°/min, and the scanning range was 5–80°.

2.5.5. Thermal Gravimetric Analysis

Thermogravimetric analysis (TA SDT 650) was employed to evaluate the thermal stability of GA-SD. The samples of about 10 mg were sealed in an aluminum plate and heated from 30 °C to 800 °C with the rate of 10 °C/min under an atmosphere of nitrogen. The weight variation of the samples was recorded in relation to temperature.

2.5.6. Stability Studies

To investigate the stability of the prepared GA-SD, we took 50 mg of the prepared GA-SD powder and dissolved it in 25 mL of deionized water. The studies were carried out at room temperature for 63 days. The change in GA content in the solid dispersion was measured by HPLC every 7 days. Meanwhile, the GA-SD were stored at 4 °C for 7 months and analyzed by X-ray crystal diffraction to determine the crystallization propensity of GA-SD over time.

2.5.7. Solubility of Formulation

The GA-SD (500 mg) was respectively added to a 15 mL centrifuge tube containing 2 mL deionized water and then shaken at 37 °C for 72 h. After the shaking, the samples were filtered with a 0.22 filter membrane and diluted with absolute ethanol. Then, the GA was quantified by HPLC (the conditions were described in Section 2.4). Each experiment was conducted in triplicates and the average solubility was obtained.

2.6. In Vitro Anti-Inflammatory Activity

The safe concentration of cell administration on RAW264.7 cells was assessed by CCK-8 assay. Briefly, cells dispersed evenly in the medium were seeded at a density of 5.0×10^3 cells/well in 96-well plates. The next day, cells were treated with different doses (0, 12.5, 25, 50, 100, 200, and 300 μM) of GA and GA-SD, respectively, for 24 h. Then, CCK-8 solution was added and the optical density (OD) at 450 nm was determined. GA was dissolved in DMSO, and the volume of DMSO used was one-thousandth of the volume of the medium [27]. The dissolved GA was configured with DMEM serum-free medium to a concentration of 50 μM. The total mass of GA-SD required for drug-loaded 50 μM GA was calculated according to the drug loading of solid dispersion of 24.8%. Then the serum-free DMEM was prepared, filtered through a 0.22 μm filter to sterilize the preparation, and then stored at 4 °C.

RAW264.7 cells in the logarithmic growth phase were collected by trypsin digestion and configured into a 1×10^5/mL cell suspension, which were inoculated in 96-well cell culture plates with 100 μL of cell suspension per well. They were incubated in a 37 °C, 5% CO_2 incubator. When the cells were spread in a monolayer across the bottom of the well, the supernatant was removed, and 100 μL of the serum-free medium was added as the normal group, 100 μL of serum-free medium containing Lipopolysaccharide (LPS) (1 μg/mL) as the model group, and 100 μL of serum-free medium containing a final concentration of 50 μM GA, GA-SD and LPS (1 μg/mL) as the experimental group [28]. The culture was continued for 24 h, and the cell supernatant was collected to assess the levels of IL-1β, IL-4, IL-6, IL-10, MCP-1, TNF-α, IL-23 and IL-17A using enzyme-linked immunosorbent assay (ELISA) kits (Abcam) following the manufacturer's instructions.

2.7. Construction of Mouse Ear Edema Model

The mice were randomly divided into 4 groups, each with 5 animals. These groups included the control group, TPA model group, GA group (20 mg/kg) and GA-SD group (20 mg/kg) (Table S2). All drugs were dissolved in DMSO, and the volume of DMSO was one-thousandth of the final solution volume and was diluted with PBS. All drugs were prepared before the assay. All mice, except the control and model mice, were administered at the same time each day, and the gavage operation lasted for one week. Normal and model mice were administered with the same volume of PBS. For ear edema, 1 h after the last gavage, TPA (0.3 μg) dissolved in 20 μL of acetone was repeatedly applied to the inner and outer surfaces of the mouse ears. The normal group was coated with an equal amount of acetone [29]. Orbital venous blood was taken from mice 6 h after the application of TPA for the detection of hepatorenal toxicity. Liver, kidney and ear tissues were taken for pathological section analysis.

2.8. Histopathology

To evaluate the therapeutic effect of GA and GA-SD on ear inflammation, ear tissues were collected from each group of mice, and to evaluate the hepatic and renal toxicity of GA and GA-SD, liver and kidney tissues were collected after perfusion and paraffin sectioning. The ear tissue and liver and kidney tissues were first fixed by immersion in 4% paraformaldehyde with gradient dehydration and paraffin embedding. They were sliced into 4 μm post-thin sections. They were stained with hematoxylin-eosin stain [30].

The sections were observed by optical microscopy, and three visual fields were randomly selected for analysis. Image analysis was performed by a pathologist who did not know the experimental conditions to evaluate the degree of tissue damage.

2.9. Analysis of Serum Biochemical Parameters

The orbital venous blood of mice in the normal group, the GA experimental group and the GA-SD experimental group were centrifuged at 3000 rpm for 10 min, and the serum was collected. According to the manufacturer's instructions, the serum total protein (TP), serum albumin (ALB), creatinine (CREA), urea (UREA), aspartate aminotransferase (AST) and alanine aminotransferase (ALT) were measured with a commercial kit (CSCN). According to the normal reference values of the biochemical indices of Kunming mice provided by Huaying Biology, the biosafety of GA and GA-SD was evaluated.

2.10. Construction of Ethanol-Induced Gastric Ulcer Model

Animals were randomly assigned to five groups (n = 5) as follows: normal control group; model group; GA group (20 mg/kg) and GA-SD group (20 mg/kg) (Table S3). Mice in the normal control group and model group were administered with PBS. The GA and GA-SD samples were prepared according to the method described herein. Mice were administered by gavage once a day for 7 days. Before ulcer induction, animals fasted for 24 h and water was also withheld for two hours to empty their stomach of food. One hour after the last administration, mice except those in the normal control group were given 85% ethanol (10 mL/kg) by gavage to establish an acute gastric ulcer model [31].

2.11. Assessment of Gastric Tissue Injury and Histopathological Examination

One hour after the ulcer induction, animals were anesthetized with isoflurane and euthanized by cervical dislocation. The excised stomach was opened along the greater curvature and rinsed completely with PBS. Then, the stomachs were blotted dry with filter paper, spread out, and photographed. For the determination of gastric lesion area, the gastric ulcer index (GUI) was calculated by analyzing the inner surface of the stomach using Image J software (v1.53c.). The gastric tissues were taken for pathological section analysis after the photoshoot. For each group, the gastric ulcer index was determined using the following equation:

$$\text{Ulcer Index} = \frac{\text{Sum of lesion areas}}{\text{Total stomach area}} \times 100 \quad (1)$$

The percentage of ulcer preventive index was calculated as follows:

$$\text{Preventive index} = \frac{\text{Ulcer index(ulcerated group)} - \text{Ulcer index(treated)}}{\text{Ulcer index(ulcerated group)}} \times 100 \quad (2)$$

After a general examination, gastric tissues were preserved in a 4% paraformaldehyde buffer solution for 24 h and then embedded in paraffin wax. Slices were prepared and stained with hematoxylin and eosin (H&E) for histological evaluation.

2.12. Immunohistochemical (IHC) Staining

IHC staining was employed to assess the expression levels of pro-inflammatory cytokines TNF-α and IL-6. For a start, tissue sections were deparaffinized, rehydrated, and then antigen retrieved. Subsequently, the sections were pretreated for 25 min with sodium citrate buffer via heat-mediated antigen retrieval followed by treatment with 3% H_2O_2 to inhibit endogenous peroxidase activity and blocking with 3% BSA for 30 min. After that, the slices were treated with primary antibodies diluted at 1:500 overnight at 4 °C, and then with peroxidase-coupled secondary antibodies for 50 min. Color development was carried out by incubating with 3,3′-diaminobenzidine tetrahydrochloride for 5 min. The results were captured by light microscopy, followed by analysis by Image J software.

2.13. Statistical Analysis

All results are presented as the mean ± standard deviation (SD). Statistical comparison was made via Student's t-test. The significance levels ($p < 0.05$) were regarded as statistically acceptable.

3. Results

3.1. Preparation and Characterization of GA-SD

GA-SDs were prepared using the co-solvent evaporation method. As described in the experimental section, the GA and L-Arg solutions were mixed thoroughly and left for 30 min to form salts. Then, Soluplus® was added, and Soluplus® formed solid dispersions of the solutions via hydrogen bonding or complexation reactions.

As shown in Figure 1A, the highest entrapment efficiency of the solid dispersion was achieved at 95.9% with a GA: L-Arg ratio of 1:1. A further increase in L-Arg resulted in decreased EE%, so the ratio of GA and L-ARG was most suitable at 1:1. The encapsulation efficiency was directly related to its bioavailability and in vivo efficacy. The highest value of entrapment efficiency (99.4%) was achieved at a mass ratio of 1:1:2 when the drug loading was 24.8% (Figure 1B). In aqueous solution, the polymer first formed hydrogen bonds with water to fully dissolve. When the GA: L-Arg: Soluplus® was less than 1:1:2 (*w*/*w*/*w*), the encapsulation efficiency gradually increased to nearly 100%. At this point, we believed that GA-L-Arg was excessive and more Soluplus® provided more loading space, leading to the increase in the encapsulation efficiency. As the Soluplus® content increased, the entrapment efficiency did not increase further but instead decreased slightly, possibly because the excess dissolved Soluplus® seized too many water molecules, resulting in there not being enough water to rehydrate with GA-Arg, making redissolving difficult [19].

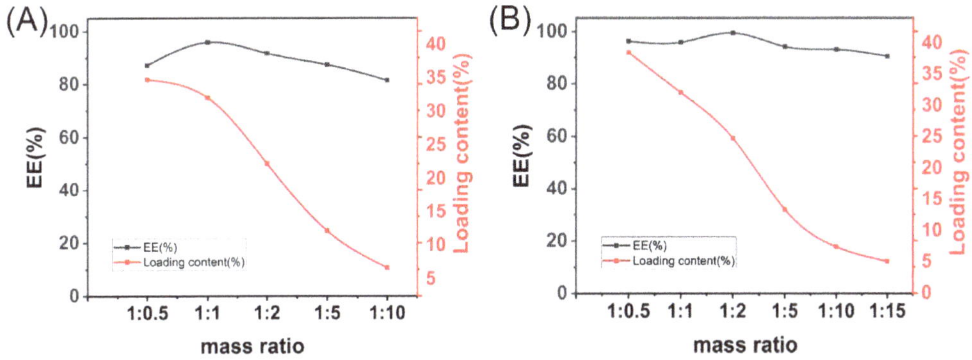

Figure 1. Formulation screening results. (**A**) The ratio of GA to Soluplus® was fixed at 1:1 (*w*/*w*), and the ratio of L-Arg was changed. The mass ratio indicates the ratio of GA to L-Arg (*w*/*w*). (**B**) In the screening results shown in (**A**), the optimal ratio of GA to L-Arg was 1:1 (*w*/*w*), and based on this result, the ratio of Soluplus® was changed; the mass ratio indicates the ratio of GA to Soluplus® (*w*/*w*).

The best mass ratio of GA, L-Arg and Soluplus® was determined to be 1:1:2.

3.2. Physicochemical Characterization

3.2.1. Particle Size and Zeta Potentials

In this experiment, the particle size and Zeta Potentials of Soluplus® and prepared GA-SD were measured by DLS. The result is demonstrated in Figure 2A,B. It was known that Soluplus® could form micelles spontaneously due to its amphipathic property. The results of zeta potential indicated that Soluplus® micelles were formed with nearly neutral charges. Therefore, the charge of GA-SD should be derived from its loading components. We tested the potential of the GA-Arg complex and found that its charge was −3.4 mV, while GA-SD loaded a large number of complexes, which made the surface charge accumulate, showing the zeta potential was approximately −4.15 mV. An important factor in measuring the performance of nanoparticles is their particle size, which affects the circulation and biodistribution of the drugs [32]. The particle size of Soluplus® was 63.17 nm, and the average particle size of GA-SD was 68 nm, which was very close to the particle size of Soluplus®. The DLS results of GA-SD showed a sharp peak, indicating single and narrow particle size distributions. Additionally, the microscopic details of GA-SD were confirmed by TEM (Figure 2C,D), and the GA-SD particles had irregular morphology, which was consistent with the basic characteristics of solid dispersions [22,32,33].

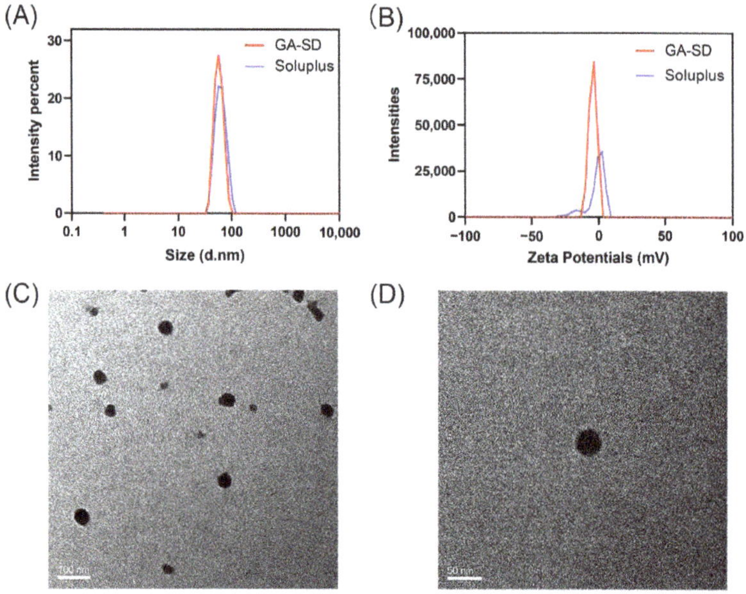

Figure 2. The particle size, Zeta Potentials and morphology of GA-SD (**A**) DLS analysis of GA-SD and Soluplus particle size. (**B**) Zeta Potentials analysis of GA-SD and Soluplus. (**C**,**D**) TEM analysis of GA-SD morphology.

It has been reported that nanoparticles with a particle size below 100 nm can escape rapid clearance by the reticuloendothelial system, prolong the in vivo circulation time, increase cell membrane permeability, and improve bioavailability [34]. Therefore, the GA-SD prepared in this experiment may have higher cell membrane permeability and bioavailability than GA. In addition, liver cells are the main cells that phagocytose particles below 100 nm, so the hepatotoxicity of GA-SD had to be subsequently verified.

3.2.2. XRD and FT-IR Analysis

XRD and FTIR were used to characterize the interaction forms and the structure of the solid dispersion. The XRD results are plotted in Figure 3A. Figure 3A shows that GA and L-Arg were in crystalline form and Soluplus® was an amorphous powder. Comparing the images, it can be seen that the characteristic peaks of both GA and L-Arg disappeared after the formation of solid dispersion, and a peak signal did not appear, suggesting an amorphous state of the powder which confirmed that GA was encapsulated in the Soluplus®. Thus, we successfully prepared GA-SD. Infrared spectroscopy can better analyze the molecular binding sites of GA, L-Arg and Soluplus®. The IR spectra of GA, L-Arg, Soluplus®, and GA-SD are plotted in Figures 3B and S1. The absorption peak at 1664 cm^{-1} represented the stretching vibration of the C = O group of ketone segment in the GA structure, and the peak at 1706 cm^{-1} belonged to the stretching vibration of the C = O group of the carboxylic acid [16]. These signals disappeared completely in GA-SD, which might have been due to the encapsulation of the amphiphilic polymer Soluplus®. For Soluplus®, peaks around 1641 cm^{-1} and 1741cm^{-1} were related to the carbonyl groups in the vinyl acetate and caprolactam segments [35]. The infrared peaks of Arg were assigned according to the literature [36,37]. The peaks at 1680 and 1623 cm^{-1} were from the guanidyl group, including the C=N stretching, which reflected the basic functional group for salt formation with acidic compounds. The other peaks were assigned as follows: amide C–N stretching (1558 cm^{-1}), COO– stretching (1420 cm^{-1}), and NH_2 deformation (1134 cm^{-1}). Carboxylate anion usually shows an absorption peak at 1650–1550 cm^{-1} due to strong asymmetric carboxylate stretching [38]. The disappearance of the O-H stretches peak (3437 cm^{-1}) of the carboxyl group in GA suggested the ionization of the carboxyl group [39–41]. There were two new peaks at 1554 cm^{-1} and 1368 cm^{-1}, attributed to the asymmetric (Vas COO−) and symmetric stretching vibration (Vs COO−) of the –COO– group [16,42,43]. This indicated that interaction between GA and L-Arg led to the formation of a structure that belonged to a carboxylate.

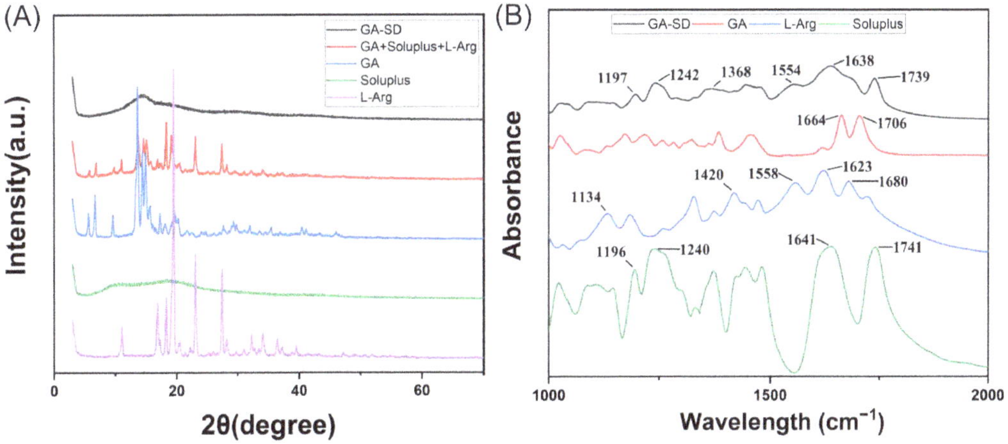

Figure 3. Structural analysis of solid dispersions. (**A**) XRD analysis of the GA-SD solid dispersion. (**B**) FT-IR spectra with the major characteristic peaks.

The strong ionic interaction between the GA and L-Arg, the formation of salts and the hydrophilic structure of Soluplus® make GA-SD extremely hydrophilic. Therefore, the water solubility of GA was greatly improved.

3.2.3. Thermogravimetric Analysis

The TGA scan of GA showed almost a constant weight until 300 °C (Figure 4). GA began to decompose and lose weight as the temperature increased to 300 °C, which was close to the inherent melting point of GA at 294 °C. The weight loss of GA-SD in the early stage of heating may have been due to residual moisture from incomplete freeze-drying. Similar to Soluplus, GA-SD had no obvious endothermic peak, which indicated that the GA-SD was amorphous. The trend of GA-SD was very similar to Soluplus, which proved that Soluplus was contained in the outside of the GA. At 308 °C, the retention rate of GA-SD was 80%, which proved its good thermal stability.

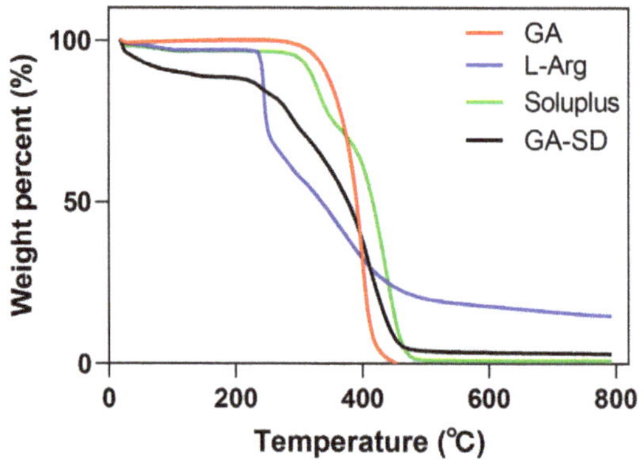

Figure 4. TGA curves of the mass loss as a function of temperature.

3.2.4. Stability of GA-SD

The stability of GA-SD is shown in Figure 5A. GA-SD was placed at room temperature for 63 days, and the GA content only decreased by 9.8%, and the degradation rate was uniform. The results confirmed that GA-SD had good stability. Changes in the crystalline content of amorphous solid dispersions over time are shown in Figure 5B. Throughout all trials, the GA-SD preparation did not undergo crystallization, and even up to 7 months after preparation, dispersions still lacked any crystalline peaks by XRD, indicating that GA-SD had good crystalline stability. This may be related to the inherent properties of Soluplus® and its crystallization inhibitory effect [44].

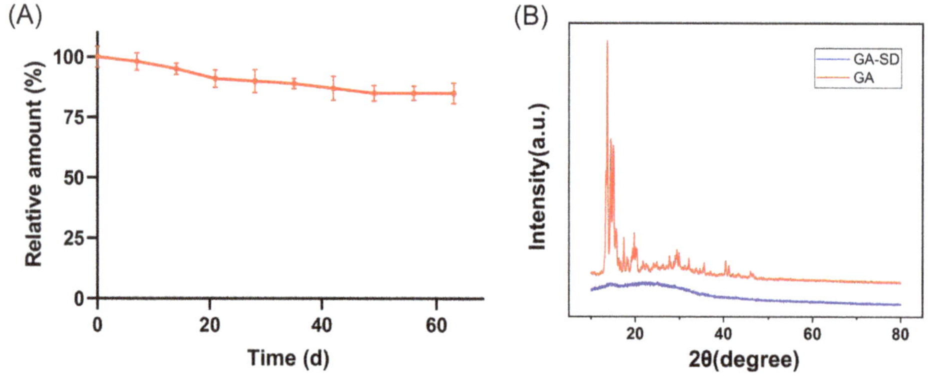

Figure 5. Stability of GA-SD. (**A**) Experimental results of GA-SD placement stability. Values are presented as the mean ± SD (n = 3). (**B**) Changes in the crystalline content of GA-SD after storage at 4 °C for 7 months.

3.2.5. Solubility GA-SD

The saturated solubility of GA in water was 6.62×10^{-3} mg/mL (Table 1), The detected saturation solubility was in good agreement with the reported $5.86 \pm 0.45 \times 10^{-3}$ mg/mL [15] and 6.36×10^{-3} mg/mL [45], and the saturated solubility of GA-SD in water was 37.6 ± 0.03 mg/mL. The dissolution phenomenon was shown in Figure S2. Compared with the GA group, the GA-SD group possessed a higher dissolving ability with a 5680-fold higher dissolving ability in water. The solubility of the drug is critical to the efficacy of the drug. The excellent solubility of GA-SD may improve the absorption and bioavailability of GA in oral administration.

Table 1. Saturated solubility of GA and GA-SD.

Group	GA	GA-SD
Saturated solubility(mg/mL)	6.62×10^{-3}	37.6 ± 0.03

Values are presented as the mean ± SD (n = 3).

3.3. *Anti-Inflammatory Effect In Vitro*

To further study the bioavailability of GA-SD in vivo, we examined the effect of this material on the anti-inflammatory activity of GA. In this study, we finally determined the safe administration concentration to be 50 μM, at which RAW 264.7 cells maintained high viability (>90%). The result of the cell viability assay is shown in Figure 6.

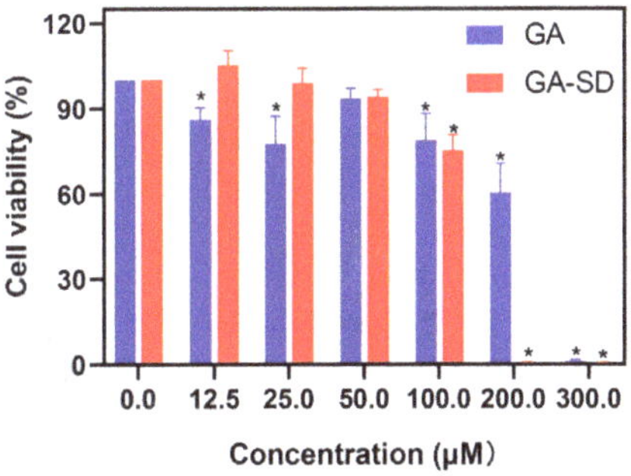

Figure 6. Cell viability at different drug concentrations on RAW 264.7 cells. The values presented are the means ± SD (n = 4). 0 μM represents the control group. * $p < 0.05$ vs. Control.

LPS stimulation of the mouse peritoneal mononuclear macrophage cell Line 264.7 was used to simulate the inflammatory response in vitro, and the cell supernatant was analyzed for inflammatory factors by ELISA. When cells are stimulated by LPS, the secretion of proinflammatory cytokines, such as IL-1β, IL-6, MCP-1, TNF-α, IL-23, and IL-17A, increases, while the secretion of anti-inflammatory cytokines such as IL-4 and IL-10 decreases. Cytokines, such as IL-1β, TNF-α, and IL-6, are key proinflammatory factors that can mediate inflammation by inducing cellular pro-inflammatory gene expression [46,47]. IL-10 and IL-4 are key anti-inflammatory factors that inhibit the production of pro-inflammatory molecules, limit excessive immune responses, and play a key role in the treatment of inflammation [48,49]. The experimental results are shown in Figure 7. After treatment with free GA and GA-SD, the release of pro-inflammatory cytokines, due to LPS stimulation, was inhibited by free GA and GA-SD. The secretion of anti-inflammatory cytokines was elevated. Moreover, the immunomodulatory effect of GA-SD treatment was superior to that of the free GA experimental group. GA-SD protects the anti-inflammatory activity of free GA itself, and the enhanced anti-inflammatory effects might be due to the presence of a solubility enhancer (Soluplus®), leading to higher solubility. Moreover, the suitable particle size of GA-SD enhanced the permeability of its cell membrane, which also improved the utilization of the drug by the cells and enhanced the anti-inflammatory effect.

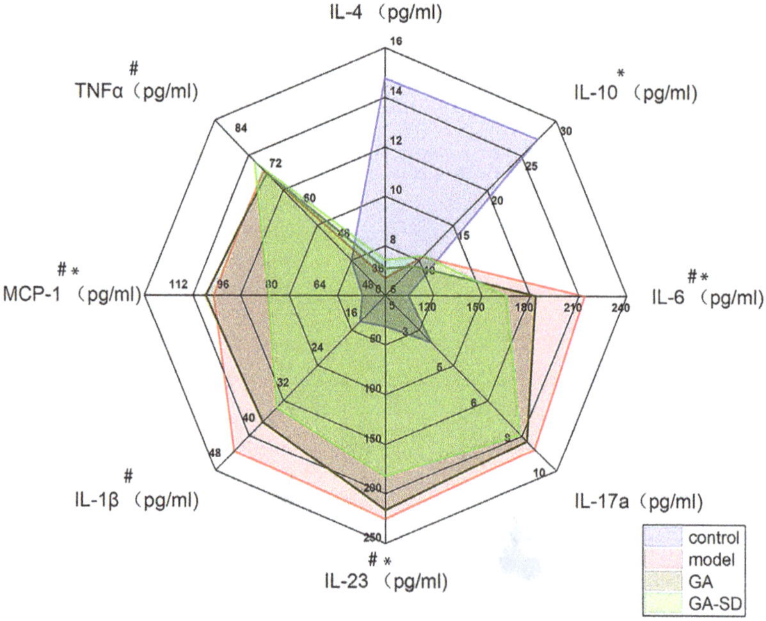

Figure 7. Effect of GA and GA-SD on LPS-induced secretion levels of cytokines such as IL-4, IL-1β, IL-6, MCP-1, TNF-α, IL-23, IL-17A, and IL-10 in RAW264.7 cells. Values are presented as the mean ± SD ($n = 3$). # $p < 0.05$ vs. model group. * $p < 0.05$ vs. LPS group.

3.4. Anti-Inflammatory Efficacy on TPA-Induced Mouse Ear Edema

Based on the current anti-inflammatory effect of solid dispersion GA-SD in vitro, this study was conducted to construct a mouse ear edema model by applying TPA to the outer part of the mouse ear, and the anti-inflammatory effect of GA-SD in vivo was evaluated by gavage administration, using free GA in the control group. The experimental scheme (Figure 8A) and the hematoxylin-eosin staining (H&E) results of the ears of mice receiving different drug treatments are shown in Figure 8. Compared with the ear tissues of the control group of mice (Figure 8B), those of the TPA model group (Figure 8C) showed increased thickness of the auricle, discrete breaks in the transverse muscle fibers, partial congestion of small blood vessels was visible, and a significant increase in inflammatory cell infiltration. In the GA-SD treatment group (Figure 8E), ear tissue edema and transverse muscle fiber breaks were significantly reduced, as was the number of infiltrating inflammatory cells. The inflammatory response induced by TPA was effectively suppressed. In the free GA-treated group (Figure 8D), transverse muscle rupture was reduced, but inflammatory cell infiltration and small vessel congestion were not effectively suppressed. The GA-SD enhanced the anti-inflammatory effect of free GA in vivo. The enhanced anti-inflammatory effect was closely related to the increased solubility of free GA by GA-SD. As a nano-drug delivery system of less than 100 nm, solid dispersions can be adsorbed by the adsorption endocytosis pathway [50,51]. The enhanced cell membrane permeability increased the absorption of GA by the gastrointestinal tract and further increased oral bioavailability for better in vivo anti-inflammatory effects.

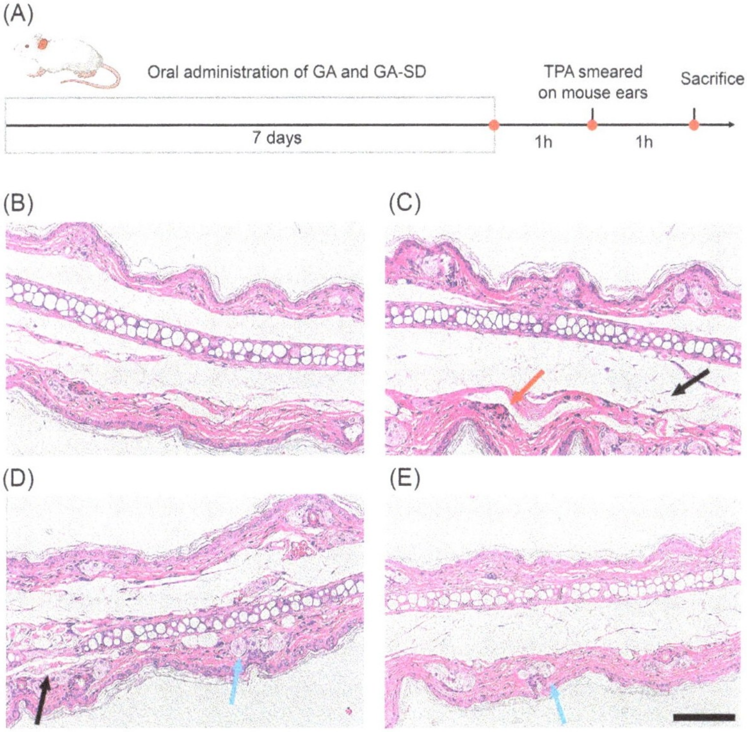

Figure 8. Histopathology of mouse ear in each experimental group. (**A**) Experimental scheme of TPA-induced mouse ear edema model. H&E staining of ear tissue slices after treatment with (**B**) PBS+ acetone, (**C**) PBS+TPA, (**D**) free GA+TPA, and (**E**) GA-SD+TPA. Scale bar: 100 μm. The black arrow marks the discrete rupture of the transverse muscle, the red arrow marks the small vessel congestion, and the blue arrow marks the inflammatory cell infiltration.

3.5. The Biosafety of GA-SD

3.5.1. Histopathological Results from the Liver and Kidney

Arg is a unique, non-toxic, and biocompatible biomolecule [52]. Parikh A, et al. [53] confirmed that histopathological examinations of all the vital organs did not reveal any treatment-related changes in a Soluplus-treated mouse group, indicating the material Soluplus® is biocompatible and could be a suitable candidate for orally administered dosage forms [54]. GA-SD possesses unique physicochemical properties and further improves in vivo cellular uptake efficiency by modifying the free GA morphology and size, but it may also affect the biosafety of the solid dispersion. Thus, a detailed evaluation of GA-SD's potential toxicity in vivo must precede any prospective applications. The results of H&E staining of the liver tissues of mice treated with different drugs are shown in Figure 9A–C. The results showed that the liver tissues of the GA-SD-treated mice were similar to those of the normal group mice. There were abundant numbers of hepatocytes with neatly arranged hepatic cords and intact structures, and no focal necrosis of hepatocytes, fat droplets, or obvious inflammatory cell infiltration was observed. A small amount of inflammatory cell infiltration was seen in the liver tissue of mice in the free GA-treated group, though there was no other obvious pathological damage. The H&E staining results of the kidney tissues of mice receiving different drug treatments are shown in Figure 9D–F. They showed that the kidney tissues of GA-SD-treated mice were similar to those of the control group, with normal glomerular size, intact basement membranes, no obvious inflammatory cell infiltration, and a small number of cellular debris visible in the renal tubules. A certain amount of cellular debris was present in the renal tubules of the mice in the free GA-treated group, though no other obvious damage was observed. This result confirmed that there was no significant histopathological difference between the GA-SD-treated and normal groups and that GA-SD had good biosafety.

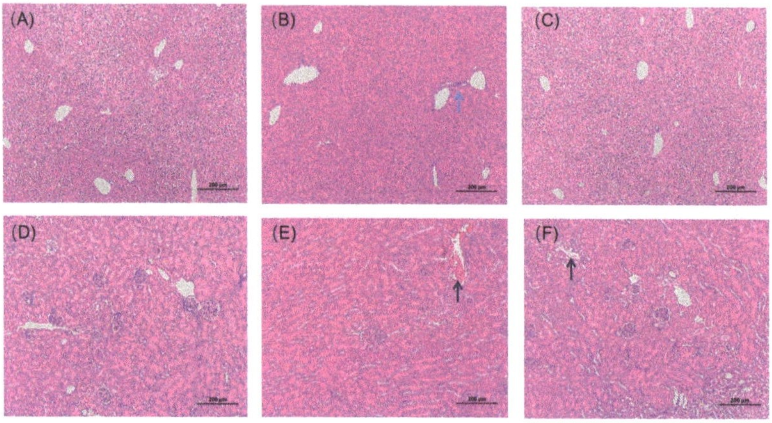

Figure 9. Histopathological studies of the liver and kidney of each group of mice after gavage administration. (**A**) Liver tissue section of the control group; (**B**) liver tissue section of the free GA administration group; (**C**) liver tissue section of the GA-SD administration group; (**D**) kidney tissue section of the normal group; (**E**) kidney tissue section of the GA administration group; (**F**) kidney tissue section of the GA-SD administration group. Scale bar: 200 μm. Black arrows mark cellular debris in the renal tubules; blue arrows mark the phenomenon of inflammatory cell infiltration.

3.5.2. Effect of GA-SD on Liver and Kidney Function

The liver is the main target organ for toxic compounds, while the kidney is a metabolic organ with multiple functions, such as eliminating blood waste and balancing body fluids. In this study, we examined alterations in liver and kidney function biomarkers (AST, ALT, TP, ALB, CREA, UREA) in male Kunming mice after oral administration of GA and GA-SD, thus, assessing the effects of GA and GA-SD on liver and kidney function. Increase in liver enzymes is related to the change in cell membrane permeability caused by liver and hepatocyte damage, so the change in liver enzyme content reflects the hepatotoxicity of the drug. Creatinine and urea are important indicators used to reflect the detoxification of the kidneys, by which the status of renal function is judged as normal [55,56]. The biochemical parameters (TP, ALB, CREA, UREA, AST and ALT) are shown in Figure 10A–F. According to the results, the serum levels of ALT, ACT, TP, ALB, CREA, and UREA in the GA-SD mice were within the normal index range [57,58], and there were no significant changes in the levels of each biochemical index compared to the normal group. The serum biochemical levels were consistent with the histopathological results of the kidney and liver. This result suggested that GA-SD administration did not cause abnormal liver and kidney functions. Therefore, GA-SD has good biosafety.

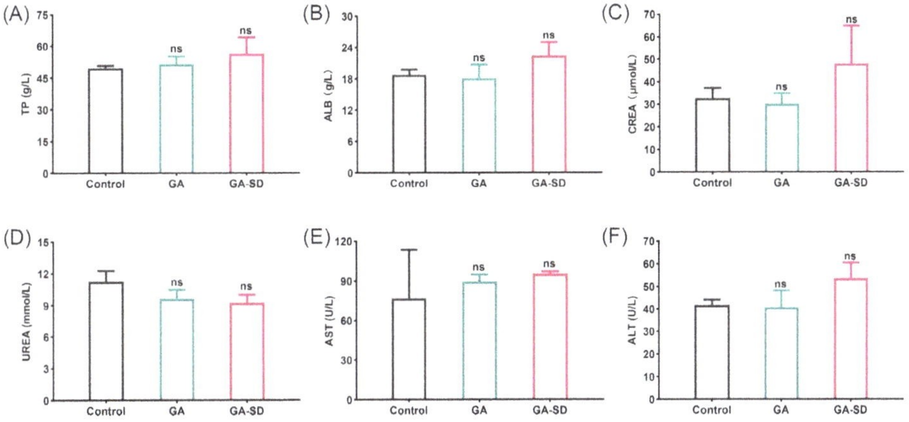

Figure 10. (**A–F**) Serum biochemical changes of drugs treated mice. Values are presented as the mean ± SD (n = 3). ns $p > 0.05$ vs. control group. Biochemical index reference values: TP (57.1 ± 19.4 g/L), ALB (22.4 ± 5.1 g/L), CREA (50.4 ± 35.4 μmol/L), UREA (8.99 ± 2.89 mmol/L), AST (<400 U/L), and ALT (<400 U/L).

3.6. Anti-Inflammatory Efficacy on Ethanol-Induced Gastric Ulcer Model

3.6.1. Effect of GA-SD on the Pathological Features of Ethanol-Induced Gastric Ulcer Model

To further evaluate the anti-inflammatory effect of GA-SD, we established an ethanol-induced gastric ulcer model (Figure 11A). One hour after EtOH gastric ulcer induction, the gastric mucosa of mice in the normal control group was smooth and light pink, also lacking submucosal edema and hemorrhage (Figures 11B and S3). In contrast, the model group gastric mucosa showed severe damage with linear and striated hemorrhagic ulceration covered with coagulated blood, submucosal edema, and erosion. Compared with the model group, bleeding of gastric mucosa was improved in the GA group, but linear hemorrhagic ulceration was still present (ulcer index: 11.94; ulcer inhibition rate %: 31.67) (Figure 11C). The gastric mucosa of GA-SD treated mice were the same as those in the normal control group, with light pink and almost no ulceration (ulcer index:1.38; ulcer inhibition rate %: 92.07). The local and systemic inflammatory response is common in patients with gastric ulcers. The degree of inflammatory response is directly related to the severity of gastric ulcers. The result shows that GA-SD could significantly improve the damage to gastric tissue and reduce the number of bleeding points, suggesting that GA-SD may have a protective effect against gastric ulcer induced by ethanol in mice. Some novel formulations are expected as anti-inflammatory agents to increase the oral uptake of GA. The GA-SD enhanced the anti-inflammatory effect of free GA in vivo.

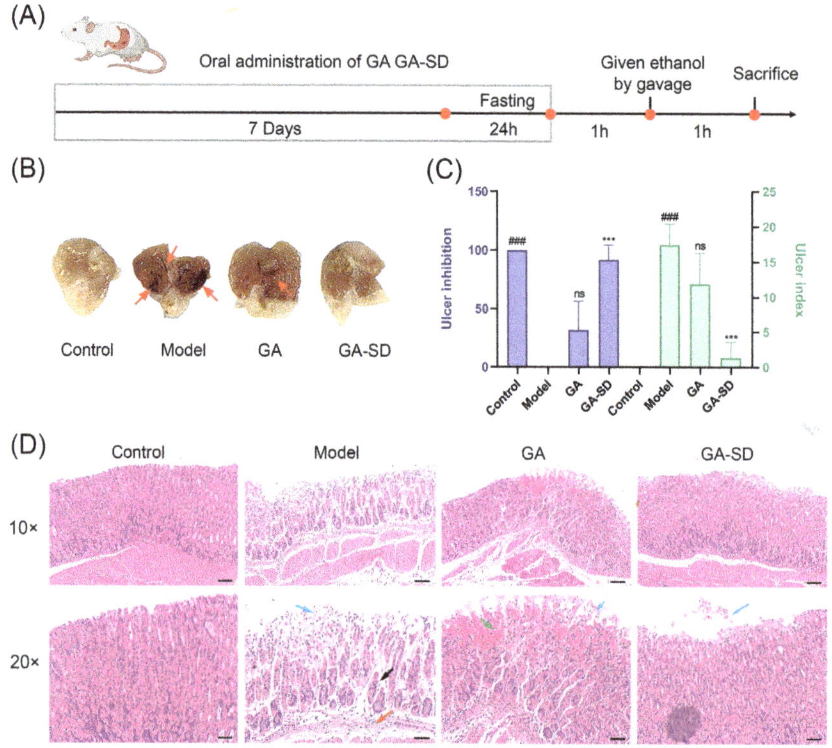

Figure 11. Effect of GA-SD on ethanol-induced gastric ulcer in mice. (**A**) Experimental protocol. (**B**) Macroscopic appearance of gastric tissues (**C**) Ulcer index and the inhibition rate. Data are presented as the mean ± SD (n = 3). Different letters indicate statistically significant differences at the level of $p < 0.05$. $^{###}$ $p < 0.001$ when compared with the control group; *** $p < 0.001$ when compared with the model group. (**D**) H&E staining of gastric tissues (magnification of 10× and 20×). Scale bar of 10×: 100 μm. Scale bar of 20×: 50 μm. Green arrow: hemorrhagic injury; blue arrow: loss of gastric epithelial cells; red arrow: inflammatory cells infiltration; black arrow: disorganized glandular structure.

3.6.2. Histopathological Examination of Gastric Tissues

The results of hematoxylin and eosin-stained (H&E) gastric sections further verified the enhanced anti-inflammatory effect of GA-SD (Figure 11D). Examination of the control group showed normal architecture with intact mucosa, submucosa, muscularis and serosa. In contrast, ethanol caused extensive damage to the gastric tissue. We observed focal areas of erosions and ulcers with epithelial loss, irregular arrangement of gastric glands, the decrease of mucosal glands, and the infiltration of submucosal inflammatory cells. In the GA group, we observed mild submucosal edema, epithelial loss, and a small area of gastric gland necrosis with hemorrhage in the gastric tissue. Stomachs of the GA-SD group showed nearly normal gastric architecture with the absence of epithelial erosion, submucosal edema, and leucocyte infiltration. Ulcered mice, treated with GA-SD demonstrated comparatively better protection of the stomach compared to those treated with GA. The better anti-ulcer and anti-inflammatory effects of GA-SD compared to GA were confirmed by histological analysis. The enhanced anti-inflammatory effect is closely related to the increased solubility of free GA by GA-SD.

3.6.3. Immunohistochemical Analysis of Gastric Tissues

Gastric mucosa damage activates the inflammatory process, which increases the secretion of inflammatory cytokines, leading to gastric mucosal damage [1,59,60]. Pro-inflammatory cytokines in the tissue may be used as biomarkers of gastric visceral damage. The overexpression of TNF-α and IL-6 is considered deleterious to the gastrointestinal system, as it promotes the accumulation of neutrophils, lymphocytes and monocytes/macrophages at inflammatory sites, thereby disrupting the mucosal barrier [61–64]. The protein expression of TNF-α and IL-6 were stained in Cytoplasm, and the positive expression of TNF-α and IL-6 in the ethanol ulcerated group was significantly higher than that in the other two groups (Figure 12). The increased levels of TNF-α and IL-6 in the gastric tissues of ethanol ulcerated mice were confirmed via IHC staining. Compared with the ethanol ulcerated group, the GA-SD group significantly reduced the release of TNF-α and IL-6. Collectively, GA-SD was more effective than free GA in preventing ethanol-induced acute gastric ulcer, which was related to the improved solubility and bioavailability of GA-SD and enhanced anti-inflammatory activity.

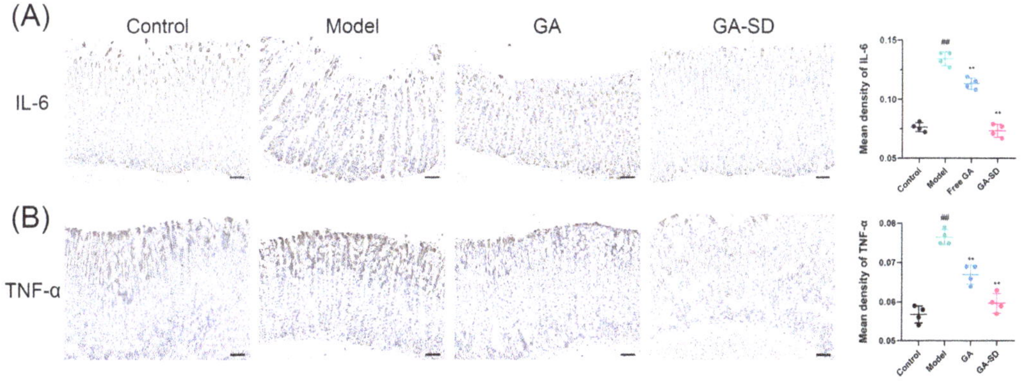

Figure 12. Immunohistochemical analysis of IL-6 and TNF-α in gastric tissues (magnification of 20×). Scale bar: 50 μm. (**A**) Representative photomicrographs of immunohistochemical staining for IL-6 among different groups. (**B**) Representative photomicrographs of immunohistochemical staining for TNF-α among different groups. Data are presented as the mean ± SD (n = 4) ## $p < 0.01$ vs. control. ** $p < 0.01$ vs. the model group.

4. Conclusions

In this study, we used the co-solvent evaporation method to make GA and L-Arg react to form salts and then added the polymer-solvent Soluplus® with an amphiphilic chemical structure. GA-SD solid dispersions with particle size less than 100 nm, irregular morphology and good stability were successfully prepared. GA-SD has a particle size below 100 nm, which allows GA-SD to avoid rapid clearance by the reticuloendothelial system and increases cytomembrane penetrability. The presence of L-Arg and Soluplus® in the solid dispersion enables GA-SD to have high solubility; therefore, many of the limitations of free GA, such as poor water solubility, low cellular utilization, and low bioavailability, have been solved. The results of anti-inflammatory effect in vitro showed that the immunomodulatory effect of GA-SD was superior to free GA and GA-SD enhanced the anti-inflammatory effect of free GA in vitro. The anti-inflammatory effect of GA-SD in vivo was evaluated by gavage administration in a TPA-induced mouse ear edema model and ethanol-induced gastric ulcer model. The results indicated that GA-SD effectively improved the anti-inflammatory effect of free GA in vivo. Furthermore, GA-SD had no significant effects on liver and kidney functions, there was no significant tissue toxicity and it displayed good biosafety. With the improvement of the solubility and utilization of GA, the application scope of GA in the treatment of many inflammatory diseases will be expanded. As a safe and effective solid dispersion, it is a promising anti-inflammatory oral formulation and may provide some references for other oral drug candidates with low bioavailability.

Supplementary Materials: The following supporting information can be downloaded at: https://www.mdpi.com/article/10.3390/pharmaceutics14091797/s1, Table S1: Relative proportions of solid dispersion components; Table S2: Grouping and sampling of mice in the ear edema model ($n = 5$). Table S3: Grouping and sampling of mice in ethanol-induced gastric ulcer model ($n = 5$); Figure S1. FT-IR analysis; Figure S2. Dissolution phenomena for 10 mg GA, GA-SD samples in 1 mL water; Figure S3. Macroscopic appearance of gastric tissues.

Author Contributions: Conceptualization, H.L., M.Q. and C.H.; Supervision, funding acquisition and writing-review and editing, H.L. and M.Q.; Investigation, data curation, formal analysis, and writing-original draft, R.L., H.W. and Y.R., S.L.; Formal analysis and validation: H.W., R.L., Y.R., S.L., Y.Z., L.M., Q.W. and Q.O. All authors have read and agreed to the published version of the manuscript.

Funding: This work was funded by the National Key Research and Development Program of China (2021YFE0103500), National Natural Science Foundation (52003021), and Beijing Municipal Science & Technology Commission (Project No. Z171100001717024).

Institutional Review Board Statement: The authors are thankful to the Committee for Care and Use of experimental animals. All experiments were conducted by the regulations of the National Institutes of Health (NIH) and the Beijing Laboratory Animal Ethics Committee.

Informed Consent Statement: Not applicable.

Data Availability Statement: The data presented in this study are available in the article or Supplementary Materials here.

Conflicts of Interest: The authors declare no conflict of interest.

References

1. Ptaschinski, C.; Lukacs, N.W. Acute and chronic inflammation induces disease pathogenesis. In *Molecular Pathology*; Elsevier: Amsterdam, The Netherlands, 2018; pp. 25–43.
2. Wang, C.-Y.; Kao, T.-C.; Lo, W.-H.; Yen, G.-C. Glycyrrhizic acid and 18β-glycyrrhetinic acid modulate lipopolysaccharide-induced inflammatory response by suppression of NF-κB through PI3K p110δ and p110γ inhibitions. *J. Agric. Food Chem.* **2011**, *59*, 7726–7733. [CrossRef] [PubMed]
3. Henderson, W.R. The role of leukotrienes in inflammation. *Ann. Intern. Med.* **1994**, *121*, 684–697. [CrossRef] [PubMed]
4. Tasneem, S.; Liu, B.; Li, B.; Choudhary, M.I.; Wang, W. Molecular pharmacology of inflammation: Medicinal plants as anti-inflammatory agents. *Pharmacol. Res.* **2019**, *139*, 126–140. [CrossRef] [PubMed]
5. Kao, T.-C.; Shyu, M.-H.; Yen, G.-C. Glycyrrhizic acid and 18β-glycyrrhetinic acid inhibit inflammation via PI3K/Akt/GSK3β signaling and glucocorticoid receptor activation. *J. Agric. Food Chem.* **2010**, *58*, 8623–8629. [CrossRef]
6. Wu, J.; Zhang, Y.-Y.; Guo, L.; Li, H.; Chen, D.-F. Bupleurum polysaccharides attenuates lipopolysaccharide-induced inflammation via modulating Toll-like receptor 4 signaling. *PLoS ONE* **2013**, *8*, e78051. [CrossRef]
7. Fong, S.Y.; Liu, M.; Wei, H.; Löbenberg, R.; Kanfer, I.; Lee, V.H.; Amidon, G.L.; Zuo, Z. Establishing the pharmaceutical quality of Chinese herbal medicine: A provisional BCS classification. *Mol. Pharm.* **2013**, *10*, 1623–1643. [CrossRef]
8. Hosseinzadeh, H.; Nassiri-Asl, M. Pharmacological effects of Glycyrrhiza spp. and its bioactive constituents: Update and review. *Phytother. Res.* **2015**, *29*, 1868–1886. [CrossRef]
9. Peng, L.-N.; Li, L.; Qiu, Y.-F.; Miao, J.-H.; Gao, X.-Q.; Zhou, Y.; Shi, Z.-X.; Xu, Y.-L.; Shao, D.-H.; Wei, J.-C. Glycyrrhetinic acid extracted from Glycyrrhiza uralensis Fisch. induces the expression of Toll-like receptor 4 in Ana-1 murine macrophages. *J. Asian Nat. Prod. Res.* **2011**, *13*, 942–950. [CrossRef]
10. Cai, J.; Luo, S.; Lv, X.; Deng, Y.; Huang, H.; Zhao, B.; Zhang, Q.; Li, G. Formulation of injectable glycyrrhizic acid-hydroxycamptothecin micelles as new generation of DNA topoisomerase I inhibitor for enhanced antitumor activity. *Int. J. Pharm.* **2019**, *571*, 118693. [CrossRef]
11. Lei, Y.; Kong, Y.; Sui, H.; Feng, J.; Zhu, R.; Wang, W.J.D.D.; Research, T. Enhanced oral bioavailability of glycyrrhetinic acid via nanocrystal formulation. *Drug Deliv. Transl. Res.* **2016**, *6*, 519–525. [CrossRef]
12. Sahoo, A.; Kumar, N.K.; Suryanarayanan, R.J. Crosslinking: An avenue to develop stable amorphous solid dispersion with high drug loading and tailored physical stability. *J. Control. Release* **2019**, *311*, 212–224. [CrossRef]
13. Vasconcelos, T.; Sarmento, B.; Costa, P. Solid dispersions as strategy to improve oral bioavailability of poor water soluble drugs. *Drug Discov. Today* **2007**, *12*, 1068–1075. [CrossRef]

14. Osman, Y.B.; Liavitskaya, T.; Vyazovkin, S. Polyvinylpyrrolidone affects thermal stability of drugs in solid dispersions. *Int. J. Pharm.* **2018**, *551*, 111–120. [CrossRef]
15. Sui, X.; Chu, Y.; Zhang, J.; Zhang, H.; Wang, H.; Liu, T.; Han, C. The Effect of PVP Molecular Weight on Dissolution Behavior and Physicochemical Characterization of Glycyrrhetinic Acid Solid Dispersions. *Adv. Polym. Technol.* **2020**, *2020*, 8859658. [CrossRef]
16. Dong, L.; Mai, Y.; Liu, Q.; Zhang, W.; Yang, J.J.P. Mechanism and improved dissolution of glycyrrhetinic acid solid dispersion by alkalizers. *Pharmaceutics* **2020**, *12*, 82. [CrossRef]
17. Hou, J.; Sun, E.; Sun, C.; Wang, J.; Yang, L.; Jia, X.-B.; Zhang, Z.-H. Improved oral bioavailability and anticancer efficacy on breast cancer of paclitaxel via Novel Soluplus®—Solutol®HS15 binary mixed micelles system. *Int. J. Pharm.* **2016**, *512*, 186–193. [CrossRef]
18. Nagy, Z.K.; Balogh, A.; Vajna, B.; Farkas, A.; Patyi, G.; Kramarics, Á.; Marosi, G. Comparison of electrospun and extruded Soluplus®-based solid dosage forms of improved dissolution. *J. Pharm. Sci.* **2012**, *101*, 322–332. [CrossRef]
19. Bonde, G.V.; Ajmal, G.; Yadav, S.K.; Mittal, P.; Singh, J.; Bakde, B.V.; Mishra, B.J.C.; Biointerfaces, S.B. Assessing the viability of Soluplus®self-assembled nanocolloids for sustained delivery of highly hydrophobic lapatinib (anticancer agent): Optimisation and in-vitro characterisation. *Colloids Surf. B Biointerfaces* **2020**, *185*, 110611. [CrossRef]
20. Grotz, E.; Tateosian, N.L.; Salgueiro, J.; Bernabeu, E.; Gonzalez, L.; Manca, M.L.; Amiano, N.; Valenti, D.; Manconi, M.; García, V.; et al. Pulmonary delivery of rifampicin-loaded soluplus micelles against Mycobacterium tuberculosis. *J. Drug Deliv. Sci. Technol.* **2019**, *53*, 101170. [CrossRef]
21. Shi, F.; Chen, L.; Wang, Y.; Liu, J.; Adu-Frimpong, M.; Ji, H.; Toreniyazov, E.; Wang, Q.; Yu, J.; Xu, X. Enhancement of oral bioavailability and anti-hyperuricemic activity of aloe emodin via novel Soluplus®—Glycyrrhizic acid mixed micelle system. *Drug Deliv. Transl. Res.* **2022**, *12*, 603–614. [CrossRef]
22. Shamma, R.N.; Basha, M. Soluplus®: A novel polymeric solubilizer for optimization of carvedilol solid dispersions: Formulation design and effect of method of preparation. *Powder Technol.* **2013**, *237*, 406–414. [CrossRef]
23. Löbmann, K.; Grohganz, H.; Laitinen, R.; Strachan, C.; Rades, T. Amino acids as co-amorphous stabilizers for poorly water soluble drugs—Part 1: Preparation, stability and dissolution enhancement. *Eur. J. Pharm. Biopharm.* **2013**, *85*, 873–881. [CrossRef]
24. Azzi, J.; Danjou, P.-E.; Landy, D.; Ruellan, S.; Auezova, L.; Greige-Gerges, H.; Fourmentin, S. The effect of cyclodextrin complexation on the solubility and photostability of nerolidol as pure compound and as main constituent of cabreuva essential oil. *Beilstein J. Org. Chem.* **2017**, *13*, 835–844. [CrossRef]
25. Zi, P.; Zhang, C.; Ju, C.; Su, Z.; Bao, Y.; Gao, J.; Sun, J.; Lu, J.; Zhang, C. Solubility and bioavailability enhancement study of lopinavir solid dispersion matrixed with a polymeric surfactant-Soluplus. *Eur. J. Pharm. Sci.* **2019**, *134*, 233–245. [CrossRef]
26. Karagianni, A.; Kachrimanis, K.; Nikolakakis, I. Co-amorphous solid dispersions for solubility and absorption improvement of drugs: Composition, preparation, characterization and formulations for oral delivery. *Pharmaceutics* **2018**, *10*, 98. [CrossRef]
27. Qi, W.; Ding, D.; Salvi, R. Cytotoxic effects of dimethyl sulphoxide (DMSO) on cochlear organotypic cultures. *Hear. Res.* **2008**, *236*, 52–60. [CrossRef]
28. Wang, S.; Cao, M.; Xu, S.; Shi, J.; Mao, X.; Yao, X.; Liu, C. Luteolin alters macrophage polarization to inhibit inflammation. *Inflammation* **2020**, *43*, 95–108. [CrossRef]
29. He, Y.; Liu, H.; Bian, W.; Liu, Y.; Liu, X.; Ma, S.; Zheng, X.; Du, Z.; Zhang, K.; Ouyang, D. Molecular interactions for the curcumin-polymer complex with enhanced anti-inflammatory effects. *Pharmaceutics* **2019**, *11*, 442. [CrossRef]
30. Clemens, M.M.; Vazquez, J.H.; Kennon-McGill, S.; McCullough, S.S.; James, L.P.; McGill, M.R. Pre-treatment twice with liposomal clodronate protects against acetaminophen hepatotoxicity through a pre-conditioning effect. *Liver Res.* **2020**, *4*, 145–152. [CrossRef] [PubMed]
31. Park, H.-S.; Seo, C.-S.; Baek, E.B.; Rho, J.-H.; Won, Y.-S.; Kwun, H.-J.; Medicine, A. Gastroprotective effect of myricetin on ethanol-induced acute gastric injury in rats. *Altern. Med.* **2021**, *2021*, 9968112. [CrossRef] [PubMed]
32. Cai, Z.; Wang, Y.; Zhu, L.-J.; Liu, Z.-Q. Nanocarriers: A general strategy for enhancement of oral bioavailability of poorly absorbed or pre-systemically metabolized drugs. *Curr. Drug Metab.* **2010**, *11*, 197–207. [CrossRef] [PubMed]
33. Al-Akayleh, F.; Al-Naji, I.; Adwan, S.; Al-Remawi, M.; Shubair, M. Enhancement of curcumin solubility using a novel solubilizing polymer Soluplus®. *J. Pharm. Innov.* **2020**, *17*, 142–154. [CrossRef]
34. Kazunori, K.; Masayuki, Y.; Teruo, O.; Yasuhisa, S. Block copolymer micelles as vehicles for drug delivery. *J. Control. Release* **1993**, *24*, 119–132. [CrossRef]
35. Albadarin, A.B.; Potter, C.B.; Davis, M.T.; Iqbal, J.; Korde, S.; Pagire, S.; Paradkar, A.; Walker, G. Development of stability-enhanced ternary solid dispersions via combinations of HPMCP and Soluplus®processed by hot melt extrusion. *Int. J. Pharm.* **2017**, *532*, 603–611. [CrossRef]
36. Löbmann, K.; Laitinen, R.; Strachan, C.; Rades, T.; Grohganz, H. Biopharmaceutics. Amino acids as co-amorphous stabilizers for poorly water-soluble drugs—Part 2: Molecular interactions. *Eur. J. Pharm. Biopharm.* **2013**, *85*, 882–888. [CrossRef]
37. Ueda, H.; Wu, W.; Löbmann, K.; Grohganz, H.; Müllertz, A.; Rades, T. Application of a salt coformer in a co-amorphous drug system dramatically enhances the glass transition temperature: A case study of the ternary system carbamazepine, citric acid, and l-arginine. *Mol. Pharm.* **2018**, *15*, 2036–2044. [CrossRef]
38. Hao, J.; Sun, Y.; Wang, Q.; Tong, X.; Zhang, H.; Zhang, Q. Effect and mechanism of penetration enhancement of organic base and alcohol on Glycyrrhetinic acid in vitro. *Int. J. Pharm.* **2010**, *399*, 102–108. [CrossRef]

39. Tian, B.; Ju, X.; Yang, D.; Kong, Y.; Tang, X. Effect of the third component on the aging and crystallization of cinnarizine-soluplus®binary solid dispersion. *Int. J. Pharm.* **2020**, *580*, 119240. [CrossRef]
40. Li, Q.; He, Q.; Xu, M.; Li, J.; Liu, X.; Wan, Z.; Yang, X. Food-grade emulsions and emulsion gels prepared by soy protein-pectin complex nanoparticles and glycyrrhizic acid nanofibrils. *J. Agric. Food Chem.* **2020**, *68*, 1051–1063. [CrossRef]
41. Selvakumar, E.; Ramasamy, P.; Devi, T.U.; Meenakshi, R.; Chandramohan, A.; Spectroscopy, B. Synthesis, growth, structure and spectroscopic characterization of a new organic nonlinear optical hydrogen bonding complex crystal: 3-Carboxyl anilinium p-toluene sulfonate. *Spectrochim. Acta Part A Mol. Biomol. Spectrosc.* **2014**, *125*, 114–119. [CrossRef]
42. Chisca, D.; Croitor, L.; Coropceanu, E.B.; Fonari, M.S. Four Cu (II) coordination polymers with biocompatible isonicotinamide and picolinate ligands in interplay with anionic and neutral linkers. *Inorg. Chem. Commun.* **2021**, *132*, 108864. [CrossRef]
43. Hamed, A.A.; Saad, G.R.; Abdelhamid, I.A.; Elwahy, A.H.; Abdel-Aziz, M.M.; Elsabee, M.Z. Chitosan Schiff bases-based polyelectrolyte complexes with graphene quantum dots and their prospective biomedical applications. *Int. J. Biol. Macromol.* **2022**, *208*, 1029–1045. [CrossRef]
44. Shi, N.-Q.; Lai, H.-W.; Zhang, Y.; Feng, B.; Xiao, X.; Zhang, H.-M.; Li, Z.-Q.; Qi, X.-R. Technology. On the inherent properties of Soluplus and its application in ibuprofen solid dispersions generated by microwave-quench cooling technology. *Pharm. Dev. Technol.* **2018**, *23*, 573–586. [CrossRef]
45. Liu, T.; Zhu, W.; Han, C.; Sui, X.; Liu, C.; Ma, X.; Dong, Y. Preparation of glycyrrhetinic acid liposomes using lyophilization monophase solution method: Preformulation, optimization, and in vitro evaluation. *Nanoscale Res. Lett.* **2018**, *13*, 1–13. [CrossRef]
46. Chan, M.; Cheung, C.; Chui, W.; Tsao, S.; Nicholls, J.; Chan, Y.; Chan, R.; Long, H.; Poon, L.; Guan, Y. Proinflammatory cytokine responses induced by influenza A (H5N1) viruses in primary human alveolar and bronchial epithelial cells. *Respir. Res.* **2005**, *6*, 1–13. [CrossRef]
47. Liu, Q.; Zhou, Y.-h.; Yang, Z.-Q. The cytokine storm of severe influenza and development of immunomodulatory therapy. *Cell. Mol. Immunol.* **2016**, *13*, 3–10. [CrossRef]
48. Iyer, S.S.; Cheng, G. Role of interleukin 10 transcriptional regulation in inflammation and autoimmune disease. *Crit. Rev.™ Immunol.* **2012**, *32*, 23–63. [CrossRef]
49. Sharma, A.; Tirpude, N.V.; Kulurkar, P.M.; Sharma, R.; Padwad, Y. Berberis lycium fruit extract attenuates oxi-inflammatory stress and promotes mucosal healing by mitigating NF-κB/c-Jun/MAPKs signalling and augmenting splenic Treg proliferation in a murine model of dextran sulphate sodium-induced ulcerative colitis. *Eur. J. Nutr.* **2020**, *59*, 2663–2681. [CrossRef]
50. Carstens, M.G.; Rijcken, C.J.; Nostrum, C.F.; Hennink, W.E. Pharmaceutical micelles: Combining longevity, stability, and stimuli sensitivity. In *Multifunctional Pharmaceutical Nanocarriers*; Springer: Berlin/Heidelberg, Germany, 2008; pp. 263–308.
51. Zhu, Y.; Peng, W.; Zhang, J.; Wang, M.; Firempong, C.K.; Feng, C.; Liu, H.; Xu, X.; Yu, J. Enhanced oral bioavailability of capsaicin in mixed polymeric micelles: Preparation, in vitro and in vivo evaluation. *J. Funct. Foods* **2014**, *8*, 358–366. [CrossRef]
52. Han, C.; Yu, Q.; Jiang, J.; Zhang, X.; Wang, F.; Jiang, M.; Yu, R.; Deng, T.; Yu, C. Bioenzyme-responsive l-arginine-based carbon dots: The replenishment of nitric oxide for nonpharmaceutical therapy. *Biomater. Sci.* **2021**, *9*, 7432–7443. [CrossRef]
53. Parikh, A.; Kathawala, K.; Li, J.; Chen, C.; Shan, Z.; Cao, X.; Wang, Y.-J.; Garg, S.; Zhou, X.-F. Self-nanomicellizing solid dispersion of edaravone: Part II: In vivo assessment of efficacy against behavior deficits and safety in Alzheimer's disease model. *Drug Des. Dev. Ther.* **2018**, *12*, 2111. [CrossRef]
54. Lian, X.; Dong, J.; Zhang, J.; Teng, Y.; Lin, Q.; Fu, Y.; Gong, T. Soluplus® based 9-nitrocamptothecin solid dispersion for peroral administration: Preparation, characterization, in vitro and in vivo evaluation. *Int. J. Pharm.* **2014**, *477*, 399–407. [CrossRef]
55. Ghosh, S.; Ghosh, I.; Chakrabarti, M.; Mukherjee, A.; Toxicology, C. Genotoxicity and biocompatibility of superparamagnetic iron oxide nanoparticles: Influence of surface modification on biodistribution, retention, DNA damage and oxidative stress. *Food Chem. Toxicol.* **2020**, *136*, 110989. [CrossRef]
56. Mossa, A.-T.H.; Mohafrash, S.M.; Chandrasekaran, N. Safety of natural insecticides: Toxic effects on experimental animals. *BioMed Res. Int.* **2018**, *2018*, 4308054. [CrossRef]
57. Silva-Santana, G.; Bax, J.C.; Fernandes, D.C.S.; Bacellar, D.T.L.; Hooper, C.; Dias, A.A.S.O.; Silva, C.B.; de Souza, A.M.; Ramos, S.; Santos, R.A. Clinical hematological and biochemical parameters in Swiss, BALB/c, C57BL/6 and B6D2F1 Mus musculus. *Anim. Model. Exp. Med.* **2020**, *3*, 304–315. [CrossRef]
58. Li, Z.; Qiao, Y.; Li, J.; An, C.; Hu, K.; Tang, M. Pharmacology. Acute and sub-chronic toxicity studies of the extract of Thunberg Fritillary Bulb. *Regul. Toxicol. Pharmacol.* **2014**, *68*, 370–377. [CrossRef]
59. Akanda, M.R.; Kim, I.-S.; Ahn, D.; Tae, H.-J.; Nam, H.-H.; Choo, B.-K.; Kim, K.; Park, B.-Y. Anti-inflammatory and gastroprotective roles of rabdosia inflexa through downregulation of pro-inflammatory cytokines and MAPK/NF-κB signaling pathways. *Int. J. Mol. Sci.* **2018**, *19*, 584. [CrossRef]
60. Tadić, V.M.; Dobrić, S.; Marković, G.M.; Đorđević, S.M.; Arsić, I.A.; Menković, N.R.; Stević, T. Anti-inflammatory, gastroprotective, free-radical-scavenging, and antimicrobial activities of hawthorn berries ethanol extract. *J. Agric. Food Chem.* **2008**, *56*, 7700–7709. [CrossRef]
61. Augusto, A.C.; Miguel, F.; Mendonça, S.; Pedrazzoli, J., Jr.; Gurgueira, S.A. Oxidative stress expression status associated to Helicobacter pylori virulence in gastric diseases. *Clin. Biochem.* **2007**, *40*, 615–622. [CrossRef]
62. Mei, X.; Xu, D.; Xu, S.; Zheng, Y.; Xu, S. Novel role of Zn (II)-curcumin in enhancing cell proliferation and adjusting proinflammatory cytokine-mediated oxidative damage of ethanol-induced acute gastric ulcers. *Chem. Interact.* **2012**, *197*, 31–39. [CrossRef]

63. Mahmoud, Y.I.; Abd El-Ghffar, E.A. Spirulina ameliorates aspirin-induced gastric ulcer in albino mice by alleviating oxidative stress and inflammation. *Biomed. Pharm.* **2019**, *109*, 314–321. [CrossRef] [PubMed]
64. Li, M.; Lv, R.; Xu, X.; Ge, Q.; Lin, S. Tricholoma matsutake-Derived Peptides Show Gastroprotective Effects against Ethanol-Induced Acute Gastric Injury. *J. Agric. Food Chem.* **2021**, *69*, 14985–14994. [CrossRef] [PubMed]

pharmaceutics

MDPI

Review

Potential Applications of Chitosan-Based Nanomaterials to Surpass the Gastrointestinal Physiological Obstacles and Enhance the Intestinal Drug Absorption

Nutthapoom Pathomthongtaweechai * and **Chatchai Muanprasat**

Chakri Naruebodindra Medical Institute, Faculty of Medicine Ramathibodi Hospital, Mahidol University, Bang Phli 10540, Samut Prakan, Thailand; chatchai.mua@mahidol.ac.th
* Correspondence: nutthapoom.pat@mahidol.edu; Tel.: +66-61-016-7343

Abstract: The small intestine provides the major site for the absorption of numerous orally administered drugs. However, before reaching to the systemic circulation to exert beneficial pharmacological activities, the oral drug delivery is hindered by poor absorption/metabolic instability of the drugs in gastrointestinal (GI) tract and the presence of the mucus layer overlying intestinal epithelium. Therefore, a polymeric drug delivery system has emerged as a robust approach to enhance oral drug bioavailability and intestinal drug absorption. Chitosan, a cationic polymer derived from chitin, and its derivatives have received remarkable attention to serve as a promising drug carrier, chiefly owing to their versatile, biocompatible, biodegradable, and non-toxic properties. Several types of chitosan-based drug delivery systems have been developed, including chemical modification, conjugates, capsules, and hybrids. They have been shown to be effective in improving intestinal assimilation of several types of drugs, e.g., antidiabetic, anticancer, antimicrobial, and anti-inflammatory drugs. In this review, the physiological challenges affecting intestinal drug absorption and the effects of chitosan on those parameters impacting on oral bioavailability are summarized. More appreciably, types of chitosan-based nanomaterials enhancing intestinal drug absorption and their mechanisms, as well as potential applications in diabetes, cancers, infections, and inflammation, are highlighted. The future perspective of chitosan applications is also discussed.

Keywords: chitosan; drug delivery; drug absorption; intestinal assimilation; oral bioavailability

Citation: Pathomthongtaweechai, N.; Muanprasat, C. Potential Applications of Chitosan-Based Nanomaterials to Surpass the Gastrointestinal Physiological Obstacles and Enhance the Intestinal Drug Absorption. *Pharmaceutics* **2021**, *13*, 887. https://doi.org/10.3390/pharmaceutics13060887

Academic Editors: Ana Isabel Fernandes and Angela Faustino Jozala

Received: 7 May 2021
Accepted: 11 June 2021
Published: 15 June 2021

1. Introduction

Oral entry route is the most favorable and frequently used pathway for drug administration owing to its simplicity, feasibility, convenience, low-cost manufacturing process, non-invasiveness, and safety for most patients [1,2]. After intake of medication, the orally administered drugs travel down to the stomach and they are majorly absorbed at the proximal part of small intestine before entering the systemic circulation. However, the drug substances have to challenge with the harsh environment of the gastrointestinal (GI) tract, including gastric pH, digestive enzymes, bile salts, GI motility, and intestinal mucosal layers, ameliorating the drug absorption or drug assimilation and leading to poor oral bioavailability [3,4]. In order to overcome these physiological obstacles, the drug delivery system has been designed and developed. The ideal characteristics of nano-drug carriers are safe, biocompatible, biodegradable, acid-tolerant, and GI enzyme-stable [5–7]. Moreover, to deliver the drugs to the systemic circulation, the carriers should help to penetrate the mucosal microenvironment and prolong the drug-mucosa contact time for extent duration of drug absorption [8,9]. In response to the fluctuation of pH along the GI tract, the suitable carriers should be able to control the drug release in each GI segment. In recent times, the investigators have taken the advantages of these properties found in the natural polymers, particularly chitosan [2,4].

Chitosan is a cationic linear heteropolysaccharide, consisting of β-(1,4)-linked D-glucosamine (GlcN, deacetylated monomer) and N-acetyl-D-glucosamine (GlcNAc, acetylated monomer) [10,11]. It is obtained from chitin, containing β-(1,4)-linked 2-acetamido-2-deoxy-β-D-glucose, which is the second-most abundant natural polymer in the world and is mostly found in the structural component of exoskeletons of crustaceans (e.g., shrimps, lobsters, and crabs), insects, and arthropods as well as in the cell wall of fungi [10,11]. The outstanding features of chitosan, including natural abundance, water solubility, non-toxicity, biodegradability, and chemical modifiability, make this natural biomaterial attractive as an ideal candidate for adopting in pharmacological and biotechnological applications [8]. In the drug delivery system, the chitosan-based nanoparticles have been formulated by several techniques, such as chemical modification, ionic gelation, and polyelectrolyte complexation methods [12,13]. These nanomaterials can boost up the oral drug absorption by improving mucoadhesion, the permeation-enhancing effect, and controlled drug release [2,4,8,9].

Herein, the aims of this review are (i) to provide the comprehensive knowledge involving GI physiological challenge-modulated intestinal drug absorption and oral bioavailability, as well as (ii), to address the implication of chitosan and various types of emerged chitosan-based nanomaterials in the improvement of intestinal drug assimilation.

2. The GI Challenges of Intestinal Drug Absorption

In any given patients, the orally taken drugs must encounter a ruthless GI environment, which is influenced by multiple determinants, such as the age, gender, and ethnicity of the treated patients [14–17]. These factors can affect the physiologically challenging variables involved in the drug absorption, including intraluminal pH, gastric emptying time, intestinal transit time, GI motility, intestinal transporter proteins, gut microbiota, and disease conditions (Figure 1).

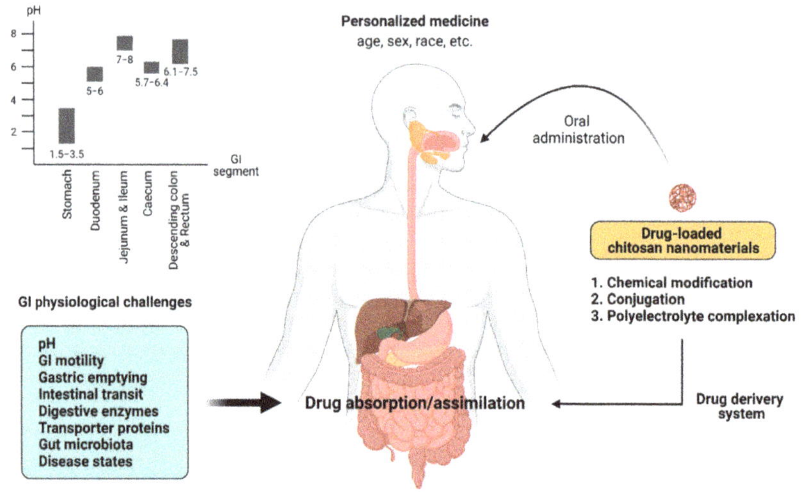

Figure 1. The schematic illustration of the GI physiological barriers affecting drug absorption. When one orally takes the drug-loaded chitosan nanomaterials (e.g., chitosan-based nanoparticles with chemical modification, conjugated chitosan, and chitosan-based polyelectrolyte complex), they encounter GI physiological challenges, including a variable pH along the GI tract, GI motility and gastric emptying, intestinal transit, digestive enzymes, transporter protein expression, gut microbiota, and disease conditions. The GI physiological challenge can be influenced by aging, gender, and ethnicity. Created with BioRender.com.

Age-dependent alteration of oral drug absorption gives rise to the adjustment of drug dosing to meet the medical requirement, particularly in childhood, due to the immaturity of the GI tract [14,18]. Therefore, tailor-made pediatric dosage at a specific age is necessary. In addition, poor cooperation in pediatric patients makes it more difficult. For the elderly, the frailty is associated with the progressive impairment of organ structures and functions, which affects the GI physiology and oral drug bioavailability [15,19]. Additionally, polypharmacy in advancing age brings about the increased risk of adverse drug reactions and poor drug compliance [19]. Gender-based changes in GI function also needs to be considered. The difference in occupational exposures, behavior, lifestyle, and medications between men and women leads to the dissimilarity in body weight, body surface area, and the amount of water, contributing to sex-divergent pharmacokinetics [20,21]. Ethnicity/race-related differences in body response to medications has been documented due to the interaction of genetic variation and the environmental factors [17,22]. In particular, the racial genetic difference is resulted from the variance in genetic polymorphisms [23,24].

The GI physiological challenges limit the capability of absorption of orally taken drugs and thus affect their oral bioavailability. The amount of drugs that are assimilated at the absorption site will reflect the alteration of the pharmacokinetics in the patients, compared with normal subjects. A synopsis of the physiological challenges impacting on oral drug bioavailability is recapitulated as below and is depicted in Figure 1. In addition, the effect of chitosan on those parameters and disease states are included.

2.1. Gastric pH

The gastric pH is acidic, with a pH between 1.5 and 3.5. When passing down to the small intestine, the pH slowly increases to 5–6 in the duodenum and 7–8 in the jejunum and terminal ileum. Meanwhile, the pH falls to 5.7–6.4 in the caecum and rises again at the range of 6.1–7.5 in the descending colon and rectum [14,25]. Therefore, the drugs have to expose to the variation of the pH along the GI tract, which may cause the deactivation of the drugs, particularly in protein and peptide drugs by the modulation of differential oxidation, hydrolysis, or deamination of these drugs [26]. In the drug delivery system, the environmental pH determines the drug dissolution and drug absorption by affecting the degree of ionization (pK_a) of the drug substrates [27]. The water-insoluble weakly alkaline drugs are ionized and dissolved in the low-pH stomach lumen, but have poor drug absorption at the small intestine [28]. Impaired drug absorption of weak basic drug can occur in the stomach of the patients with achlorhydria or hypochlorhydria, which have no or decreased gastric acid secretion, respectively [29]. In addition, the patients who took weakly basic drugs with antacids, which could cause a rise in gastric pH, were reported to reduce the drug absorption of those basic drugs by the chelation with polyvalent cations (e.g., Ca^{2+}, Mg^{2+}, and Al^{3+}) and subsequent formation of insoluble complex [30,31].

At birth, the gastric pH is neutral due to the presence of amniotic fluid in the stomach. It then gradually decreases until the age of two years, reaching to the adult-equivalent pH [32,33]. In the elderly, the gastric pH is increased, resulting in the slight decrease in drug absorption [19,33]. In women, smaller gastric secretion is found with pH ~ 0.5 units higher than in men. Therefore, the drugs that require the acidic gastric pH have a poorer bioavailability in women [20,34,35].

Chitosan has the amino group with the pK_a of ~6.5, relating to the degree of N-deacetylation, and is fully protonated at the pH of ~4, resulting in the increase in acidity of chitosan [36,37]. Therefore, the chitosan-loaded drug has better mucoadhesive and permeation-enhancing properties, promoting drug absorption at proximal part of GI tract, including stomach and duodenum, when compared with the chitosan-free group [4,8,37,38]. The problem is that chitosan precipitates at the pH of >6.5 in the jejunum, ileum, and colon, and thus chitosan has less adhesion to the mucus layer of GI tract, leading to the ineffective drug absorption [38,39]. Interestingly, this drawback is solved by the modification of chitosan, such as thiolated chitosan, which will be addressed in a later section [40–42].

2.2. GI Motility

The GI motility is defined as the contraction and relaxation of GI smooth muscles to propel the contents along the GI tract with the change in intraluminal pressure and it is a causal determinant for the drug absorption. The gastric emptying, which is a process of removing the content from the stomach and moving it into the duodenum, also has an impact on the intestinal assimilation [43,44]. The increasing rate of gastric emptying, found in the case of solutions or suspensions, may lead to a rise in the drug absorption rate [25,45,46]. However, medications for gastric ulcer need delayed gastric emptying in order to prolong in the stomach. After reaching the small intestine, the content of drugs in the bowel needs a sufficient residence time and a long intestinal transit time in order to facilitate the opportunity of drug absorption at this site, owing to the enormous surface area of the small intestine [47–49]. Peristaltic contraction also enhances the capacity of drug absorption, as it promotes drug dissolution and membrane–drug contact [50]. In addition, the volume of GI luminal fluids may contribute to drug assimilation by affecting drug dissolution and providing the driving force for drug permeation [51,52]. In adults, the rate of gastric emptying is varied, relating to fasted and fed conditions [33,53]. At the age of 6–8 months, the gastric emptying is much slower than that in adults, owing to the immature development of neural control for GI motility [54]. Moreover, in the elderly, there is the delayed gastric emptying and a decrease in GI motility [19]. Indeed, women have slower gastric emptying than men, which gives rise to a longer gastric retention time and attenuates drug absorption [34,55,56]. Therefore, in women, a longer interval between having meals and taking drugs is required [56].

Chitosan-poly(acrylic) acid (PAA) polyionic complex was fabricated and was shown to prolong gastric retention of ampicillin, an antibiotic used for the treatment of *Helicobacter pylori* infection-induced gastric ulcer, in swelling and drug release studies, suggesting a role in drug absorption enhancement of this complex [57]. Furthermore, chitosan-based nanoparticles using sodium tripolyphosphate (TPP) as a cross-linking agent were revealed to delay gastric emptying, as well as to improve the absorption and oral bioavailability of ketoconazole, an antifungal drug with poor absorption due to rapid gastric emptying and a short gastric residence time [58]. In addition, in ex vivo porcine gastric mucosa, ketoconazole-loaded chitosan/TPP was demonstrated to adhere to negatively charged mucin layers, implicating good mucoadhesive properties of this nanoparticle formulation [58].

2.3. Transport Proteins and Enzymes

The drug substances reaching to the small intestine, where the major site for drug absorption is taken, can be transported across the enterocytes by several mechanisms, such as simple diffusion, active transport, facilitated transport, and pinocytosis, via the paracellular or transcellular route. However, the drugs can be pumped out of enterocytes by the ATP-binding cassette (ABC) efflux transporters, which are a major hindrance for the drug assimilation. The drug transporter proteins located at the apical side of the intestinal epithelial cells include P-glycoprotein (P-gp) multidrug resistance protein-2 (MRP-2) and breast cancer resistance protein (BCRP) [59–63]. These transporters are responsible for the drug efflux into the intestinal lumen. In addition, they can bind to some unspecific compounds other than drug substrates; therefore, they may attenuate the absorption of some drugs, such as antibiotics, lipid-lowering agents, and anti-cancer drugs. Meanwhile, the other transporters located at basolateral side of enterocytes comprise MRP-1, -3, and -5, which are for pumping the drug into the blood circulation [63–68]. In the small bowel, the drugs also encounter bile salts and pancreatic enzymes secreted into the intestinal lumen. These bile salts and pancreatic enzymes contribute to the drug dissolution and solubility in the GI tract [69,70]. The intestine-absorbed drugs will pass into the liver via the portal vein in order to undergo drug metabolism. The drug-metabolizing enzymes (DMEs), including cytochrome P450 (CYP450) and CYP3A, also modulate the drug absorption and oral bioavailability [71–73]. The immaturity of the GI function in pediatric patients causes the increase in epithelial permeability [33,74]. The intestinal drug absorption in newborns might be variable due to irregular peristalsis. The expressions and functions of efflux transporter protein (i.e., P-gp) and tight junction may increase with age, as the early infancy relies on the passive diffusion [75,76]. However, Toornvliet and colleagues revealed the decreased activity of P-gp efflux transporter in the elderly [77]. For ethnicity-based drug assimilation, the genetic polymorphisms are variedly distributed to a gene product related to drug metabolism enzymes, including CYP450 superfamilies, and transport proteins, including P-gp and organic anion transporting polypeptides [OATPs] [17,78,79]. Several studies have suggested that the P-gp expression is abundantly found in Africans, compared with Caucasians [80–83].

Interestingly, chitosan can attenuate the P-gp expression in dose-dependent manner, and thereby enhance the oral bioavailability of norfloxacin, an antibacterial agent used for the treatment of gram-negative bacteria infection, in Grass Carp [84]. For the chitosan conjugates, curcumin-carboxymethyl chitosan was developed, serving as an inhibitor of P-gp and an enhancer of drug absorption [85]. In addition, quercetin-chitosan (QT-CS) conjugate was synthesized as an enhancer of drug absorption of doxorubicin by inhibiting P-gp, opening tight junction, and enhancing the water solubility [86]. Carboxymethyl chitosan-quercetin conjugate also helped to improve oral drug delivery and oral bioavailability of paclitaxel by inhibiting P-gp and increasing its water solubility [87].

2.4. Gut Microbiota

The human gut microbiota, containing $>10^{14}$ microbes and their genome, resides in the distal segment of the GI tract, particularly in the ileum and colon [88]. For the small intestine, there is less gut microbiota due to its lower luminal pH, higher levels of oxygen delivery, and higher concentrations of antimicrobial agents [89–92]. The gut microbiota helps to regulate the immune system and to maintain physiological conditions. Importantly, it can ferment the indigested carbohydrates and proteins, giving rise to the byproducts as short-chain fatty acids (SCFAs) [93,94]. Moreover, the gut microbiota and microbial metabolites can metabolize endogenous substances such as amino acids, cholesterol, and bile acids, by various enzymes (e.g., glucuronidases and glucosidases), and modulate the pharmacokinetics (i.e., drug absorption and drug metabolism) [95]. The study of the drugs affected by gut microbiota sheds the light on personalized medicine to predict the drug pharmacokinetics for individual patients. The human microbiome can alter drug-induced pharmacological and toxicological effects. For example, the gut microbiota can alter the oral bioavailability and activity of insulin, as it is susceptible to proteolysis [92,96]. Additionally, it may increase acetaminophen-induced hepatotoxicity, involved with p-cresol, a microbial metabolite [97]. The enhanced toxicity of diclofenac by gut microbiota is associated with the deglucuronidation and delayed excretion [98]. The decrease in firs pass a metabolism effect and high levels of intestinal β-glucuronidase activity were documented in neonates [99]. The gender difference contributing to the gut microbiota compositions has not been well-addressed due to its inconsistency. However, several lines of evidence related to the sex difference in gut microbiota have been documented [100]. Ethnicity-, dietary-, and lifestyle-specific variations in gut microbiota composition are also observed [101,102].

Several studies have reported that chitosan and its derivatives can modulate the gut microbiota imbalance. For instance, carboxymethyl chitosan has revealed to alter the gut microbiota in *Escherichia coli* (*E. coli*)-treated mice, affecting to fat and glucose metabolism, as well as the inflammatory profile [103,104]. It was also found that chitosan-chelated zinc has reduced the intestinal inflammatory process and mucosal injury in *E. coli*-infected rats by reversing the gut bacterial composition [105]. In addition, chitosan oligosaccharide (COS), a derivative of chitosan, has been exhibited to restore the gut microbial imbalance in diabetic mice [106].

2.5. Disease Conditions

The disease conditions can influence the drug absorption of orally administered drugs, as they impact on the structures and functions of GI tract organs, including esophagus, stomach, small intestine, and large intestine. The change in drug absorption is associated with the alteration of the aforementioned physiological characteristics.

In diabetic patients, they secrete less gastric acid than healthy individuals [107]. Therefore, the gastric pH is increased, resulting in the poor absorption of basic drugs. However, the delayed gastric emptying and prolonged transit times have been impressed in diabetes [108–110]. Importantly, owing to the microvascular complications, the gastric blood flow is declined, leading to further delayed gastric emptying and affect to the drug absorption in the small bowel. The alterations of P-gp expression and function under diabetic conditions were decreased in diabetic rats [111]. However, some evidence has mentioned that the P-gp expression is temporally induced and then restored to a baseline level [112]. In addition, it has been shown that the level of the CYP3A4 enzyme is reduced, leading to the change in the oral bioavailability of some drugs related to CYP3A4 activity, such as carbamazepine, anti-retroviral drugs and some statins [113,114]. In obesity, a larger gastric volumes and lower gastric pH have been reported, compared with lean subjects [115]. The gastric emptying time in obese patients is controversial [25]. For the intestinal transporter proteins, the inhibition of P-gp could result in hepatic steatosis and obesity using P-gp deficiency mice fed a high-fat diet model [116]. The CYP34A enzyme activity was found to be reduced in obese individuals; therefore, it needs to be cautious when using CYP3A4 substrates, inhibitors, or inducers in these patients [117]. For the treatment of diabetic patients, oral insulin is applied due to its greater convenience and its less adverse drug reaction than subcutaneously injected insulin. However, it still interferes with proteolytic degradation and mucosal layers in the GI tract. Insulin-loaded chitosan nanoparticles increase residence time to retain in the GI tract and enhance mucoadhesion, therefore promoting drug assimilation [118,119].

In patients with gastric cancer, the gastric pH is 6–7, which results from the gastric atrophy and decreased gastric secretion [120,121]. The gastric emptying is slower than in healthy subjects, and is further decreased after gastrectomy [122,123]. However, the oral anticancer drugs may improve their efficacy as they retain in the stomach for a longer duration, thus providing sufficient time for gastric tumor to expose with drugs [124]. For colorectal cancer, the transit time is not clear, although the colon motility change in this type of cancer is well-known [25]. Of note, the efflux transporters (e.g., P-gp, MRP-2, BCRP) were reported to be altered in cancer cells and were still the big concern for the drug resistance in the cancers [125,126]. Doxorubicin is an oral chemotherapy used in the treatment of considerable cancers, including lung, gastric, breast, thyroid, and ovarian cancers, by acting on the nucleus of target cells [127–129]. Doxorubicin was documented to have a low bioavailability because it was abolished by the first-pass metabolism of CYP450 and the overexpression of P-gp [130–133]. It was shown that doxorubicin-loaded chitosan nanoparticles increased the permeation across intestinal epithelium. Moreover, when conjugating with quercetin, it inhibited the P-gp efflux transporter. Collectively, chitosan was claimed to relieve the poor absorption of doxorubicin [87,131].

The effect of GI tract infections on oral drug assimilation is unpredictable, as the GI membrane damage induced by infections can cause both the increase and decrease in drug intestinal absorption. The delayed gastric emptying may be associated with an increasing chance of experiencing nausea and vomiting and a longer onset of medications, resulting in uncontrolled drug plasma concentrations. *H. pylori* infection leads to the decrease in gastric secretion and the impairment of drug absorption. The poor absorption of some antibacterial drugs (e.g., gentamicin, metronidazole) were alleviated by the drug-chitosan complex [134,135]. For pain and stress, the alterations of GI physiology are relevant to the gut–brain axis, such as the reduction in GI motility, gastric secretion, and mucosal blood being low [136]. It was demonstrated that chitosan-based hydrogels could manipulate the drug release of paracetamol in the intestine [137]. Besides, a chitosan complex could regulate the drug release properties of ibuprofen, a non-steroidal anti-inflammatory drug (NSAID) [138].

The altered kinetics of drug absorption in these disease states have been partially acknowledged. Further investigations involving pharmacokinetics towards personalized and precision medicines should be considered.

3. Chitosan-Based Nanomaterials for Improving Intestinal Drug Absorption and Their Pharmacological Applications

Since one of our goals of this review is to summarize the types of fabricated chitosan-based nanomaterials in the aspect of the drug absorption enhancer, the literature search was performed on the full-text articles published in English, with date limits of 2010 up to 8 February 2021, assessed in the PubMed database by using the search term of "chitosan" AND "intestine" AND "drug delivery". As a result, a total of 106 articles were collected by EndNote and further selected for relevant topics. Additional articles that provided specific evidence and information (e.g., diabetes, cancers, infections, inflammation, polyelectrolyte complex, thiolated chitosan, trimethyl chitosan, carboxymethyl chitosan, alginate, Eudragit etc.) were included.

Chitosan-based nanomaterials have received tremendous attention from many investigators over the past decade as the enhancer of drug delivery, particularly drug absorption, based on their marvelous properties, which are (i) protection against GI luminal degradation (ii) mucoadhesion, (iii) permeation enhancement, (iv) controlled drug release, and (v) efflux inhibition (Figure 2). The significance of chitosan-based nanomaterials is indicated and discussed in detail as below. In addition, the types of chitosan-based nanomaterials are summarized in Table 1.

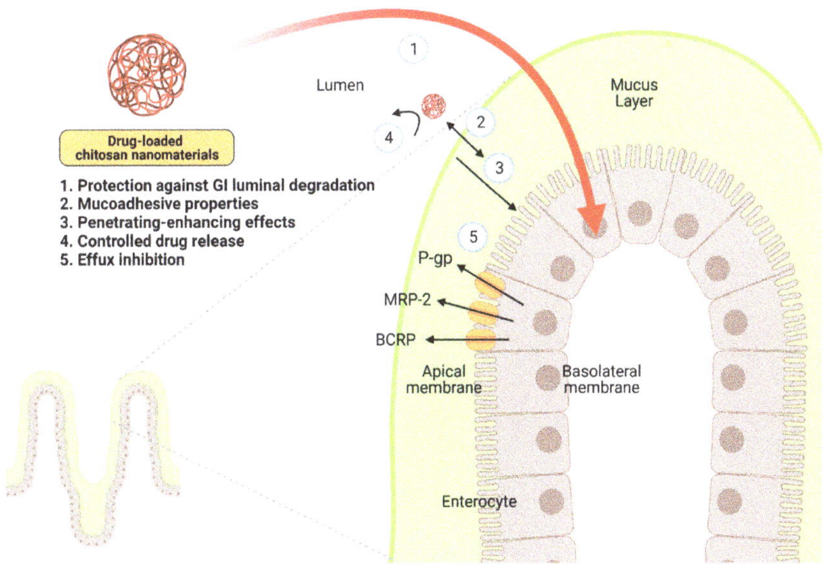

Figure 2. The mechanistic insights of the enhancement of drug absorption by drug-loaded chitosan nanomaterials in the intestine. The ideal properties of these nanomaterials include (i) protection against GI luminal degradation, (ii) mucoadhesion, (iii) permeation enhancement, (iv) controlled drug release, and (v) inhibition of P-gp, MRP-2, or BCRP. Abbreviation: P-gp, P-glycoprotein; MRP-2, multidrug resistance protein-2; BCRP, breast cancer resistance protein. Created with BioRender.com.

3.1. Chitosan-Based Polymeric Nanoparticles with Chemical Modifications

Although chitosan is well-soluble in acidic medium, it has poor solubility in the basic environment, as in the duodenum. Fortunately, chitosan is easy to chemically modify at its functional groups, including an amino group (-NH_2) and two hydroxyl groups (-OH), in order to improve its physical and biological properties [139].

Thiolated chitosan is a favorable derivative of chitosan with the immobilized sulfhydryl- or thiol-bearing groups onto the primary amine groups of chitosan. The disulfide bond formation with cysteine-rich subdomains of mucus glycoprotein by a thiol-disulfide interchange reaction leads to the close contact between the thiomer and mucosal layers, hence making this modified chitosan have a better mucus entrapment efficiency, compared with conventional chitosan [139]. The increased mucoadhesivity retains the nanoparticles at the site of absorption, giving rise to the enhanced drug oral bioavailability. Fabiano and colleagues revealed the importance of thiol groups on drug oral bioavailability by comparing quaternary ammonium-chitosan with S-protected thiol groups (NP QA-Ch-S-pro) and without thiol ones (NP QA-Ch) [140]. Moreover, thiolated chitosan provides a beneficial effect as a permeation enhancer by inhibiting the protein tyrosine phosphatase (PTP) enzyme, which in turn dephosphorylates the tyrosine subunits of occluding protein and further promotes the opening of tight junctions [141,142]. The enhancement of permeation depends on the degree of the thiolation and the physiochemical properties of the drug [143]. The utilizations of thiolated chitosan were denoted in diabetes treatment. In the insulin delivery, oral insulin-loaded thiolated chitosan nanoparticles (Ins-TCNPs) could be prepared with pentaerythritol tetrakis (3-mercaptoproprionate) or PETMP, which was used for penetrating the cell membrane, while the thiomer inhibited the PTP enzyme and enhanced the opening tight junctions, promoting the drug absorption [118]. In addition, Ins-TCNPs was shown to reduce blood glucose as well as enhance the level of plasma insulin and prolong its duration in rats [118,144]. Insulin was released from thiolated chitosan-based nanoparticles at two phases, which were a rapid initial release or burst release at pH 2 and a sustained release at pH 5.3 [145,146]. It also improved the mucus adhesion between the polymer and the intestinal mucosa and prolonged drug gastric residence time, improving the oral bioavailability and thus implicating the potential role of thiolated chitosan in oral delivery of insulin [118]. Besides mucoadhesive and permeation-enhancing features, thiomers could inhibit the ATP-dependent drug efflux pumps, including P-gp and MRP-2, which were able to pump the drug molecules out of the cells, causing the attenuated drug efficiency and the poor oral drug bioavailability. Recently, it has been shown that both anionic and cationic thiolated chitosans could inhibit these efflux pumps and promote intestinal transcellular drug uptake [147]. For their applications in cancers, docetaxel (DTX), an anticancer drug for metastatic breast, lung, and gastric cancers, was carried by thiolated chitosan with the improvement of cellular internalization, the augmentation of mucoadhesivity, and the inhibition of P-gp [148]. Aside from DTX, α-mangostin, a natural xanthonoid extracted from mangosteen, was loaded by thiolated chitosan with pH-dependent Eudragit L100 and cross-linking genipin and this xanthonoid-bearing nanoparticle exhibited the mucoadhesive and controlled drug release properties in colorectal cancer [149]. Besides, thiolated chitosan could provide to increase the stability of low-molecular weight heparin (LMWH) in a gastric environment by ionic cross-linking with hydroxypropyl methylcellulose phthalate (HPMCP) [150]. Mechanistically, thiolated chitosan improved mucoadhesion, increased paracellular permeability of LMWH at the absorption site, and controlled the release of LMWH in the circulation [150]. Moreover, S-protected chitosan-thioglycolic acid using 6-mercaptonicotinamide (TGA-MNA) had better mucoadhesive, permeation-enhancing, and efflux pump-inhibiting properties than chitosan-thioglycolic acid (chitosan-TGA) with thiol-free groups [151–153]. Thiolated chitosan with reduced glutathione (GSH) enhanced the oral drug delivery of leuprolide, a poor-permeable peptide drug using as a gonadotropin-releasing hormone (GnRH) analogue, by preventing it from enzyme degradation and promoting its absorption [154,155].

Trimethyl chitosan (TMC) is a water-soluble quaternized chitosan derivative produced from the methylation of chitosan with iodomethane in the presence of sodium hydroxide (NaOH) at the elevated temperature [156,157]. TMC has the potential for augmenting the membrane-penetrating features for hydrophilic macromolecular drugs, which are poorly absorbed owing to rapid hydrolytic degradation by gastrointestinal juices [158]. For the treatment of diabetes, encapsulated insulin-incorporated TMCs exerted mucoadhesive and permeation-enhancing effects and stimulated the intestinal absorption by mediating the intestinal barrier integrity and promoted the insulin transport via the paracellular route. The self-assembly of chitosan nanoparticles with negatively charged fucoidan was anticipated to have the hypoglycemic effects and avoid diabetic complications [159]. Moreover, it was documented that oral insulin-loaded TMC nanoparticles provided a better therapeutic outcome, compared with injected insulin in type 1 diabetes (T1D) [160]. In the field of cancers, TMC could be applied in the drug delivery of paclitaxel (PTX), an anti-microtubule agent using the treatment of gastrointestinal tumors. TMC-loaded PTX enhanced the internalization of the nanoparticles and exerted the cytotoxic effect to cancer cells without the systemic adverse effects [161]. Interestingly, when TMC-loaded peptides were coated with liposome, they prolonged the residence time and increased the mucoadhesivity in the GI tract [162]. TMCs were also utilized in peptide drug delivery in cancer immunotherapy. For instance, the Oral PD-L1 Binding Peptide 1 (OPBP-1)-loaded TMC was shown to increase the oral bioavailability of the peptide drug and impede the tumor cell growth [163]. In addition, it has been reported that TMCs could carry curcumin, which plays a vital role in the signaling cascades related to cancers and inflammation, as curcumin-loaded TMC provided the controlled release and enhanced the oral bioavailability of curcumin [164,165]. Interestingly, TMC-coated solid lipid nanoparticles (SLNs) incorporated the curcumin displayed in the sustained release of curcumin and elevated its oral bioavailability, compared with free curcumin and non-coating chitosan nanoparticles [166].

Carboxymethyl chitosan (CMS or CMCS) is a pH-sensitive chitosan derivative with the carboxymethyl substituent that improves the water solubility in a neutral and basic pH, based on the degree of substitution, as well as enhancing the mucoadhesive properties [167]. CMCS can be produced by direct or reductive alkylation. For the treatment of diabetes, insulin-loaded chitosan/CMCS nanogels increased mucoadhesion and permeation in a rat jejunal ex vivo model, even though it had no differences in the duodenum [168]. CMCS has a negative charge, which can interact with positively charged chitosan to obtain the polyelectrolyte complex through electrostatic interaction, which provides the pH responsive stability and thus controls the drug release [133]. This will be included in the later section "chitosan-based polyelectrolyte complex nanoparticles". Several lines of evidence have shown that doxorubicin, an anti-neoplastic drug used for treating solid tumors, can be loaded with chitosan/*O*-carboxymethyl chitosan (OCMCS) by simple ionic gelation. Doxorubicin-loaded chitosan/CMCS nanoparticles had better mucoadhesive properties and helped to improve oral bioavailability in ex vivo intestine [133,169,170]. Furthermore, CMCS was employed in the delivery of clarithromycin for the treatment of *H. pylori.* infection in the gastric environment. CMCS was grafted with stearic acid and conjugated with urea to obtain ureido-modified CMCS-graft-stearic acid (U-CMCS-g-SA). This nanopolymer was claimed to have a gastric retention property and a drug-controlled release with a target specificity [171]. For the inflammation, pH-responsive OCMCS/fucoidan nanoparticles were potentially used for the delivery of curcumin, as they controlled the release of curcumin and promoted the cellular uptake and endocytosis of curcumin Caco-2 cells [165]. In addition, gum Arabic (GA)-CMCS microcapsules enhanced the oral bioavailability of omeprazole, an antacid and a proton-pump inhibitor, to augment GI-targeted delivery [172].

3.2. Conjugated Chitosan

Chitosan can conjugate or form the complex with other superporous networks and (SPNs)-based polymers, which have numerous interconnected pores in three-dimensional structures with water-soluble agents, such as poly(vinyl alcohol) (PVA) and alginate [173]. The rapid swelling of SPNs could occur since the porous space of SPNs provide the water absorption, extending the gastric retention of the drug in the GI tract [174]. For the applications of conjugated chitosan, cross-linked chitosan/PVA was revealed to enhance the delivery of ascorbic acid with the formulated hydroxypropyl methylcellulose (HPMC), a hydrophilic and polymer and glyoxal, which was used for a crosslinking reagent, by prolonging the gastric retention time and promoting sustained release [173]. Additionally, for the diabetes therapy, the conjugation of cationic charged chitosan and anionic charged poly(γ-glutamic acid) (PGA) ameliorated the oral insulin delivery to adhere to the GI mucosal surface and transiently stimulated to open the tight junctions of the intestinal epithelial cells [175,176]. Moreover, in the treatment of cancer, Caco-2 cell monolayers treated with antiangiogenic, protein-loaded chitosan-*N*-arginine/PGA-taurine conjugated nanoparticles exhibited the enhancement of the cell permeation of antiangiogenic protein [177]. Not only chitosan alone, but chemically modified chitosans could take part in the conjugation process. For example, CMCS was prepared with poly(ethylene glycol) (PEG) to load doxorubicin hydrochloride in tumor cells. This nanoparticle was able to serve as a candidate for drug delivery of the antitumor drug [178]. Besides, thiolated chitosan could be conjugated with PEG to generate the thiol group bearing PEGylated chitosan (Chito-PEG-SH) with magnified mucoadhesive and permeation-enhancing properties, in isolated porcine and rat intestines [179]. In addition to drug delivery, chitosan-based nanoparticles are employed in a protein delivery system by inventing spherical PEG-grafted (chitosan-g-PEG), using TPP or PGA as a cross-linking agent [180].

3.3. *Chitosan-Based Polyelectrolyte Complex Nanoparticles/Nanocapsules*

To improve the drug stability in the GI tract and to lessen the systemic toxicity, the nanoencapsulation of the drugs is generated as the drug molecule loading into nanocarriers (e.g., nanoparticles, liposomes, micelles, and microemulsions) [130,132,181–184]. However, the encapsulated drugs confront the site-dependent pH change along the GI tract as the pH increases from the stomach (pH 1.2–3.7) to the small intestine (pH 6–7.4). Therefore, pH-sensitive/responsive polymers containing ionizable acidic and basic residues regarding the environmental pH are produced. The formations of the polyelectrolytes by non-covalent electrostatic interactions between polycations and polyanions are known as polyelectrolyte complex nanoparticles (PECNs). In response to the pH variation, these complex polymers could be adapted as swelling or shrinking, relying on the different degree of ionization of functional groups of PECNs [185]. The multishell structures in hollow nanocapsules were made from the dissolution of the core from the epitaxial core-shell structure of the nanoparticles [185,186]. A polyelectrolyte sphere was developed by the layer-by-layer (LbL) assembly method, employing a positively charged chitosan as the pH-responsive outer layer. The shrinking process of the chitosan-based nanoparticle might occur in the acidic surroundings [187,188].

Apart from chitosan, other biocompatible polymers, such as alginate, tripolyphosphate (TPP), and Eudragit, can serve as the outer membrane of nanocapsules. Alginate, consisting of 1,4-linked β-D-mannuronic acid and α-L-guluronic acid, was also a water-soluble and biodegradable natural polymer derived from seaweed [137,189]. It was able to crosslink with divalent/polyvalent cations (e.g., calcium, zinc, and copper) to form a network structure for use in sustaining drug release [137,189]. The carboxyl groups of alginate provided the negative charge and interact with the positively charged amino group of chitosan in the polyelectrolyte complex gel. Methoxy poly(ethylene glycol) or poly(ethylene glycol) monomethyl ether (mPEG)-grafted-CMCS (mPEG-g-CMCS) was synthesized with alginate to increase the loading capacity and provide a well-controlled drug release, particularly in the basic environment. In other words, mPEG-g-CMCS was a promising pH-sensitive nanoparticle for site-specific drug delivery in the intestine [190]. It was demonstrated that the fabricated core-shell nanoparticles, containing the curcumin at the core and the chitosan/alginate multilayer shell, could exhibit controlled release of the curcumin nanocrystal to target the inflamed colon in mice with ulcerative colitis (UC) [191]. In addition to alginate, TPP has been well-recognized. It had a negative charge and was used as a cross-linking agent with chitosan for the application of a chitosan-based hybrid system, such as quercetin-loaded and 5-Flurouracil (5-FU)-encapsulated chitosan/TPP nanoparticles [192–194]. Apart from that, a Eudragit polymer could be used for coating the nanoparticles in order to prevent the rapid release of curcumin and theophylline in the stomach and small intestine [195,196].

Chitosan-based PECNs are prepared from the interaction between the opposite charges of copolymers. For instance, chitosan/insulin PECNs could be obtained by positively charged chitosan-g-mPEG copolymers and negatively charged insulin [197]. These PECNs were used for improving the oral insulin to cross the mucus and epithelial membrane barriers in the GI tract [197,198]. mPEGylation is the process to enhance mucus-penetrating properties of chitosan-based nanomaterials. Recently, $mPEG_{10\%}$-chitosan glyceryl monocaprylate $(GMC)_{10\%}$ copolymers have been modified to add the feature of hydrophobicity onto their surface, which helped to impale the epithelial membrane [197]. However, the differential advantages of hydrophilicity/hydrophobicity were still controversial for preferable usage of nanoparticles, since the hydrophilic surface was better permeable in the mucus layer, while the hydrophobic exterior was preferred to penetrate the cell membrane.

In addition, pH-sensitive PECNs were generated for improving doxorubicin to overcome the obstacles both in the GI tract and the intracellular tumor cell regulation, such as multidrug resistance (MDR) [199]. Chitosan/doxorubicin PECNs contained two polyelectrolytes, including positively charged chitosan and negatively charged poly(L-glutamic acid) grafted polyethylene glycol-doxorubicin conjugate nanoparticles (PG-g-PEG-hyd-DOX NPs) [132]. These PECNs prolonged duration in the blood circulation and tumor tissue accumulation with rapid drug release at target cells; therefore, these PECNs might serve as the ideal nanocarriers for the anticancer field [132]. Additionally, chitosan-based PECNs could be synthesized by the electrostatic interactions between positively charged chitosan and negatively charged CMCS, which was a water soluble derivative of chitosan, as previously mentioned, and produce the nanoparticles by the ionic gelation using $CaCl_2$ as a cross-linking agent [131]. Doxorubicin was also prepared as DOX-loaded chitosan/carboxymethyl chitosan-based nanoparticles (DOX:CS/CMCS-NPs) with the porous-core nanoparticle and coacervate microcapsules-immobilized multilayer sodium alginate beads (NPs-M-ALG-Beads and CMs-M-ALG-Beads) in order to stabilize the drug in the GI tract [133,169,170].

Furthermore, the delivery of several antimicrobial agents was enhanced by the PECNs. For example, delafloxacin, a broad-spectrum fluoroquinolone used for both Gram-positive and negative aerobic and anaerobic bacteria, was loaded with positively charged chitosan and negatively charged stearic acid. The hybrid nanoparticles could increase the bioavailability and sustain the drug release via the electrostatic interaction of the polymer and lipid [200]. Another fluoroquinolone ciprofloxacin was carried by an embelin-chitosan gold nanoparticle (Emb-Chi-Au). This complex nanoparticle could enhance antipseudomonal activities by inhibiting the MDR efflux pump [201]. Tobramycin, an aminoglycoside antibiotic used for inhibiting biofilm formation by *Pseudomonas aeruginosa*, also relied on PECNs using *N*,*O*-[*N*,*N*-diethylaminomethyl(diethyldimethylene ammonium)$_n$ methyl]chitosan (QAL) nanoparticles and GENUVISCO type CSW-2 carrageenin (CG) [202]. Moreover, to achieve a better anti-inflammatory effect, curcumin was loaded with chitosan/GA and it was found that this nanoparticle helped control the release of curcumin [165]. Another example of CMCS-based application was the drug delivery of omeprazole using gum Arabic (GA)-*O*-carboxymethyl chitosan LbL microcapsules, which were able to enhance the oral bioavailability of omeprazole [172].

Table 1. Summary of chitosan-based nanocarriers used for improving the absorption of indicated drugs and their pharmacologic effects. This table summarizes the chitosan-based nanomaterials that carry the considerable drugs for better drug assimilation. The nanocarriers, loading drugs, and their exerting pharmacological effects are listed with their attainable references. Abbreviations: LMWH, low-molecular weight heparin; OPBP-1, Oral PD-L1 Binding Peptide 1; 5-FU, 5-flurouracil; BSA, bovine serum albumin.

Nanocarrier	Drug	Pharmacological Effect(s)	Reference(s)
1. Chemical modification			
1.1 Thiolated chitosan	Insulin	mucoadhesion, permeation enhancement, controlled drug release	[118]
	Docetaxel	mucoadhesion, permeation enhancement, controlled drug release, efflux inhibition	[148]
	α-mangostin	mucoadhesion, controlled drug release	[149]
	LMWH	protection against GI luminal degradation, mucoadhesion, permeation enhancement, controlled drug release	[150]
	Leuprolide	mucoadhesion, permeation enhancement	[154]
1.2 Trimethyl chitosan (TMC)	Insulin	mucoadhesion, permeation enhancement, controlled drug release	[160]
	Paclitaxel	mucoadhesion, permeation enhancement, controlled drug release	[161]
	Calcitonin	mucoadhesion, permeation enhancement, prolongation of residence time	[162]
	OPBP-1	mucoadhesion, permeation enhancement, controlled drug release	[163]
	Curcumin	mucoadhesion, permeation enhancement, controlled drug release	[164–166]
1.3 Carboxymethyl chitosan	Doxorubicin	mucoadhesion, permeation enhancement, controlled drug release, efflux inhibition	[131–133,169,170]
	Clarithromycin	controlled drug release, prolongation of residence time	[171]
	5-FU	controlled drug release	[192]
	Curcumin	mucoadhesion, controlled drug release, efflux inhibition	[85,165]
	Omeprazole	protection against gastric degradation, controlled drug release	[172]
2. Conjugation			
Poly(vinyl alcohol) (PVA)	Ascorbic acid	controlled drug release	[173]
Poly(γ-glutamic acid) (PGA)	Insulin	protection against GI luminal degradation, mucoadhsion, permeation enhancement	[175,176]
Poly(ethylene glycol) (PEG)	Insulin	mucoadhsion, permeation enhancement, controlled drug release	[197]
	BSA	mucoadhsion, permeation enhancement, controlled drug release	[190]
3. Polyelectrolyte complexation	Insulin	protection against GI luminal degradation, mucoadhesion, permeation enhancement, controlled drug release	[119,197]
	Doxorubicin	mucoadhesion, permeation enhancement, controlled drug release, efflux inhibition	[131–133,169,170]
	5-FU	controlled drug release	[192]

Table 1. *Cont.*

Nanocarrier	Drug	Pharmacological Effect(s)	Reference(s)
	Quercetin	protection against GI luminal degradation, controlled drug release	[193]
	Curcumin	mucoadhesion, controlled drug release	[165,191,195]
	Rutin	mucoadhesion, permeation enhancement, controlled drug release	[194]
	Gentamicin	mucoadhesion, permeation enhancement, controlled drug release	[134]
	Paracetamol	permeation enhancement, controlled drug release	[137]
	Ibuprofen	controlled drug release	[138]
	Omeprazole	protection against GI luminal degradation, controlled drug release	[172]
	Furosemide	mucoadhesion, permeation enhancement, controlled drug release	[189]
	Theophylline	controlled drug release	[196]
	Delafloxacin	controlled drug release	[200]
	Ciprofloxacin	efflux inhibition	[201]
	Tobramycin	mucoadhesion, permeation enhancement	[202]

4. Future Perspectives and Conclusions

The oral route is the most promising for drug administration; however, it is essential to overcome various physiological barriers along the GI tract (i.e., gastric pH, GI enzymes, mucus layer, efflux pump) before reaching the systemic circulation and exerting its effects at the action site. These challenges limit the absorption of multitudinous drugs, including antidiabetic, anticancer, antimicrobial, and anti-inflammatory drugs and hence their oral drug bioavailability. To surpass these GI obstacles, the drug delivery carriers have been designed and developed. Chitosan is chosen to be a potentially unique candidate that meets the ideal properties for bioinspired drug delivery. Chitosan is a natural origin-based polymer with its versatile functional groups, and hence it is feasible to be chemically modified to improve the chitosan's physiochemical properties, including mucoadhesive capabilities, the permeating-enhancing effect, controlled drug release, and efflux inhibition. Several types of chitosan-based nanomaterials are fabricated and they are investigated for the potential to be the enhancer for drug assimilation. Even though the drug can reach the blood circulation, the fluctuations in drug concentrations can occur and may result in the increased incidence of either the drug adverse reaction or subtherapeutic treatment. Therefore, the sustained delivery system has been introduced to solve this problem [9,203]. Thiolated chitosan can be applied for the sustained delivery, but the maintenance of the drug remaining for longer period of time is required. Moreover, particularly in the elderly, polypharmacy is increasingly occupied in many cases. For the effective treatment, the co-delivery systems will assist to carry multiple drugs to differential targets at the same time [204–206]. Aging-, gender-, and race-dependent physiological factors related to drug absorption are still unclear. A better understanding in the study of personalized medicine will help to clarify these variations. The state-of-art technology related to personalized medicine is needed to be developed. Considering the novelty of theranostics, the combination of the therapeutics and diagnostics, chitosan and chitosan-based nanocarriers have been emerged in the biomedical engineering field. The large varieties of chitosan derivatives and modifications, as well as their versatilities, allow them to be the ideal carriers that can reach the specific site of such diseases. Theranostics and imaging-guided therapies will help instantaneously keep track of chitosan-based drug delivery and direct them to the target site [207]. The development of personalized nanomedicine will provide the information of an individualized drug response in order to adjust it to an optimal dosage and proper management for each patient [208]. Moreover, since chitosan could be applied with other polymers to fabricate various chitosan formulations, the studies of toxicity and safety of chitosan-based nanoparticles need to be further explored in vivo to ascertain the appropriate dose selection in humans [209]. The in-depth in vivo studies for chitosan nanoparticles may include the types of utilized polymer, size, shape, surface, morphology, and electrokinetic potential, which are significant determinants for the toxicity and safety and are associated with the nanotoxicity of these nanoparticles [207]. It is possible that the cytotoxicity of chitosan-based nanocarriers is resulted from the electrostatic interaction between chitosan and cell membrane, as well as the cellular uptake of chitosan and subsequent activation of intracellular signaling cascades [210]. Unfortunately, for the biocompatibility studies in the animal models, the short duration after the intravenous injection of nanoparticles might be insufficient [207]. Therefore, the clinical efficiency and in vivo efficacy of these nanoparticles should be stepped up. Another concern in the use of chitosan-based nanomaterials is that the antimicrobial activity of chitosan may be disrupted by interaction with food (e.g., fruits and vegetables). Besides, the patients who take warfarin, an anticoagulant, with chitosan, may have a potential risk of bleeding due to the effect of chitosan on intrinsic coagulation and fat-soluble vitamin absorption [211]. In addition, for the pharmaceutically industrial and commercial scales, the technology for the high-throughput level may be integrated. Recent advances in the development and application of chitosan-based nanomaterials have been brought up in this review. The implementations of the nanomaterials in diabetes, cancers, infections, and inflammation are specific; therefore, the further research for polymeric drug delivery in such individual diseases are encouraged toward a new paradigm in the future treatment based on nanotechnology.

Author Contributions: Conceptualization, N.P. and C.M.; writing, N.P.; review and editing, N.P. and C.M., supervision, C.M.; project administration, N.P. and C.M.; funding acquisition, N.P. and C.M. All authors have read and agreed to the published version of the manuscript.

Funding: This research was funded by Mahidol University, Thailand Research Fund and National Research Council of Thailand (grant number DBG6180029 and grant number NFS6300233).

Institutional Review Board Statement: Not applicable.

Informed Consent Statement: Not applicable.

Data Availability Statement: Not applicable.

Conflicts of Interest: The authors declare no conflict of interest.

References

1. Khafagy, E.-S.; Morishita, M. Oral biodrug delivery using cell-penetrating peptide. *Adv. Drug Deliv. Rev.* **2012**, *64*, 531–539. [CrossRef]
2. Chen, M.C.; Mi, F.L.; Liao, Z.X.; Hsiao, C.W.; Sonaje, K.; Chung, M.F.; Hsu, L.W.; Sung, H.W. Recent advances in chitosan-based nanoparticles for oral delivery of macromolecules. *Adv. Drug Deliv. Rev.* **2013**, *65*, 865–879. [CrossRef]
3. Hatton, G.B.; Madla, C.M.; Rabbie, S.C.; Basit, A.W. Gut reaction: Impact of systemic diseases on gastrointestinal physiology and drug absorption. *Drug Discov. Today* **2019**, *24*, 417–427. [CrossRef]
4. Lang, X.; Wang, T.; Sun, M.; Chen, X.; Liu, Y. Advances and applications of chitosan-based nanomaterials as oral delivery carriers: A review. *Int. J. Biol. Macromol.* **2020**, *154*, 433–445. [CrossRef] [PubMed]
5. Patra, J.K.; Das, G.; Fraceto, L.F.; Campos, E.V.R.; Rodriguez-Torres, M.D.P.; Acosta-Torres, L.S.; Diaz-Torres, L.A.; Grillo, R.; Swamy, M.K.; Sharma, S.; et al. Nano based drug delivery systems: Recent developments and future prospects. *J. Nanobiotechnol.* **2018**, *16*, 71. [CrossRef] [PubMed]
6. Bajracharya, R.; Song, J.G.; Back, S.Y.; Han, H.K. Recent Advancements in Non-Invasive Formulations for Protein Drug Delivery. *Comput. Struct. Biotechnol. J.* **2019**, *17*, 1290–1308. [CrossRef]
7. Sung, Y.K.; Kim, S.W. Recent advances in polymeric drug delivery systems. *Biomater. Res.* **2020**, *24*, 12. [CrossRef] [PubMed]
8. Bernkop-Schnürch, A.; Dünnhaupt, S. Chitosan-based drug delivery systems. *Eur. J. Pharm. Biopharm. Off. J. Arb. Pharm. Verfahr. EV* **2012**, *81*, 463–469. [CrossRef] [PubMed]
9. Homayun, B.; Lin, X.; Choi, H.J. Challenges and Recent Progress in Oral Drug Delivery Systems for Biopharmaceuticals. *Pharmaceutics* **2019**, *11*, 129. [CrossRef]

10. Thadathil, N.; Velappan, S.P. Recent developments in chitosanase research and its biotechnological applications: A review. *Food Chem.* **2014**, *150*, 392–399. [CrossRef]
11. Muanprasat, C.; Chatsudthipong, V. Chitosan oligosaccharide: Biological activities and potential therapeutic applications. *Pharmacol. Ther.* **2017**, *170*, 80–97. [CrossRef] [PubMed]
12. Grenha, A. Chitosan nanoparticles: A survey of preparation methods. *J. Drug Target.* **2012**, *20*, 291–300. [CrossRef] [PubMed]
13. Hu, L.; Sun, Y.; Wu, Y. Advances in chitosan-based drug delivery vehicles. *Nanoscale* **2013**, *5*, 3103–3111. [CrossRef]
14. Debotton, N.; Dahan, A. A mechanistic approach to understanding oral drug absorption in pediatrics: An overview of fundamentals. *Drug Discov. Today* **2014**, *19*, 1322–1336. [CrossRef] [PubMed]
15. Khan, M.S.; Roberts, M.S. Challenges and innovations of drug delivery in older age. *Adv. Drug Deliv. Rev.* **2018**, *135*, 3–38. [CrossRef]
16. Soldin, O.P.; Chung, S.H.; Mattison, D.R. Sex differences in drug disposition. *J. Biomed. Biotechnol.* **2011**, *2011*, 187103. [CrossRef] [PubMed]
17. Cazzola, M.; Calzetta, L.; Matera, M.G.; Hanania, N.A.; Rogliani, P. How does race/ethnicity influence pharmacological response to asthma therapies? *Expert Opin. Drug Metab. Toxicol.* **2018**, *14*, 435–446. [CrossRef]
18. Williams, K.; Thomson, D.; Seto, I.; Contopoulos-Ioannidis, D.G.; Ioannidis, J.P.; Curtis, S.; Constantin, E.; Batmanabane, G.; Hartling, L.; Klassen, T. Standard 6: Age groups for pediatric trials. *Pediatrics* **2012**, *129* (Suppl. 3), S153–S160. [CrossRef]
19. Klotz, U. Pharmacokinetics and drug metabolism in the elderly. *Drug Metab. Rev.* **2009**, *41*, 67–76. [CrossRef] [PubMed]
20. Soldin, O.P.; Mattison, D.R. Sex differences in pharmacokinetics and pharmacodynamics. *Clin. Pharmacokinet.* **2009**, *48*, 143–157. [CrossRef]
21. Messing, K.; Mager Stellman, J. Sex, gender and women's occupational health: The importance of considering mechanism. *Environ. Res.* **2006**, *101*, 149–162. [CrossRef]
22. Yasuda, S.U.; Zhang, L.; Huang, S.M. The role of ethnicity in variability in response to drugs: Focus on clinical pharmacology studies. *Clin. Pharmacol. Ther.* **2008**, *84*, 417–423. [CrossRef]
23. Huang, T.; Shu, Y.; Cai, Y.D. Genetic differences among ethnic groups. *BMC Genom.* **2015**, *16*, 1093. [CrossRef]
24. Pontoriero, A.C.; Trinks, J.; Hulaniuk, M.L.; Caputo, M.; Fortuny, L.; Pratx, L.B.; Frías, A.; Torres, O.; Nuñez, F.; Gadano, A.; et al. Influence of ethnicity on the distribution of genetic polymorphisms associated with risk of chronic liver disease in South American populations. *BMC Genet.* **2015**, *16*, 93. [CrossRef]
25. Stillhart, C.; Vučićević, K.; Augustijns, P.; Basit, A.W.; Batchelor, H.; Flanagan, T.R.; Gesquiere, I.; Greupink, R.; Keszthelyi, D.; Koskinen, M.; et al. Impact of gastrointestinal physiology on drug absorption in special populations—An UNGAP review. *Eur. J. Pharm. Sci. Off. J. Eur. Fed. Pharm. Sci.* **2020**, *147*, 105280. [CrossRef]
26. Liu, L.; Yao, W.; Rao, Y.; Lu, X.; Gao, J. pH-Responsive carriers for oral drug delivery: Challenges and opportunities of current platforms. *Drug Deliv.* **2017**, *24*, 569–581. [CrossRef] [PubMed]
27. Manallack, D.T. The pK(a) Distribution of Drugs: Application to Drug Discovery. *Perspect. Med. Chem.* **2007**, *1*, 25–38.
28. Kataoka, M.; Fukahori, M.; Ikemura, A.; Kubota, A.; Higashino, H.; Sakuma, S.; Yamashita, S. Effects of gastric pH on oral drug absorption: In vitro assessment using a dissolution/permeation system reflecting the gastric dissolution process. *Eur. J. Pharm. Biopharm. Off. J. Arb. Pharm. Verfahr. EV* **2016**, *101*, 103–111. [CrossRef] [PubMed]
29. Mitra, A.; Kesisoglou, F. Impaired drug absorption due to high stomach pH: A review of strategies for mitigation of such effect to enable pharmaceutical product development. *Mol. Pharm.* **2013**, *10*, 3970–3979. [CrossRef] [PubMed]
30. Patel, D.; Bertz, R.; Ren, S.; Boulton, D.W.; Någård, M. A Systematic Review of Gastric Acid-Reducing Agent-Mediated Drug-Drug Interactions with Orally Administered Medications. *Clin. Pharmacokinet.* **2020**, *59*, 447–462. [CrossRef] [PubMed]
31. Zhang, L.; Wu, F.; Lee, S.C.; Zhao, H.; Zhang, L. pH-dependent drug-drug interactions for weak base drugs: Potential implications for new drug development. *Clin. Pharmacol. Ther.* **2014**, *96*, 266–277. [CrossRef] [PubMed]
32. Neal-Kluever, A.; Fisher, J.; Grylack, L.; Kakiuchi-Kiyota, S.; Halpern, W. Physiology of the Neonatal Gastrointestinal System Relevant to the Disposition of Orally Administered Medications. *Drug Metab. Dispos. Biol. Fate Chem.* **2019**, *47*, 296–313. [CrossRef]
33. van den Anker, J.; Reed, M.D.; Allegaert, K.; Kearns, G.L. Developmental Changes in Pharmacokinetics and Pharmacodynamics. *J. Clin. Pharmacol.* **2018**, *58* (Suppl. 10), S10–S25. [CrossRef] [PubMed]
34. Donovan, M.D. Sex and racial differences in pharmacological response: Effect of route of administration and drug delivery system on pharmacokinetics. *J. Women Health* **2005**, *14*, 30–37. [CrossRef] [PubMed]
35. Sansone-Parsons, A.; Krishna, G.; Simon, J.; Soni, P.; Kantesaria, B.; Herron, J.; Stoltz, R. Effects of age, gender, and race/ethnicity on the pharmacokinetics of posaconazole in healthy volunteers. *Antimicrob. Agents Chemother.* **2007**, *51*, 495–502. [CrossRef] [PubMed]
36. Yuan, Y.; Chesnutt, B.M.; Haggard, W.O.; Bumgardner, J.D. Deacetylation of Chitosan: Material Characterization and in vitro Evaluation via Albumin Adsorption and Pre-Osteoblastic Cell Cultures. *Materials* **2011**, *4*, 1399–1416. [CrossRef] [PubMed]
37. Mohammed, M.A.; Syeda, J.T.M.; Wasan, K.M.; Wasan, E.K. An Overview of Chitosan Nanoparticles and Its Application in Non-Parenteral Drug Delivery. *Pharmaceutics* **2017**, *9*, 53. [CrossRef]
38. TM, M.W.; Lau, W.M.; Khutoryanskiy, V.V. Chitosan and Its Derivatives for Application in Mucoadhesive Drug Delivery Systems. *Polymers* **2018**, *10*, 267. [CrossRef]

39. Botelho da Silva, S.; Krolicka, M.; van den Broek, L.A.M.; Frissen, A.E.; Boeriu, C.G. Water-soluble chitosan derivatives and pH-responsive hydrogels by selective C-6 oxidation mediated by TEMPO-laccase redox system. *Carbohydr. Polym.* **2018**, *186*, 299–309. [CrossRef]
40. Dhaliwal, S.; Jain, S.; Singh, H.P.; Tiwary, A.K. Mucoadhesive microspheres for gastroretentive delivery of acyclovir: In vitro and in vivo evaluation. *AAPS J.* **2008**, *10*, 322–330. [CrossRef]
41. Bonengel, S.; Bernkop-Schnürch, A. Thiomers—From bench to market. *J. Control Release Off. J. Control Release Soc.* **2014**, *195*, 120–129. [CrossRef] [PubMed]
42. Islam, M.A.; Park, T.E.; Reesor, E.; Cherukula, K.; Hasan, A.; Firdous, J.; Singh, B.; Kang, S.K.; Choi, Y.J.; Park, I.K.; et al. Mucoadhesive Chitosan Derivatives as Novel Drug Carriers. *Curr. Pharm. Des.* **2015**, *21*, 4285–4309. [CrossRef]
43. Kuo, P.; Rayner, C.K.; Jones, K.L.; Horowitz, M. Pathophysiology and management of diabetic gastropathy: A guide for endocrinologists. *Drugs* **2007**, *67*, 1671–1687. [CrossRef]
44. Huang, W.; Lee, S.L.; Yu, L.X. Mechanistic approaches to predicting oral drug absorption. *AAPS J.* **2009**, *11*, 217–224. [CrossRef]
45. Shekhawat, P.B.; Pokharkar, V.B. Understanding peroral absorption: Regulatory aspects and contemporary approaches to tackling solubility and permeability hurdles. *Acta Pharm. Sin. B* **2017**, *7*, 260–280. [CrossRef] [PubMed]
46. Back, H.M.; Song, B.; Pradhan, S.; Chae, J.W.; Han, N.; Kang, W.; Chang, M.J.; Zheng, J.; Kwon, K.I.; Karlsson, M.O.; et al. A mechanism-based pharmacokinetic model of fenofibrate for explaining increased drug absorption after food consumption. *BMC Pharmacol. Toxicol.* **2018**, *19*, 4. [CrossRef] [PubMed]
47. Sarosiek, I.; Selover, K.H.; Katz, L.A.; Semler, J.R.; Wilding, G.E.; Lackner, J.M.; Sitrin, M.D.; Kuo, B.; Chey, W.D.; Hasler, W.L.; et al. The assessment of regional gut transit times in healthy controls and patients with gastroparesis using wireless motility technology. *Aliment. Pharmacol. Ther.* **2010**, *31*, 313–322. [CrossRef] [PubMed]
48. Roland, B.C.; Ciarleglio, M.M.; Clarke, J.O.; Semler, J.R.; Tomakin, E.; Mullin, G.E.; Pasricha, P.J. Small Intestinal Transit Time Is Delayed in Small Intestinal Bacterial Overgrowth. *J. Clin. Gastroenterol.* **2015**, *49*, 571–576. [CrossRef]
49. Koziolek, M.; Grimm, M.; Garbacz, G.; Kühn, J.P.; Weitschies, W. Intragastric volume changes after intake of a high-caloric, high-fat standard breakfast in healthy human subjects investigated by MRI. *Mol. Pharm.* **2014**, *11*, 1632–1639. [CrossRef]
50. Koziolek, M.; Garbacz, G.; Neumann, M.; Weitschies, W. Simulating the postprandial stomach: Physiological considerations for dissolution and release testing. *Mol. Pharm.* **2013**, *10*, 1610–1622. [CrossRef]
51. Grimm, M.; Koziolek, M.; Kühn, J.P.; Weitschies, W. Interindividual and intraindividual variability of fasted state gastric fluid volume and gastric emptying of water. *Eur. J. Pharm. Biopharm. Off. J. Arb. Pharm. Verfahr. EV* **2018**, *127*, 309–317. [CrossRef]
52. Mudie, D.M.; Murray, K.; Hoad, C.L.; Pritchard, S.E.; Garnett, M.C.; Amidon, G.L.; Gowland, P.A.; Spiller, R.C.; Amidon, G.E.; Marciani, L. Quantification of gastrointestinal liquid volumes and distribution following a 240 mL dose of water in the fasted state. *Mol. Pharm.* **2014**, *11*, 3039–3047. [CrossRef] [PubMed]
53. Yu, G.; Zheng, Q.S.; Li, G.F. Similarities and differences in gastrointestinal physiology between neonates and adults: A physiologically based pharmacokinetic modeling perspective. *AAPS J.* **2014**, *16*, 1162–1166. [CrossRef] [PubMed]
54. Allegaert, K.; van den Anker, J. Neonatal drug therapy: The first frontier of therapeutics for children. *Clin. Pharmacol. Ther.* **2015**, *98*, 288–297. [CrossRef] [PubMed]
55. Moyer, A.M.; Matey, E.T.; Miller, V.M. Individualized medicine: Sex, hormones, genetics, and adverse drug reactions. *Pharmacol. Res. Perspect.* **2019**, *7*, e00541. [CrossRef] [PubMed]
56. Whitley, H.; Lindsey, W. Sex-based differences in drug activity. *Am. Fam. Phys.* **2009**, *80*, 1254–1258.
57. Torrado, S.; Prada, P.; de la Torre, P.M.; Torrado, S. Chitosan-poly(acrylic) acid polyionic complex: In vivo study to demonstrate prolonged gastric retention. *Biomaterials* **2004**, *25*, 917–923. [CrossRef]
58. Modi, J.; Joshi, G.; Sawant, K. Chitosan based mucoadhesive nanoparticles of ketoconazole for bioavailability enhancement: Formulation, optimization, in vitro and ex vivo evaluation. *Drug Dev. Ind. Pharm.* **2013**, *39*, 540–547. [CrossRef] [PubMed]
59. Leslie, E.M.; Deeley, R.G.; Cole, S.P. Multidrug resistance proteins: Role of P-glycoprotein, MRP1, MRP2, and BCRP (ABCG2) in tissue defense. *Toxicol. Appl. Pharmacol.* **2005**, *204*, 216–237. [CrossRef]
60. Gutmann, H.; Hruz, P.; Zimmermann, C.; Beglinger, C.; Drewe, J. Distribution of breast cancer resistance protein (BCRP/ABCG2) mRNA expression along the human GI tract. *Biochem. Pharmacol.* **2005**, *70*, 695–699. [CrossRef]
61. Stappaerts, J.; Annaert, P.; Augustijns, P. Site dependent intestinal absorption of darunavir and its interaction with ketoconazole. *Eur. J. Pharm. Sci. Off. J. Eur. Fed. Pharm. Sci.* **2013**, *49*, 51–56. [CrossRef] [PubMed]
62. Peters, S.A.; Jones, C.R.; Ungell, A.L.; Hatley, O.J. Predicting Drug Extraction in the Human Gut Wall: Assessing Contributions from Drug Metabolizing Enzymes and Transporter Proteins using Preclinical Models. *Clin. Pharmacokinet.* **2016**, *55*, 673–696. [CrossRef]
63. Gameiro, M.; Silva, R.; Rocha-Pereira, C.; Carmo, H.; Carvalho, F.; Bastos, M.L.; Remião, F. Cellular Models and In Vitro Assays for the Screening of modulators of P-gp, MRP1 and BCRP. *Molecules* **2017**, *22*, 600. [CrossRef] [PubMed]
64. Estudante, M.; Morais, J.G.; Soveral, G.; Benet, L.Z. Intestinal drug transporters: An overview. *Adv. Drug Deliv. Rev.* **2013**, *65*, 1340–1356. [CrossRef]
65. Hilgendorf, C.; Ahlin, G.; Seithel, A.; Artursson, P.; Ungell, A.L.; Karlsson, J. Expression of thirty-six drug transporter genes in human intestine, liver, kidney, and organotypic cell lines. *Drug Metab. Dispos. Biol. Fate Chem.* **2007**, *35*, 1333–1340. [CrossRef]
66. Murakami, T.; Takano, M. Intestinal efflux transporters and drug absorption. *Expert Opin. Drug Metab. Toxicol.* **2008**, *4*, 923–939. [CrossRef]

67. Grandvuinet, A.S.; Steffansen, B. Interactions between organic anions on multiple transporters in Caco-2 cells. *J. Pharm. Sci.* **2011**, *100*, 3817–3830. [CrossRef] [PubMed]
68. Fu, D.; Arias, I.M. Intracellular trafficking of P-glycoprotein. *Int. J. Biochem. Cell Biol.* **2012**, *44*, 461–464. [CrossRef] [PubMed]
69. Li, X.; Lindquist, S.; Lowe, M.; Noppa, L.; Hernell, O. Bile salt-stimulated lipase and pancreatic lipase-related protein 2 are the dominating lipases in neonatal fat digestion in mice and rats. *Pediatric Res.* **2007**, *62*, 537–541. [CrossRef]
70. Ianiro, G.; Pecere, S.; Giorgio, V.; Gasbarrini, A.; Cammarota, G. Digestive Enzyme Supplementation in Gastrointestinal Diseases. *Curr. Drug Metab.* **2016**, *17*, 187–193. [CrossRef] [PubMed]
71. Shi, S.; Li, Y. Interplay of Drug-Metabolizing Enzymes and Transporters in Drug Absorption and Disposition. *Curr. Drug Metab.* **2014**, *15*, 915–941. [CrossRef] [PubMed]
72. Chen, Y.T.; Trzoss, L.; Yang, D.; Yan, B. Ontogenic expression of human carboxylesterase-2 and cytochrome P450 3A4 in liver and duodenum: Postnatal surge and organ-dependent regulation. *Toxicology* **2015**, *330*, 55–61. [CrossRef]
73. Brussee, J.M.; Yu, H.; Krekels, E.H.J.; de Roos, B.; Brill, M.J.E.; van den Anker, J.N.; Rostami-Hodjegan, A.; de Wildt, S.N.; Knibbe, C.A.J. First-Pass CYP3A-Mediated Metabolism of Midazolam in the Gut Wall and Liver in Preterm Neonates. *CPT Pharmacomet. Syst. Pharmacol.* **2018**, *7*, 374–383. [CrossRef]
74. Kearns, G.L.; Abdel-Rahman, S.M.; Alander, S.W.; Blowey, D.L.; Leeder, J.S.; Kauffman, R.E. Developmental pharmacology–drug disposition, action, and therapy in infants and children. *N. Engl. J. Med.* **2003**, *349*, 1157–1167. [CrossRef]
75. Takashima, T.; Yokoyama, C.; Mizuma, H.; Yamanaka, H.; Wada, Y.; Onoe, K.; Nagata, H.; Tazawa, S.; Doi, H.; Takahashi, K.; et al. Developmental changes in P-glycoprotein function in the blood-brain barrier of nonhuman primates: PET study with R-11C-verapamil and 11C-oseltamivir. *J. Nucl. Med. Off. Publ. Soc. Nucl. Med.* **2011**, *52*, 950–957. [CrossRef]
76. Lam, J.; Koren, G. P-glycoprotein in the developing human brain: A review of the effects of ontogeny on the safety of opioids in neonates. *Ther. Drug Monit.* **2014**, *36*, 699–705. [CrossRef]
77. Toornvliet, R.; van Berckel, B.N.; Luurtsema, G.; Lubberink, M.; Geldof, A.A.; Bosch, T.M.; Oerlemans, R.; Lammertsma, A.A.; Franssen, E.J. Effect of age on functional P-glycoprotein in the blood-brain barrier measured by use of (R)-[(11)C]verapamil and positron emission tomography. *Clin. Pharmacol. Ther.* **2006**, *79*, 540–548. [CrossRef]
78. Marzolini, C.; Tirona, R.G.; Kim, R.B. Pharmacogenomics of the OATP and OAT families. *Pharmacogenomics* **2004**, *5*, 273–282. [CrossRef]
79. Shah, R.R.; Gaedigk, A.; LLerena, A.; Eichelbaum, M.; Stingl, J.; Smith, R.L. CYP450 genotype and pharmacogenetic association studies: A critical appraisal. *Pharmacogenomics* **2016**, *17*, 259–275. [CrossRef]
80. Hoffmeyer, S.; Burk, O.; von Richter, O.; Arnold, H.P.; Brockmöller, J.; Johne, A.; Cascorbi, I.; Gerloff, T.; Roots, I.; Eichelbaum, M.; et al. Functional polymorphisms of the human multidrug-resistance gene: Multiple sequence variations and correlation of one allele with P-glycoprotein expression and activity in vivo. *Proc. Natl. Acad. Sci. USA* **2000**, *97*, 3473–3478. [CrossRef] [PubMed]
81. Cascorbi, I.; Gerloff, T.; Johne, A.; Meisel, C.; Hoffmeyer, S.; Schwab, M.; Schaeffeler, E.; Eichelbaum, M.; Brinkmann, U.; Roots, I. Frequency of single nucleotide polymorphisms in the P-glycoprotein drug transporter MDR1 gene in white subjects. *Clin. Pharmacol. Ther.* **2001**, *69*, 169–174. [CrossRef] [PubMed]
82. Sansone-Parsons, A.; Krishna, G.; Calzetta, A.; Wexler, D.; Kantesaria, B.; Rosenberg, M.A.; Saltzman, M.A. Effect of a nutritional supplement on posaconazole pharmacokinetics following oral administration to healthy volunteers. *Antimicrob. Agents Chemother.* **2006**, *50*, 1881–1883. [CrossRef]
83. Vendelbo, J.; Olesen, R.H.; Lauridsen, J.K.; Rungby, J.; Kleinman, J.E.; Hyde, T.M.; Larsen, A. Increasing BMI is associated with reduced expression of P-glycoprotein (ABCB1 gene) in the human brain with a stronger association in African Americans than Caucasians. *Pharm. J.* **2018**, *18*, 121–126. [CrossRef]
84. Hu, K.; Xie, X.; Zhao, Y.N.; Li, Y.; Ruan, J.; Li, H.R.; Jin, T.; Yang, X.L. Chitosan Influences the Expression of P-gp and Metabolism of Norfloxacin in Grass Carp. *J. Aquat. Anim. Health* **2015**, *27*, 104–111. [CrossRef]
85. Ni, J.; Tian, F.; Dahmani, F.Z.; Yang, H.; Yue, D.; He, S.; Zhou, J.; Yao, J. Curcumin-carboxymethyl chitosan (CNC) conjugate and CNC/LHR mixed polymeric micelles as new approaches to improve the oral absorption of P-gp substrate drugs. *Drug Deliv.* **2016**, *23*, 3424–3435. [CrossRef] [PubMed]
86. Mu, Y.; Fu, Y.; Li, J.; Yu, X.; Li, Y.; Wang, Y.; Wu, X.; Zhang, K.; Kong, M.; Feng, C.; et al. Multifunctional quercetin conjugated chitosan nano-micelles with P-gp inhibition and permeation enhancement of anticancer drug. *Carbohydr. Polym.* **2019**, *203*, 10–18. [CrossRef]
87. Wang, X.; Chen, Y.; Dahmani, F.Z.; Yin, L.; Zhou, J.; Yao, J. Amphiphilic carboxymethyl chitosan-quercetin conjugate with P-gp inhibitory properties for oral delivery of paclitaxel. *Biomaterials* **2014**, *35*, 7654–7665. [CrossRef] [PubMed]
88. Thursby, E.; Juge, N. Introduction to the human gut microbiota. *Biochem. J.* **2017**, *474*, 1823–1836. [CrossRef] [PubMed]
89. Donaldson, G.P.; Lee, S.M.; Mazmanian, S.K. Gut biogeography of the bacterial microbiota. *Nat. Rev. Microbiol.* **2016**, *14*, 20–32. [CrossRef]
90. Kim, S.; Covington, A.; Pamer, E.G. The intestinal microbiota: Antibiotics, colonization resistance, and enteric pathogens. *Immunol. Rev.* **2017**, *279*, 90–105. [CrossRef]
91. Noh, K.; Kang, Y.R.; Nepal, M.R.; Shakya, R.; Kang, M.J.; Kang, W.; Lee, S.; Jeong, H.G.; Jeong, T.C. Impact of gut microbiota on drug metabolism: An update for safe and effective use of drugs. *Arch. Pharmacal Res.* **2017**, *40*, 1345–1355. [CrossRef]
92. Zhang, J.; Zhang, J.; Wang, R. Gut microbiota modulates drug pharmacokinetics. *Drug Metab. Rev.* **2018**, *50*, 357–368. [CrossRef]

93. Morrison, D.J.; Preston, T. Formation of short chain fatty acids by the gut microbiota and their impact on human metabolism. *Gut Microbes* **2016**, *7*, 189–200. [CrossRef]
94. Parada Venegas, D.; De la Fuente, M.K.; Landskron, G.; González, M.J.; Quera, R.; Dijkstra, G.; Harmsen, H.J.M.; Faber, K.N.; Hermoso, M.A. Short Chain Fatty Acids (SCFAs)-Mediated Gut Epithelial and Immune Regulation and Its Relevance for Inflammatory Bowel Diseases. *Front. Immunol.* **2019**, *10*, 277. [CrossRef]
95. Zhang, S.H.; Wang, Y.Z.; Meng, F.Y.; Li, Y.L.; Li, C.X.; Duan, F.P.; Wang, Q.; Zhang, X.T.; Zhang, C.N. Studies of the microbial metabolism of flavonoids extracted from the leaves of Diospyros kaki by intestinal bacteria. *Arch. Pharmacal Res.* **2015**, *38*, 614–619. [CrossRef] [PubMed]
96. Tozaki, H.; Emi, Y.; Horisaka, E.; Fujita, T.; Yamamoto, A.; Muranishi, S. Degradation of insulin and calcitonin and their protection by various protease inhibitors in rat caecal contents: Implications in peptide delivery to the colon. *J. Pharm. Pharmacol.* **1997**, *49*, 164–168. [CrossRef] [PubMed]
97. Clayton, T.A.; Baker, D.; Lindon, J.C.; Everett, J.R.; Nicholson, J.K. Pharmacometabonomic identification of a significant host-microbiome metabolic interaction affecting human drug metabolism. *Proc. Natl. Acad. Sci. USA* **2009**, *106*, 14728–14733. [CrossRef]
98. Saitta, K.S.; Zhang, C.; Lee, K.K.; Fujimoto, K.; Redinbo, M.R.; Boelsterli, U.A. Bacterial β-glucuronidase inhibition protects mice against enteropathy induced by indomethacin, ketoprofen or diclofenac: Mode of action and pharmacokinetics. *Xenobiotica Fate Foreign Compd. Biol. Syst.* **2014**, *44*, 28–35. [CrossRef]
99. Fujiwara, R.; Maruo, Y.; Chen, S.; Tukey, R.H. Role of extrahepatic UDP-glucuronosyltransferase 1A1: Advances in understanding breast milk-induced neonatal hyperbilirubinemia. *Toxicol. Appl. Pharmacol.* **2015**, *289*, 124–132. [CrossRef]
100. Kim, Y.S.; Unno, T.; Kim, B.Y.; Park, M.S. Sex Differences in Gut Microbiota. *World J. Men Health* **2020**, *38*, 48–60. [CrossRef]
101. Gupta, V.K.; Paul, S.; Dutta, C. Geography, Ethnicity or Subsistence-Specific Variations in Human Microbiome Composition and Diversity. *Front. Microbiol.* **2017**, *8*, 1162. [CrossRef]
102. Dwiyanto, J.; Hussain, M.H.; Reidpath, D.; Ong, K.S.; Qasim, A.; Lee, S.W.H.; Lee, S.M.; Foo, S.C.; Chong, C.W.; Rahman, S. Ethnicity influences the gut microbiota of individuals sharing a geographical location: A cross-sectional study from a middle-income country. *Sci. Rep.* **2021**, *11*, 2618. [CrossRef]
103. Stojančević, M.; Bojić, G.; Salami, H.A.; Mikov, M. The Influence of Intestinal Tract and Probiotics on the Fate of Orally Administered Drugs. *Curr. Issues Mol. Biol.* **2014**, *16*, 55–68.
104. Matuskova, Z.; Anzenbacherova, E.; Vecera, R.; Tlaskalova-Hogenova, H.; Kolar, M.; Anzenbacher, P. Administration of a probiotic can change drug pharmacokinetics: Effect of *E. coli* Nissle 1917 on amidarone absorption in rats. *PLoS ONE* **2014**, *9*, e87150. [CrossRef]
105. Feng, D.; Zhang, M.; Tian, S.; Wang, J.; Zhu, W. Chitosan-chelated zinc modulates cecal microbiota and attenuates inflammatory response in weaned rats challenged with *Escherichia coli*. *J. Microbiol.* **2020**, *58*, 780–792. [CrossRef]
106. Zheng, J.; Yuan, X.; Cheng, G.; Jiao, S.; Feng, C.; Zhao, X.; Yin, H.; Du, Y.; Liu, H. Chitosan oligosaccharides improve the disturbance in glucose metabolism and reverse the dysbiosis of gut microbiota in diabetic mice. *Carbohydr. Polym.* **2018**, *190*, 77–86. [CrossRef]
107. Owu, D.U.; Obembe, A.O.; Nwokocha, C.R.; Edoho, I.E.; Osim, E.E. Gastric ulceration in diabetes mellitus: Protective role of vitamin C. *ISRN Gastroenterol.* **2012**, *2012*, 362805. [CrossRef]
108. Eliasson, B.; Björnsson, E.; Urbanavicius, V.; Andersson, H.; Fowelin, J.; Attvall, S.; Abrahamsson, H.; Smith, U. Hyperinsulinaemia impairs gastrointestinal motility and slows carbohydrate absorption. *Diabetologia* **1995**, *38*, 79–85. [CrossRef]
109. Marathe, C.S.; Rayner, C.K.; Jones, K.L.; Horowitz, M. Relationships between gastric emptying, postprandial glycemia, and incretin hormones. *Diabetes Care* **2013**, *36*, 1396–1405. [CrossRef]
110. Zhao, M.; Liao, D.; Zhao, J. Diabetes-induced mechanophysiological changes in the small intestine and colon. *World J. Diabetes* **2017**, *8*, 249–269. [CrossRef]
111. Redan, B.W.; Buhman, K.K.; Novotny, J.A.; Ferruzzi, M.G. Altered Transport and Metabolism of Phenolic Compounds in Obesity and Diabetes: Implications for Functional Food Development and Assessment. *Adv. Nutr.* **2016**, *7*, 1090–1104. [CrossRef] [PubMed]
112. Kobori, T.; Harada, S.; Nakamoto, K.; Tokuyama, S. Functional alterations of intestinal P-glycoprotein under diabetic conditions. *Biol. Pharm. Bull.* **2013**, *36*, 1381–1390. [CrossRef] [PubMed]
113. Dostalek, M.; Sam, W.J.; Paryani, K.R.; Macwan, J.S.; Gohh, R.Y.; Akhlaghi, F. Diabetes mellitus reduces the clearance of atorvastatin lactone: Results of a population pharmacokinetic analysis in renal transplant recipients and in vitro studies using human liver microsomes. *Clin. Pharmacokinet.* **2012**, *51*, 591–606. [CrossRef]
114. Zhelyazkova-Savova, M.; Gancheva, S.; Sirakova, V. Potential statin-drug interactions: Prevalence and clinical significance. *SpringerPlus* **2014**, *3*, 168. [CrossRef]
115. Mahajan, V.; Hashmi, J.; Singh, R.; Samra, T.; Aneja, S. Comparative evaluation of gastric pH and volume in morbidly obese and lean patients undergoing elective surgery and effect of aspiration prophylaxis. *J. Clin. Anesth.* **2015**, *27*, 396–400. [CrossRef]
116. Foucaud-Vignault, M.; Soayfane, Z.; Ménez, C.; Bertrand-Michel, J.; Martin, P.G.; Guillou, H.; Collet, X.; Lespine, A. P-glycoprotein dysfunction contributes to hepatic steatosis and obesity in mice. *PLoS ONE* **2011**, *6*, e23614. [CrossRef]

117. Rodríguez-Morató, J.; Goday, A.; Langohr, K.; Pujadas, M.; Civit, E.; Pérez-Mañá, C.; Papaseit, E.; Ramon, J.M.; Benaiges, D.; Castañer, O.; et al. Short- and medium-term impact of bariatric surgery on the activities of CYP2D6, CYP3A4, CYP2C9, and CYP1A2 in morbid obesity. *Sci. Rep.* **2019**, *9*, 20405. [CrossRef]
118. Sudhakar, S.; Chandran, S.V.; Selvamurugan, N.; Nazeer, R.A. Biodistribution and pharmacokinetics of thiolated chitosan nanoparticles for oral delivery of insulin in vivo. *Int. J. Biol. Macromol.* **2020**, *150*, 281–288. [CrossRef]
119. Li, L.; Jiang, G.; Yu, W.; Liu, D.; Chen, H.; Liu, Y.; Tong, Z.; Kong, X.; Yao, J. Preparation of chitosan-based multifunctional nanocarriers overcoming multiple barriers for oral delivery of insulin. *Mater. Sci. Eng. C Mater. Biol. Appl.* **2017**, *70*, 278–286. [CrossRef]
120. Lu, P.J.; Hsu, P.I.; Chen, C.H.; Hsiao, M.; Chang, W.C.; Tseng, H.H.; Lin, K.H.; Chuah, S.K.; Chen, H.C. Gastric juice acidity in upper gastrointestinal diseases. *World J. Gastroenterol.* **2010**, *16*, 5496–5501. [CrossRef]
121. Ghosh, T.; Lewis, D.I.; Axon, A.T.; Everett, S.M. Review article: Methods of measuring gastric acid secretion. *Aliment. Pharmacol. Ther.* **2011**, *33*, 768–781. [CrossRef]
122. Chang, F.Y.; Chen, C.Y.; Lu, C.L.; Luo, J.C.; Jiun, K.L.; Lee, S.D.; Wu, C.W. Undisturbed water gastric emptying in patients of stomach cancer. *Hepato-Gastroenterology* **2004**, *51*, 1219–1224.
123. Kim, D.H.; Yun, H.Y.; Song, Y.J.; Ryu, D.H.; Han, H.S.; Han, J.H.; Kim, K.B.; Yoon, S.M.; Youn, S.J. Clinical features of gastric emptying after distal gastrectomy. *Ann. Surg. Treat. Res.* **2017**, *93*, 310–315. [CrossRef]
124. Joshi, G.; Kumar, A.; Sawant, K. Enhanced bioavailability and intestinal uptake of Gemcitabine HCl loaded PLGA nanoparticles after oral delivery. *Eur. J. Pharm. Sci. Off. J. Eur. Fed. Pharm. Sci.* **2014**, *60*, 80–89. [CrossRef]
125. Louisa, M.; Soediro, T.M.; Suyatna, F.D. In vitro modulation of P-glycoprotein, MRP-1 and BCRP expression by mangiferin in doxorubicin-treated MCF-7 cells. *Asian Pac. J. Cancer Prev. APJCP* **2014**, *15*, 1639–1642. [CrossRef]
126. Nanayakkara, A.K.; Follit, C.A.; Chen, G.; Williams, N.S.; Vogel, P.D.; Wise, J.G. Targeted inhibitors of P-glycoprotein increase chemotherapeutic-induced mortality of multidrug resistant tumor cells. *Sci. Rep.* **2018**, *8*, 967. [CrossRef]
127. Weiss, R.B. The anthracyclines: Will we ever find a better doxorubicin? *Semin. Oncol.* **1992**, *19*, 670–686.
128. Cortés-Funes, H.; Coronado, C. Role of anthracyclines in the era of targeted therapy. *Cardiovasc. Toxicol.* **2007**, *7*, 56–60. [CrossRef]
129. Thorn, C.F.; Oshiro, C.; Marsh, S.; Hernandez-Boussard, T.; McLeod, H.; Klein, T.E.; Altman, R.B. Doxorubicin pathways: Pharmacodynamics and adverse effects. *Pharm. Genom.* **2011**, *21*, 440–446. [CrossRef]
130. Kalaria, D.R.; Sharma, G.; Beniwal, V.; Ravi Kumar, M.N. Design of biodegradable nanoparticles for oral delivery of doxorubicin: In vivo pharmacokinetics and toxicity studies in rats. *Pharm. Res.* **2009**, *26*, 492–501. [CrossRef]
131. Feng, C.; Li, J.; Mu, Y.; Kong, M.; Li, Y.; Raja, M.A.; Cheng, X.J.; Liu, Y.; Chen, X.G. Multilayer micro-dispersing system as oral carriers for co-delivery of doxorubicin hydrochloride and P-gp inhibitor. *Int. J. Biol. Macromol.* **2017**, *94*, 170–180. [CrossRef]
132. Deng, L.; Dong, H.; Dong, A.; Zhang, J. A strategy for oral chemotherapy via dual pH-sensitive polyelectrolyte complex nanoparticles to achieve gastric survivability, intestinal permeability, hemodynamic stability and intracellular activity. *Eur. J. Pharm. Biopharm. Off. J. Arb. Pharm. Verfahr. EV* **2015**, *97*, 107–117. [CrossRef]
133. Feng, C.; Wang, Z.; Jiang, C.; Kong, M.; Zhou, X.; Li, Y.; Cheng, X.; Chen, X. Chitosan/o-carboxymethyl chitosan nanoparticles for efficient and safe oral anticancer drug delivery: In vitro and in vivo evaluation. *Int. J. Pharm.* **2013**, *457*, 158–167. [CrossRef]
134. Iannuccelli, V.; Montanari, M.; Bertelli, D.; Pellati, F.; Coppi, G. Microparticulate polyelectrolyte complexes for gentamicin transport across intestinal epithelia. *Drug Deliv.* **2011**, *18*, 26–37. [CrossRef]
135. Eftaiha, A.F.; Qinna, N.; Rashid, I.S.; Al Remawi, M.M.; Al Shami, M.R.; Arafat, T.A.; Badwan, A.A. Bioadhesive controlled metronidazole release matrix based on chitosan and xanthan gum. *Mar. Drugs* **2010**, *8*, 1716–1730. [CrossRef]
136. Konturek, P.C.; Brzozowski, T.; Konturek, S.J. Stress and the gut: Pathophysiology, clinical consequences, diagnostic approach and treatment options. *J. Physiol. Pharmacol. Off. J. Pol. Physiol. Soc.* **2011**, *62*, 591–599.
137. Treenate, P.; Monvisade, P. In vitro drug release profiles of pH-sensitive hydroxyethylacryl chitosan/sodium alginate hydrogels using paracetamol as a soluble model drug. *Int. J. Biol. Macromol.* **2017**, *99*, 71–78. [CrossRef]
138. Ofokansi, K.C.; Kenechukwu, F.C. Formulation Development and Evaluation of Drug Release Kinetics from Colon-Targeted Ibuprofen Tablets Based on Eudragit RL 100-Chitosan Interpolyelectrolyte Complexes. *ISRN Pharm.* **2013**, *2013*, 838403. [CrossRef]
139. Ahmed, T.A.; Aljaeid, B.M. Preparation, characterization, and potential application of chitosan, chitosan derivatives, and chitosan metal nanoparticles in pharmaceutical drug delivery. *Drug Des. Dev. Ther.* **2016**, *10*, 483–507. [CrossRef]
140. Fabiano, A.; Piras, A.M.; Uccello-Barretta, G.; Balzano, F.; Cesari, A.; Testai, L.; Citi, V.; Zambito, Y. Impact of mucoadhesive polymeric nanoparticulate systems on oral bioavailability of a macromolecular model drug. *Eur. J. Pharm. Biopharm. Off. J. Arb. Pharm. Verfahr. EV* **2018**, *130*, 281–289. [CrossRef]
141. Blanquet, S.; Zeijdner, E.; Beyssac, E.; Meunier, J.P.; Denis, S.; Havenaar, R.; Alric, M. A dynamic artificial gastrointestinal system for studying the behavior of orally administered drug dosage forms under various physiological conditions. *Pharm. Res.* **2004**, *21*, 585–591. [CrossRef]
142. Bernkop-Schnürch, A.; Kast, C.E.; Guggi, D. Permeation enhancing polymers in oral delivery of hydrophilic macromolecules: Thiomer/GSH systems. *J. Control Release Off. J. Control Release Soc.* **2003**, *93*, 95–103. [CrossRef]
143. Lipinski, C.A.; Lombardo, F.; Dominy, B.W.; Feeney, P.J. Experimental and computational approaches to estimate solubility and permeability in drug discovery and development settings. *Adv. Drug Deliv. Rev.* **2001**, *46*, 3–26. [CrossRef]
144. Hu, Q.; Luo, Y. Recent advances of polysaccharide-based nanoparticles for oral insulin delivery. *Int. J. Biol. Macromol.* **2018**, *120*, 775–782. [CrossRef] [PubMed]

145. Bayat, A.; Larijani, B.; Ahmadian, S.; Junginger, H.E.; Rafiee-Tehrani, M. Preparation and characterization of insulin nanoparticles using chitosan and its quaternized derivatives. *Nanomed. Nanotechnol. Biol. Med.* **2008**, *4*, 115–120. [CrossRef] [PubMed]
146. Arbit, E. The physiological rationale for oral insulin administration. *Diabetes Technol. Ther.* **2004**, *6*, 510–517. [CrossRef] [PubMed]
147. Menzel, C.; Silbernagl, J.; Laffleur, F.; Leichner, C.; Jelkmann, M.; Huck, C.W.; Hussain, S.; Bernkop-Schnürch, A. 2,2′Dithiodinicotinyl ligands: Key to more reactive thiomers. *Int. J. Pharm.* **2016**, *503*, 199–206. [CrossRef]
148. Sajjad, M.; Khan, M.I.; Naveed, S.; Ijaz, S.; Qureshi, O.S.; Raza, S.A.; Shahnaz, G.; Sohail, M.F. Folate-Functionalized Thiomeric Nanoparticles for Enhanced Docetaxel Cytotoxicity and Improved Oral Bioavailability. *AAPS PharmSciTech* **2019**, *20*, 81. [CrossRef]
149. Samprasit, W.; Opanasopit, P.; Chamsai, B. Mucoadhesive chitosan and thiolated chitosan nanoparticles containing alpha mangostin for possible Colon-targeted delivery. *Pharm. Dev. Technol.* **2021**, *26*, 362–372. [CrossRef]
150. Fan, B.; Xing, Y.; Zheng, Y.; Sun, C.; Liang, G. pH-responsive thiolated chitosan nanoparticles for oral low-molecular weight heparin delivery: In vitro and in vivo evaluation. *Drug Deliv.* **2016**, *23*, 238–247. [CrossRef]
151. Gradauer, K.; Vonach, C.; Leitinger, G.; Kolb, D.; Fröhlich, E.; Roblegg, E.; Bernkop-Schnürch, A.; Prassl, R. Chemical coupling of thiolated chitosan to preformed liposomes improves mucoadhesive properties. *Int. J. Nanomed.* **2012**, *7*, 2523–2534. [CrossRef]
152. Dünnhaupt, S.; Barthelmes, J.; Rahmat, D.; Leithner, K.; Thurner, C.C.; Friedl, H.; Bernkop-Schnürch, A. S-protected thiolated chitosan for oral delivery of hydrophilic macromolecules: Evaluation of permeation enhancing and efflux pump inhibitory properties. *Mol. Pharm.* **2012**, *9*, 1331–1341. [CrossRef]
153. Dünnhaupt, S.; Barthelmes, J.; Iqbal, J.; Perera, G.; Thurner, C.C.; Friedl, H.; Bernkop-Schnürch, A. In vivo evaluation of an oral drug delivery system for peptides based on S-protected thiolated chitosan. *J. Control. Release Off. J. Control Release Soc.* **2012**, *160*, 477–485. [CrossRef]
154. Iqbal, J.; Shahnaz, G.; Perera, G.; Hintzen, F.; Sarti, F.; Bernkop-Schnürch, A. Thiolated chitosan: Development and in vivo evaluation of an oral delivery system for leuprolide. *Eur. J. Pharm. Biopharm. Off. J. Arb. Pharm. Verfahr. EV* **2012**, *80*, 95–102. [CrossRef]
155. Dünnhaupt, S.; Barthelmes, J.; Hombach, J.; Sakloetsakun, D.; Arkhipova, V.; Bernkop-Schnürch, A. Distribution of thiolated mucoadhesive nanoparticles on intestinal mucosa. *Int. J. Pharm.* **2011**, *408*, 191–199. [CrossRef]
156. Mourya, V.K.; Inamdar, N.N. Trimethyl chitosan and its applications in drug delivery. *J. Mater. Sci. Mater. Med.* **2009**, *20*, 1057–1079. [CrossRef] [PubMed]
157. Kulkarni, A.D.; Patel, H.M.; Surana, S.J.; Vanjari, Y.H.; Belgamwar, V.S.; Pardeshi, C.V. *N,N,N*-Trimethyl chitosan: An advanced polymer with myriad of opportunities in nanomedicine. *Carbohydr. Polym.* **2017**, *157*, 875–902. [CrossRef]
158. Sheng, J.; Han, L.; Qin, J.; Ru, G.; Li, R.; Wu, L.; Cui, D.; Yang, P.; He, Y.; Wang, J. *N*-trimethyl chitosan chloride-coated PLGA nanoparticles overcoming multiple barriers to oral insulin absorption. *ACS Appl. Mater. Interfaces* **2015**, *7*, 15430–15441. [CrossRef]
159. Tsai, L.C.; Chen, C.H.; Lin, C.W.; Ho, Y.C.; Mi, F.L. Development of mutlifunctional nanoparticles self-assembled from trimethyl chitosan and fucoidan for enhanced oral delivery of insulin. *Int. J. Biol. Macromol.* **2019**, *126*, 141–150. [CrossRef]
160. Ghavimishamekh, A.; Ziamajidi, N.; Dehghan, A.; Goodarzi, M.T.; Abbasalipourkabir, R. Study of Insulin-Loaded Chitosan Nanoparticle Effects on TGF-β1 and Fibronectin Expression in Kidney Tissue of Type 1 Diabetic Rats. *Indian J. Clin. Biochem. IJCB* **2019**, *34*, 418–426. [CrossRef]
161. Song, R.F.; Li, X.J.; Cheng, X.L.; Fu, A.R.; Wang, Y.H.; Feng, Y.J.; Xiong, Y. Paclitaxel-loaded trimethyl chitosan-based polymeric nanoparticle for the effective treatment of gastroenteric tumors. *Oncol. Rep.* **2014**, *32*, 1481–1488. [CrossRef]
162. Huang, A.; Makhlof, A.; Ping, Q.; Tozuka, Y.; Takeuchi, H. *N*-trimethyl chitosan-modified liposomes as carriers for oral delivery of salmon calcitonin. *Drug Deliv.* **2011**, *18*, 562–569. [CrossRef]
163. Li, W.; Zhu, X.; Zhou, X.; Wang, X.; Zhai, W.; Li, B.; Du, J.; Li, G.; Sui, X.; Wu, Y.; et al. An orally available PD-1/PD-L1 blocking peptide OPBP-1-loaded trimethyl chitosan hydrogel for cancer immunotherapy. *J. Control Release Off. J. Control Release Soc.* **2021**, *334*, 376–388. [CrossRef]
164. Martins, A.F.; Bueno, P.V.; Almeida, E.A.; Rodrigues, F.H.; Rubira, A.F.; Muniz, E.C. Characterization of *N*-trimethyl chitosan/alginate complexes and curcumin release. *Int. J. Biol. Macromol.* **2013**, *57*, 174–184. [CrossRef]
165. Saheb, M.; Fereydouni, N.; Nemati, S.; Barreto, G.E.; Johnston, T.P.; Sahebkar, A. Chitosan-based delivery systems for curcumin: A review of pharmacodynamic and pharmacokinetic aspects. *J. Cell. Physiol.* **2019**, *234*, 12325–12340. [CrossRef]
166. Ramalingam, P.; Ko, Y.T. Enhanced oral delivery of curcumin from *N*-trimethyl chitosan surface-modified solid lipid nanoparticles: Pharmacokinetic and brain distribution evaluations. *Pharm. Res.* **2015**, *32*, 389–402. [CrossRef]
167. Kalliola, S.; Repo, E.; Srivastava, V.; Zhao, F.; Heiskanen, J.P.; Sirviö, J.A.; Liimatainen, H.; Sillanpää, M. Carboxymethyl Chitosan and Its Hydrophobically Modified Derivative as pH-Switchable Emulsifiers. *Langmuir ACS J. Surf. Colloids* **2018**, *34*, 2800–2806. [CrossRef]
168. Wang, J.; Xu, M.; Cheng, X.; Kong, M.; Liu, Y.; Feng, C.; Chen, X. Positive/negative surface charge of chitosan based nanogels and its potential influence on oral insulin delivery. *Carbohydr. Polym.* **2016**, *136*, 867–874. [CrossRef]
169. Li, J.; Jiang, C.; Lang, X.; Kong, M.; Cheng, X.; Liu, Y.; Feng, C.; Chen, X. Multilayer sodium alginate beads with porous core containing chitosan based nanoparticles for oral delivery of anticancer drug. *Int. J. Biol. Macromol.* **2016**, *85*, 1–8. [CrossRef]
170. Feng, C.; Song, R.; Sun, G.; Kong, M.; Bao, Z.; Li, Y.; Cheng, X.; Cha, D.; Park, H.; Chen, X. Immobilization of coacervate microcapsules in multilayer sodium alginate beads for efficient oral anticancer drug delivery. *Biomacromolecules* **2014**, *15*, 985–996. [CrossRef]

171. Cong, Y.; Geng, J.; Wang, H.; Su, J.; Arif, M.; Dong, Q.; Chi, Z.; Liu, C. Ureido-modified carboxymethyl chitosan-graft-stearic acid polymeric nano-micelles as a targeted delivering carrier of clarithromycin for *Helicobacter pylori*: Preparation and in vitro evaluation. *Int. J. Biol. Macromol.* **2019**, *129*, 686–692. [CrossRef]
172. Huang, G.Q.; Zhang, Z.K.; Cheng, L.Y.; Xiao, J.X. Intestine-targeted delivery potency of O-carboxymethyl chitosan-coated layer-by-layer microcapsules: An in vitro and in vivo evaluation. *Mater. Sci. Eng. C Mater. Biol. Appl.* **2019**, *105*, 110129. [CrossRef]
173. Le, T.N.; Her, J.; Sim, T.; Jung, C.E.; Kang, J.K.; Oh, K.T. Preparation of Gastro-retentive Tablets Employing Controlled Superporous Networks for Improved Drug Bioavailability. *AAPS PharmSciTech* **2020**, *21*, 320. [CrossRef]
174. Park, H.; Park, K.; Kim, D. Preparation and swelling behavior of chitosan-based superporous hydrogels for gastric retention application. *J. Biomed. Mater. Res. Part A* **2006**, *76*, 144–150. [CrossRef]
175. Su, F.Y.; Lin, K.J.; Sonaje, K.; Wey, S.P.; Yen, T.C.; Ho, Y.C.; Panda, N.; Chuang, E.Y.; Maiti, B.; Sung, H.W. Protease inhibition and absorption enhancement by functional nanoparticles for effective oral insulin delivery. *Biomaterials* **2012**, *33*, 2801–2811. [CrossRef]
176. Sung, H.W.; Sonaje, K.; Liao, Z.X.; Hsu, L.W.; Chuang, E.Y. pH-responsive nanoparticles shelled with chitosan for oral delivery of insulin: From mechanism to therapeutic applications. *Acc. Chem. Res.* **2012**, *45*, 619–629. [CrossRef] [PubMed]
177. Lu, K.Y.; Lin, C.W.; Hsu, C.H.; Ho, Y.C.; Chuang, E.Y.; Sung, H.W.; Mi, F.L. FRET-based dual-emission and pH-responsive nanocarriers for enhanced delivery of protein across intestinal epithelial cell barrier. *ACS Appl. Mater. Interfaces* **2014**, *6*, 18275–18289. [CrossRef] [PubMed]
178. Jeong, Y.I.; Jin, S.G.; Kim, I.Y.; Pei, J.; Wen, M.; Jung, T.Y.; Moon, K.S.; Jung, S. Doxorubicin-incorporated nanoparticles composed of poly(ethylene glycol)-grafted carboxymethyl chitosan and antitumor activity against glioma cells in vitro. *Colloids Surf. B Biointerfaces* **2010**, *79*, 149–155. [CrossRef] [PubMed]
179. Hauptstein, S.; Bonengel, S.; Griessinger, J.; Bernkop-Schnürch, A. Synthesis and characterization of pH tolerant and mucoadhesive (thiol-polyethylene glycol) chitosan graft polymer for drug delivery. *J. Pharm. Sci.* **2014**, *103*, 594–601. [CrossRef] [PubMed]
180. Papadimitriou, S.A.; Achilias, D.S.; Bikiaris, D.N. Chitosan-g-PEG nanoparticles ionically crosslinked with poly(glutamic acid) and tripolyphosphate as protein delivery systems. *Int. J. Pharm.* **2012**, *430*, 318–327. [CrossRef]
181. Mo, R.; Jin, X.; Li, N.; Ju, C.; Sun, M.; Zhang, C.; Ping, Q. The mechanism of enhancement on oral absorption of paclitaxel by N-octyl-O-sulfate chitosan micelles. *Biomaterials* **2011**, *32*, 4609–4620. [CrossRef] [PubMed]
182. Jain, A.K.; Swarnakar, N.K.; Das, M.; Godugu, C.; Singh, R.P.; Rao, P.R.; Jain, S. Augmented anticancer efficacy of doxorubicin-loaded polymeric nanoparticles after oral administration in a breast cancer induced animal model. *Mol. Pharm.* **2011**, *8*, 1140–1151. [CrossRef] [PubMed]
183. Gaucher, G.; Satturwar, P.; Jones, M.C.; Furtos, A.; Leroux, J.C. Polymeric micelles for oral drug delivery. *Eur. J. Pharm. Biopharm. Off. J. Arb. Pharm. Verfahr. EV* **2010**, *76*, 147–158. [CrossRef] [PubMed]
184. Nornoo, A.O.; Zheng, H.; Lopes, L.B.; Johnson-Restrepo, B.; Kannan, K.; Reed, R. Oral microemulsions of paclitaxel: In situ and pharmacokinetic studies. *Eur. J. Pharm. Biopharm. Off. J. Arb. Pharm. Verfahr. EV* **2009**, *71*, 310–317. [CrossRef]
185. Al-Hilal, T.A.; Alam, F.; Byun, Y. Oral drug delivery systems using chemical conjugates or physical complexes. *Adv. Drug Deliv. Rev.* **2013**, *65*, 845–864. [CrossRef]
186. Soares, S.F.; Fernandes, T.; Daniel-da-Silva, A.L.; Trindade, T. The controlled synthesis of complex hollow nanostructures and prospective applications(†). *Proc. Math. Phys. Eng. Sci.* **2019**, *475*, 20180677. [CrossRef] [PubMed]
187. Sultan, Y.; DeRosa, M.C. Target binding influences permeability in aptamer-polyelectrolyte microcapsules. *Small* **2011**, *7*, 1219–1226. [CrossRef]
188. Sultan, Y.; Walsh, R.; Monreal, C.; DeRosa, M.C. Preparation of functional aptamer films using layer-by-layer self-assembly. *Biomacromolecules* **2009**, *10*, 1149–1154. [CrossRef]
189. Radwan, S.E.; Sokar, M.S.; Abdelmonsif, D.A.; El-Kamel, A.H. Mucopenetrating nanoparticles for enhancement of oral bioavailability of furosemide: In vitro and in vivo evaluation/sub-acute toxicity study. *Int. J. Pharm.* **2017**, *526*, 366–379. [CrossRef]
190. Yang, J.; Chen, J.; Pan, D.; Wan, Y.; Wang, Z. pH-sensitive interpenetrating network hydrogels based on chitosan derivatives and alginate for oral drug delivery. *Carbohydr. Polym.* **2013**, *92*, 719–725. [CrossRef]
191. Oshi, M.A.; Lee, J.; Naeem, M.; Hasan, N.; Kim, J.; Kim, H.J.; Lee, E.H.; Jung, Y.; Yoo, J.W. Curcumin Nanocrystal/pH-Responsive Polyelectrolyte Multilayer Core-Shell Nanoparticles for Inflammation-Targeted Alleviation of Ulcerative Colitis. *Biomacromolecules* **2020**, *21*, 3571–3581. [CrossRef] [PubMed]
192. Jain, A.; Jain, S.K. Optimization of chitosan nanoparticles for colon tumors using experimental design methodology. *Artif. Cells Nanomed. Biotechnol.* **2016**, *44*, 1917–1926. [CrossRef]
193. Caddeo, C.; Díez-Sales, O.; Pons, R.; Carbone, C.; Ennas, G.; Puglisi, G.; Fadda, A.M.; Manconi, M. Cross-linked chitosan/liposome hybrid system for the intestinal delivery of quercetin. *J. Colloid Interface Sci.* **2016**, *461*, 69–78. [CrossRef]
194. Konecsni, K.; Low, N.H.; Nickerson, M.T. Chitosan-tripolyphosphate submicron particles as the carrier of entrapped rutin. *Food Chem.* **2012**, *134*, 1775–1779. [CrossRef]
195. Sareen, R.; Jain, N.; Rajkumari, A.; Dhar, K.L. pH triggered delivery of curcumin from Eudragit-coated chitosan microspheres for inflammatory bowel disease: Characterization and pharmacodynamic evaluation. *Drug Deliv.* **2016**, *23*, 55–62. [CrossRef]

196. Pandey, S.; Mishra, A.; Raval, P.; Patel, H.; Gupta, A.; Shah, D. Chitosan-pectin polyelectrolyte complex as a carrier for colon targeted drug delivery. *J. Young Pharm. JYP* **2013**, *5*, 160–166. [CrossRef]
197. Liu, C.; Kou, Y.; Zhang, X.; Dong, W.; Cheng, H.; Mao, S. Enhanced oral insulin delivery via surface hydrophilic modification of chitosan copolymer based self-assembly polyelectrolyte nanocomplex. *Int. J. Pharm.* **2019**, *554*, 36–47. [CrossRef]
198. Liu, C.; Kou, Y.; Zhang, X.; Cheng, H.; Chen, X.; Mao, S. Strategies and industrial perspectives to improve oral absorption of biological macromolecules. *Expert Opin. Drug Deliv.* **2018**, *15*, 223–233. [CrossRef] [PubMed]
199. Meng, F.; Zhong, Y.; Cheng, R.; Deng, C.; Zhong, Z. pH-sensitive polymeric nanoparticles for tumor-targeting doxorubicin delivery: Concept and recent advances. *Nanomedicine* **2014**, *9*, 487–499. [CrossRef]
200. Anwer, M.K.; Iqbal, M.; Muharram, M.M.; Mohammad, M.; Ezzeldin, E.; Aldawsari, M.F.; Alalaiwe, A.; Imam, F. Development of Lipomer Nanoparticles for the Enhancement of Drug Release, Anti-microbial Activity and Bioavailability of Delafloxacin. *Pharmaceutics* **2020**, *12*, 252. [CrossRef]
201. Khare, T.; Mahalunkar, S.; Shriram, V.; Gosavi, S.; Kumar, V. Embelin-loaded chitosan gold nanoparticles interact synergistically with ciprofloxacin by inhibiting efflux pumps in multidrug-resistant *Pseudomonas aeruginosa* and *Escherichia coli*. *Environ. Res.* **2021**, *199*, 111321. [CrossRef]
202. Maisetta, G.; Piras, A.M.; Motta, V.; Braccini, S.; Mazzantini, D.; Chiellini, F.; Zambito, Y.; Esin, S.; Batoni, G. Antivirulence Properties of a Low-Molecular-Weight Quaternized Chitosan Derivative against *Pseudomonas aeruginosa*. *Microorganisms* **2021**, *9*, 912. [CrossRef]
203. Traverso, G.; Langer, R. Perspective: Special delivery for the gut. *Nature* **2015**, *519*, S19. [CrossRef]
204. Pan, J.; Rostamizadeh, K.; Filipczak, N.; Torchilin, V.P. Polymeric Co-Delivery Systems in Cancer Treatment: An Overview on Component Drugs' Dosage Ratio Effect. *Molecules* **2019**, *24*, 1035. [CrossRef] [PubMed]
205. Tang, Y.; Liang, J.; Wu, A.; Chen, Y.; Zhao, P.; Lin, T.; Zhang, M.; Xu, Q.; Wang, J.; Huang, Y. Co-Delivery of Trichosanthin and Albendazole by Nano-Self-Assembly for Overcoming Tumor Multidrug-Resistance and Metastasis. *ACS Appl. Mater. Interfaces* **2017**, *9*, 26648–26664. [CrossRef] [PubMed]
206. Chen, A.M.; Zhang, M.; Wei, D.; Stueber, D.; Taratula, O.; Minko, T.; He, H. Co-delivery of doxorubicin and Bcl-2 siRNA by mesoporous silica nanoparticles enhances the efficacy of chemotherapy in multidrug-resistant cancer cells. *Small* **2009**, *5*, 2673–2677. [CrossRef] [PubMed]
207. Jhaveri, J.; Raichura, Z.; Khan, T.; Momin, M.; Omri, A. Chitosan Nanoparticles-Insight into Properties, Functionalization and Applications in Drug Delivery and Theranostics. *Molecules* **2021**, *26*, 272. [CrossRef]
208. Jo, S.D.; Ku, S.H.; Won, Y.Y.; Kim, S.H.; Kwon, I.C. Targeted Nanotheranostics for Future Personalized Medicine: Recent Progress in Cancer Therapy. *Theranostics* **2016**, *6*, 1362–1377. [CrossRef]
209. Hong, S.C.; Yoo, S.Y.; Kim, H.; Lee, J. Chitosan-Based Multifunctional Platforms for Local Delivery of Therapeutics. *Mar. Drugs* **2017**, *15*, 60. [CrossRef]
210. Liu, Y.; Kong, M.; Cheng, X.J.; Wang, Q.Q.; Jiang, L.M.; Chen, X.G. Self-assembled nanoparticles based on amphiphilic chitosan derivative and hyaluronic acid for gene delivery. *Carbohydr. Polym.* **2013**, *94*, 309–316. [CrossRef]
211. Tan, C.S.S.; Lee, S.W.H. Warfarin and food, herbal or dietary supplement interactions: A systematic review. *Br. J. Clin. Pharmacol.* **2021**, *87*, 352–374. [CrossRef] [PubMed]

pharmaceutics MDPI

Article

Oromucosal Alginate Films with Zein Nanoparticles as a Novel Delivery System for Digoxin

Daniela A. Rodrigues [1], Sónia P. Miguel [1,2], Jorge Loureiro [1], Maximiano Ribeiro [1,2], Fátima Roque [1,2] and Paula Coutinho [1,2,*]

[1] Center of Potential and Innovation in Natural Resources, Research Unit for Inland Development, Polytechnic Institute of Guarda (CPIRN-UDI/IPG), Avenida Dr. Francisco de Sá Carneiro, No. 50, 6300-559 Guarda, Portugal; danielaalmeidar@ipg.pt (D.A.R.); spmiguel@ipg.pt (S.P.M.); jcloureiro97@gmail.com (J.L.); mribeiro@ipg.pt (M.R.); froque@ipg.pt (F.R.)
[2] Health Sciences Research Centre, University of Beira Interior (CICS-UBI), Avenida Infante D. Henrique, 6200-506 Covilhã, Portugal
* Correspondence: coutinho@ipg.pt; Tel.: +351-965544187

Abstract: Digoxin is a hydrophobic drug used for the treatment of heart failure that possesses a narrow therapeutic index, which raises safety concerns for toxicity. This is of utmost relevance in specific populations, such as the elderly. This study aimed to demonstrate the potential of the sodium alginate films as buccal drug delivery system containing zein nanoparticles incorporated with digoxin to reduce the number of doses, facilitating the administration with a quick onset of action. The film was prepared using the solvent casting method, whereas nanoparticles by the nanoprecipitation method. The nanoparticles incorporated with digoxin (0.25 mg/mL) exhibited a mean size of 87.20 ± 0.88 nm, a polydispersity index of 0.23 ± 0.00, and a zeta potential of 21.23 ± 0.07 mV. Digoxin was successfully encapsulated into zein nanoparticles with an encapsulation efficiency of 91% (±0.00). Films with/without glycerol and with different concentrations of ethanol were produced. The sodium alginate (SA) films with 10% ethanol demonstrated good performance for swelling (maximum of 1474%) and mechanical properties, with a mean tensile strength of 0.40 ± 0.04 MPa and an elongation at break of 27.85% (±0.58), compatible with drug delivery application into the buccal mucosa. The current study suggests that SA films with digoxin-loaded zein nanoparticles can be an effective alternative to the dosage forms available on the market for digoxin administration.

Keywords: oromucosal films; sodium alginate; nanoparticle drug carriers; digoxin; zein; heart failure

Citation: Rodrigues, D.A.; Miguel, S.P.; Loureiro, J.; Ribeiro, M.; Roque, F.; Coutinho, P. Oromucosal Alginate Films with Zein Nanoparticles as a Novel Delivery System for Digoxin. *Pharmaceutics* **2021**, *13*, 2030. https://doi.org/10.3390/pharmaceutics13122030

Academic Editors: Ana Isabel Fernandes, Angela Faustino Jozala and Andrea Cappelli

Received: 4 October 2021
Accepted: 25 November 2021
Published: 29 November 2021

1. Introduction

Heart failure is a pathological condition with an estimated worldwide prevalence of 64.34 million cases representing the most significant burden after 60 years of age [1,2]. The incidence in European countries and the USA ranges from 1 to 9 cases per 1000 person-years [1]. Digoxin is a hydrophobic drug with a positive inotropic effect that reduces heart rate in supraventricular tachyarrhythmias associated with heart failure, improving the dynamic capacity of the heart [3]. It is one of the most used drugs to improve symptoms and reduce hospitalization in patients with heart failure and atrial fibrillation [4]. These conditions are highly prevalent in older adults [5]; therefore, digoxin is a widely prescribed drug at this age group [3,6]. However, this drug has a narrow therapeutic index, wide individual variability in dosage requirements, and complex metabolic pathways, which raises concern since digitalis toxicity is not only a medical emergency but can also be lethal [7]. This is of utmost relevance for the geriatric population considering the pharmacodynamic and pharmacokinetic change. The older patient's high sensitivity to glycosides and consequent risk of intoxication [8] highlights the need of developing new delivery systems for improving safety.

Digoxin is currently only available on the market in conventional dosage forms, which are a limitation for narrow therapeutic index drugs since these have several limitations, such as reduced patient compliance, shorter half-life of drugs, and high peak, failure to control the drug release ratio, poor stability, and lack on the therapeutic target [9].

The use of mucosal administration has recently received attention by researchers on the drug administration by mucosal route since it avoids the hepatic first-pass effect and the degradation by gastrointestinal enzymes [10–12]. Besides that, the sublingual mucosa is very permeable with large veins, and high blood flow provides instantaneous drug absorption and high bioavailability [13]. Therefore, oral mucoadhesive drug delivery systems can be a good solution as they provide more comfort and flexibility during the administration process [14–16]. Moreover, mucoadhesive forms may be designed to enable prolonged retention at the site of application, providing a controlled rate of drug release for improved therapeutic outcomes [17]. Oromucosal films are alternative dosage forms to traditional solid oral dosage forms [18], which are essentially prepared through the casting method [19].

Different polymers have been used in film preparations since they achieve rapid disintegration, good mouthfeel, and mechanical properties [20] and are an easy way to enhance bioavailability [21]. In addition, the use of natural and biocompatible polymers reduces the side effects of a given drug, and biodegradable biomaterials minimizes the inflammatory effect, possesses good permeability, and good therapeutic properties [9], which overcome the toxicity and non-degradability associated with synthetic polymers used in the production of commercial dosage forms. Herein, sodium alginate (SA) was selected since it is a hydrophilic, biocompatible, and antioxidant polysaccharide [22] with mucoadhesive properties [23,24]. In fact the promising properties of SA propelled the development and commercialization of oral films for the food and pharmaceutical industries [25–27].

Since polymeric nanoparticles have numerous potentialities as carrier systems for bioactive compounds, it is possible to control the drug release profile and reduce drug degradation and toxicity [28,29]. Polymers are the most common materials for constructing nanoparticle-based drug carriers and among different polymers used in nanoparticle production, zein is a natural and biodegradable polymer belonging to the group of prolamins, and it is one of the few alcohol-soluble biopolymers with more than 50% hydrophobic amino acids [30]. Besides, zein has unique characteristics, such as high coating capacity, biocompatibility, low toxicity [31,32], and its mucoadhesive character can be used for mucosal delivery of drugs and vaccines [33]. This polymer was widely described as a pharmaceutical excipient in oral solid dosage forms [34]. A significant advantage of zein-based nanoparticles is their amphiphilic character, which encapsulates both hydrophilic and hydrophobic compounds like digoxin [35]. Indeed, they have been proposed to encapsulate phenolic compounds due to their ability to increase the dispersibility of drugs in an aqueous medium, as well as to promote chemical stability [36]. This polymer has been used in modified release systems for the delivery of enzymes, drugs, essential oils, and other substances [32,33]. In fact, different studies have reported the ability of zein nanoparticles to encapsulate different drugs, such as lovastatin [37], artemether [38], gambogenic acid [39], doxorubicin [40], 5-fluorouracil [41], docetaxel [42], carvacrol [43], and maytansine [44]. These studies demonstrated the utility of zein nanoparticles as a viable drug-delivery and in a recent work, PEG-coated zein nanoparticles demonstrated to be adequate carriers for promoting the oral bioavailability of biomacromolecules [45].

Herein, the zein nanoparticles were produced through the nanoprecipitation technique, also known as solvent displacement, or antisolvent method, which consists of the interfacial interaction of zein after displacement of a semi-polar solvent, miscible in water. The rapid diffusion of the organic solvent results in the reduction of the interfacial tension between the two phases, increasing the surface area, inducing supersaturation, leading to precipitation of the solute and the formation of nanoparticles [46]. This method employs the addition of zein solution to an anti-solvent (water), which allows the controlled protein precipitation due to the reduction of solubility in the medium, promoting the nanoparticles' formation.

However, it is important to notice that the physicochemical properties of the nanoparticles (e.g., size, surface properties, and polydispersity index (PDI)) are dependent on the materials and technique used for the nanoparticles production. In this case, the production of zein nanoparticles through the nanoprecipitation technique enables the production of the reproducible and positively charged zein nanoparticles that will promote electrostatic interactions with negatively sialic acid residues in mucin, which will prolong the residence time in the buccal mucosa and consequently increase the drug bioavailability [47–49].

In turn, the oromucosal films will act as a matrix to support the incorporation of the digoxin-loaded zein nanoparticles since they are flexible, comfortable, and easy to administer, prolonging the stability of the system [50]. Herein, this study aimed to develop a sodium-alginate mucoadhesive film containing zein nanoparticles with embedded digoxin to be used as a buccal drug delivery system. The films were produced using the casting method from aqueous solutions and the nanoparticles were obtained through the nanoprecipitation method.

2. Materials and Methods

2.1. Materials

Standard digoxin 96% was purchased from Alfa Aesar (Haverhill, MA, USA). SA (molecular weight 10,000–600,000 g/mol) was obtained from AppliChem GmbH (Darmstadt, Germany). Glycerol was acquired from Guinama S.L.U (Valencia, Spain. Ethanol 100% was purchased from Carlo Erba Reagents (Cornaredo, Italy) with a density at 20 °C of 0.7893:0.7899. Zein was obtained from Acros Organics (Waltham, MA, USA). Sodium chloride 99.5% was obtained from Honeywell Fluka (Charlotte, NC, USA), potassium phosphate monobasic and sodium phosphate dibasic and High-Performance Liquid Chromatography (HPLC)-gradient grade acetonitrile 99.9% were obtained from VWR Chemicals (Radnor, PA, USA). HPLC-gradient grade methanol 99.9% was obtained from Chem-Lab NV (Zedelgem, Belgium). Deionized water was used for all sample preparation.

2.2. Preparation of Sodium Alginate Films

Films were prepared using the casting method from aqueous solutions, as previously reported [51]. An aqueous solution of SA (3% w/v), was placed under magnetic stirring at 25 °C and 400 rpm, for 6 h. After that, the ethanol was added at different concentrations (0, 10 and 20% v/v) to promote the gelation of the film [51]. Then, the glycerol (12 g/L) was added as a plasticizer for the film optimization due to its texture and mechanical properties [52]. The polymeric solution was deposited into Petri plates (55 mm) and was dried at 30 °C overnight (Incubator Hood TH 15-Edmund, Bühler GmbH, Uzwill, Switzerland). The final composition of the oromucosal films is shown in Table 1. Posteriorly, SA films with embedded zein-digoxin nanoparticles were also produced. The production process of nanoparticles is described in Section 2.4.

Table 1. Film's composition (SA: Sodium alginate, EtOH: Ethanol, and Glyc: Glycerol).

Formulation	Film Composition			
	3% SA Solution (mL)	Ethanol (mL)	Water (mL)	Glycerol (g/L)
SA $_{EtOH0}$	15.00	0.00	0.00	0.00
SA $_{EtOH10}$	10.00	1.50	3.50	0.00
SA $_{EtOH20}$	10.00	3.00	2.00	0.00
SA_Glyc $_{EtOH0}$	15.00	0.00	0.00	12.00
SA_Glyc $_{EtOH10}$	10.00	1.50	3.50	12.00
SA_Glyc $_{EtOH20}$	10.00	3.00	2.00	12.00

2.3. Characterization of Films

2.3.1. Scanning Electron Microscopy Analysis

The morphology and structure of the surface films were characterized through scanning electron microscopy analysis. The samples were mounted onto aluminum stubs with

Araldite glue and sputter-coated with gold using a Quorum Q150R ES sputter coater (Quorum Technologies Ltd., Laughton, Lewes, UK). Then the images acquired with different magnifications were acquired in a Hitachi S-3400N Scanning Electron Microscope (Hitachi, Tokyo, Japan) at an acceleration voltage of 20 kV.

2.3.2. Fourier Transform Infrared Spectroscopy (FTIR)

Fourier Transform Infrared Spectroscopy (FTIR) measurements were performed to evaluate the effect of ethanol addition in SA structure by a Nicolet iS10 FTIR spectrophotometer (Thermo Scientific, Waltham, MA, USA). The analysis was performed with an average of 128 scans, a spectral width ranging from 4000 and 400 cm^{-1}, and a spectral resolution of 4 cm^{-1}. At least three replicates were run for each sample.

2.3.3. Thickness

The film thickness was measured using a Digimatic Caliper (0.01 mm, Mitutoyo Corporation, Sakado, Japan) at 10 different film positions. At least three replicates for each formulation were considered.

2.3.4. Mechanical Properties

Tensile strength (TS) and elongation at break (EAB) were measured using a Texture Analyser (TA-XT Plus, Stable Micro Systems, Godalming, UK). All measurements were performed in three replicates for each formulation. Each test strip was cut into a specific size (3 × 1 × 0.1 cm) and placed longitudinally in a tensile grip probe (A/MTG). Initial grip separation was 5 mm and crosshead speed was 10 mm/min. The test was considered concluded at the film break. The TS was evaluated using the Equation below (1). Results were expressed in MPa.

$$\text{TS} = \frac{\text{Force at break}}{\text{Thickness} \times \text{width}} \tag{1}$$

The EAB was calculated according to the following Equation (2):

$$\text{EAB (\%)} = \frac{\text{Increase in length}}{\text{Original length}} \times 100 \tag{2}$$

2.3.5. Swelling Profile

The swelling profile of the films was measured by a method previously proposed [51]. The samples (2 × 2 cm) were immersed in 1 mL of a simulated saliva solution prepared with sodium chloride (8.00 g/L), potassium phosphate monobasic (0.19 g/L), and sodium phosphate dibasic (2.38 g/L), setting pH to 6.8 [53], at 25 °C and stirred at 120 rpm for 5 min. The samples were evaluated after 0, 30, 60, 120, 180, 240, and 300 s of the beginning of the test. The excess of simulated saliva solution was removed with a filter paper and their wet weight was immediately determined to calculate the swelling ratio by the following Equation (3), where W_t is the final weight, and W_0 is the initial weight of the films:

$$\text{Swelling (\%)} = \frac{W_t}{W_0} \times 100 \tag{3}$$

2.3.6. Dissolution Time

To investigate the dissolution time of the films, the samples (1 × 1 cm) were immersed in 5 mL of simulated saliva solution at 37 °C and at 120 rpm. The test was considered concluded when the film was completely dissolved. Measurements were performed in triplicate for each formulation.

2.4. Preparation of Zein Nanoparticles with Embedded Digoxin

Zein (2.5 mg/mL) was dissolved in ethanol (80% *v*/*v*). Nanoparticles were prepared by the nanoprecipitation method through confined impingement jets with dilution (CIJ-D) mixer, as previously described [54]. CIJ-D mixer is made of a high-density polyethylene, with two inlets and adapters fitted with threaded syringes, and one outlet adapter. The dimensions and operating mode is described in more detail in work conducted by Han et al. [54]. One of the syringes contains 2.50 mL zein solution and digoxin at different concentrations (0.00, 0.25, 0.50, and 1.00 mg/mL), and the second syringe contains 2.50 mL of deionized water. Nanoparticles without digoxin were also produced as a control. The two syringes were then attached to the two vertical openings on the CIJ-D mixer. A beaker containing 45 mL of deionized water was placed at the exit of the CIJ-D mixer. The exit stream outlet was submerged in the water. The two syringes were then pushed rapidly and simultaneously by hand to inject the liquids into the CIJ-D mixer at equal rates, where the two streams were rapidly mixed and collected in water solution.

2.5. Particle Size, Zeta Potential and Polydispersity Index (PDI)

After production, zein nanoparticles with and without digoxin, size distribution, zeta potential, and PDI were determined by dynamic scattering technique using Zetasizer Nano ZS, Malvern Instruments, Malvern, UK. Such parameters were also measured over time, for 26 days, at room temperature, to evaluate the stability of the nanoparticles.

2.6. Determination of Standard Calibration Curve and Encapsulation Efficiency of Digoxin into Nanoparticles

Encapsulation efficiency (EE) of digoxin was determined by HPLC. A standard calibration curve was previously obtained ($y = 292.67x + 17.595$, $R^2 = 0.999$). HPLC chromatography was performed according to the conditions described previously [55], with a column C18 (Acclaim™ 120 Reversed-Phase Columns C18, 5 µm, 4.6 × 150 mm, Thermo Scientific) at a temperature of 35 °C and the mobile phase (mixture of water and acetonitrile, 72:28% (*v*/*v*)) was pumped at a flow rate of 0.8 mL/min. The run time cycle was completed in 20 min. Peak areas registered at 218 nm were used for digoxin quantification. All experiments were carried out in triplicate.

The EE indicates the drug amount into nanoparticles and was determined after ultrafiltration-centrifugation (Amicon® Ultra Centrifugal Filters, 30k; Merck Millipore, Billerica, MA, USA). The filtrate, containing the unencapsulated drug, which can pass through the filter membrane during centrifugation (4000× *g*; 10 min), was analyzed by HPLC. Encapsulation efficiency was calculated using the following Equation (4):

$$EE\ (\%) = \frac{\text{Actual amount of drug} - \text{loaded in nanoparticles}}{\text{Theory amount of drug} - \text{loaded in nanoparticles}} \times 100 \quad (4)$$

2.7. Statistical Analysis

The statistical analysis of the obtained results was performed using one-way analysis of variance (ANOVA), with Tukey's test for post hoc analysis, using GraphPad Prism software version 8.0.1 (Dr Harvey Motulsky, San Diego, CA, USA). All of the results were expressed as the mean value ± standard error of the mean (SEM). A *p*-value lower than 0.05 ($p < 0.05$) was considered statistically significant.

3. Results and Discussion

3.1. Scanning Electron Microscopy Analysis

Scanning electron microscopy analysis was performed to characterize the film's surface, as previously reported in other studies [56,57]. The images indicate that the morphology of all selected films is dense, homogeneous, and has no pores and cracks (Figure S1). The addition of glycerol and ethanol did not change the surface of the developed films. These characteristics, namely the absence of pores and surface uniformity, represent good film quality and are appropriate for buccal drug delivery systems [19,58]. In fact, other authors also state that the oral films must be homogeneous and smooth, not presenting with bubbles, cracks, or aggregates, which aims to improve its acceptability [59].

3.2. Fourier Transform Infrared Spectroscopy (FTIR) Analysis

FTIR spectra of SA films are presented in Figure 1. For native SA film, the peaks at 3253 cm^{-1} and 1023 cm^{-1} were assigned to stretching vibrations of –OH and –C–O–C– bonds and asymmetric and symmetric –COO– stretching at 1590 cm^{-1} and 1413 cm^{-1}, respectively [51,60,61]. In this work, ethanol was used for gelation of SA chains. Although ionic crosslinking is commonly used in SA films, another study observed that when the SA films were crosslinked with Ca^{2+} ions, the peaks become broader. Thus, different non-conventional crosslinking methods have been used, such as the non-solvent method, which commonly uses ethanol. In fact, it has been described that the gelation of polysaccharides induced by ethanol can occur due to the low water activity, wherein the polysaccharide-water interactions are minimized and the hydrophobic interactions between polysaccharide chains are promoted [62,63]. Since the gelation occurred directly in ethanol there was no need for the solvent-exchange step and the process occurred without additional crosslinkers.

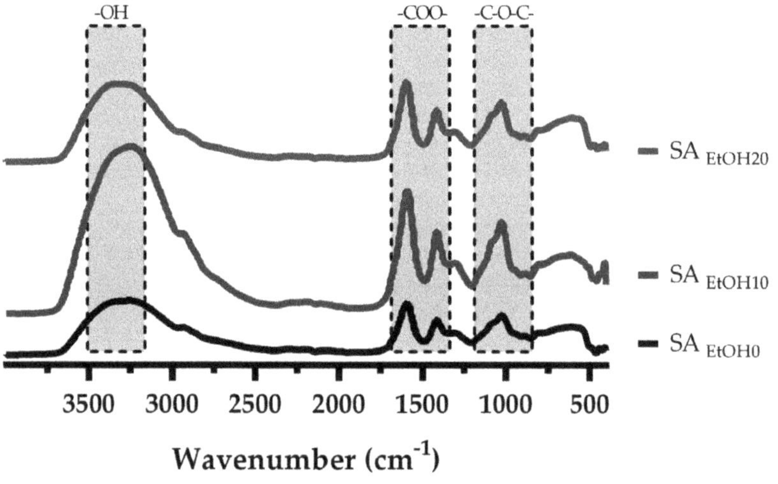

Figure 1. FTIR spectra (SA: Sodium alginate, EtOH: Ethanol).

It is possible to verify that both the asymmetric and symmetric –COO– peaks of the films did not change with increasing the ethanol proportion. Thus, ethanol fulfilled its purpose without changing the SA structure, as seen in another study [51].

3.3. Thickness

Apart from ethanol, the SA films were also composed of glycerol. Such a plasticizer has been commonly used since it improves the flexibility of films [64]. The thickness of SA films changed depending on the ethanol content and glycerol addition, as shown in Figure 2. The addition of ethanol changed the thickness of films leading to thicker films. This may be related to the structural modification in the polypeptide chain that the gelation process imposes since the three-dimensional structure assumes a conformation that takes up more space and, therefore, the greater thickness of the reticulated films [65]. It was possible to verify that the addition of glycerol does not affect film thickness (Figure 2). Despite some minor changes on the films' thickness, all formulations presented values within the suitable range (0.05–1 mm), which is considered ideal to reduce side effects and extensive metabolism of drugs in buccal films [66]. In turn, the thickness values maintain along the surface of the film, assuring the thickness uniformity, which is important for film dose accuracy [19].

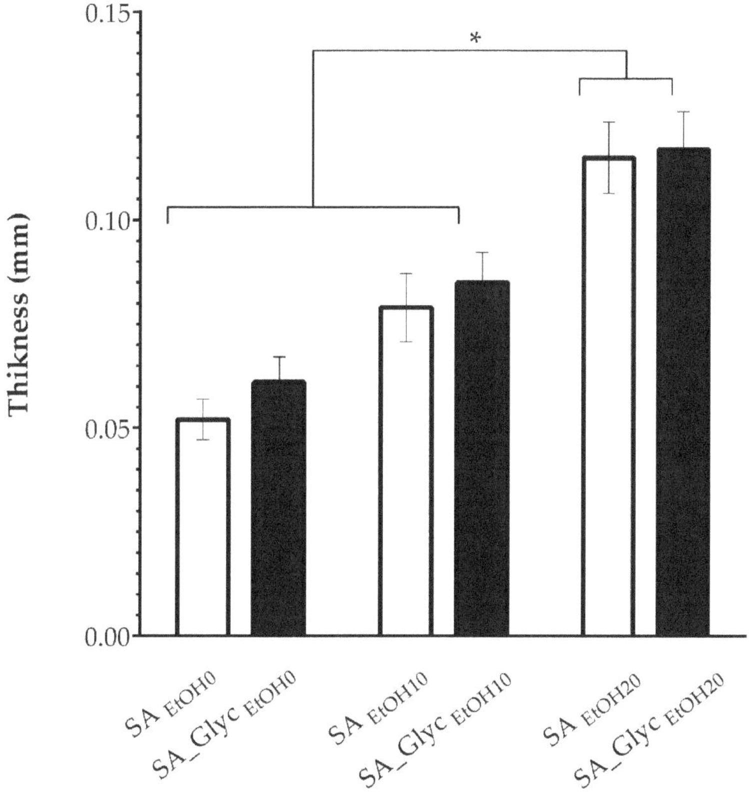

Figure 2. Thickness of the films with and without glycerol considering the gelling agent (ethanol) (SA: Sodium alginate, EtOH: Ethanol, and Glyc: Glycerol, * $p < 0.05$).

3.4. Mechanical Properties

TS is defined as a measurement of the maximum amount of force applied at which the film breaks and is used to characterize the mechanical strength of the films [67]. In turn, the percentage increase in EAB is the length that a material can be extended/stretched before it breaks. It is related to the elasticity of the material and the ability of a plastic specimen to resist changes of shape without cracking. An ideal oromucosal film dosage form should be flexible, elastic, and soft, but strong enough to resist breaking caused by stress from mouth movements [13].

Through the analysis of results presented in Table 2, it is possible to notice that the addition of glycerol promoted a decrease in TS values and an increase in EAB. It is widely reported that the plasticizers interfere with polymer chains, promoting a decrease in intermolecular forces, soften the rigidity of the film's structure, and increase the polymer mobility. Thus, the presence of glycerol leads to a ductile and flexible material [64]. The increase in ethanol led to an increase in the TS and a decrease in EAB values, except for films without glycerol (Figure 3). A significant decrease in TS was noticed in another study for gelatin films incorporated with the highest curcuma ethanol extract content [68]. The increase in the EAB values can be explained by the good physical gelation process between the polymeric matrix and the incorporated ethanol, leading to more cohesive and flexible matrices [68].

Table 2. The mechanical characterization of oromucosal films (n = 3) is expressed as mean ± SEM (SA: Sodium alginate, EtOH: Ethanol, and Glyc: Glycerol).

Formulation	Tensile Strength (MPa)	Elongation at Break (%)
SA $_{EtOH0}$	0.07 ± 0.01	5.15 ± 0.70
SA_Glyc $_{EtOH0}$	0.35 ± 0.02	41.97 ± 0.72
SA $_{EtOH10}$	0.04 ± 0.00	7.83 ± 1.27
SA_Glyc $_{EtOH10}$	0.42 ± 0.01	27.85 ± 4.59
SA $_{EtOH20}$	0.02 ± 0.00	6.38 ± 1.17
SA_Glyc $_{EtOH20}$	0.72 ± 0.03	26.19 ± 1.96

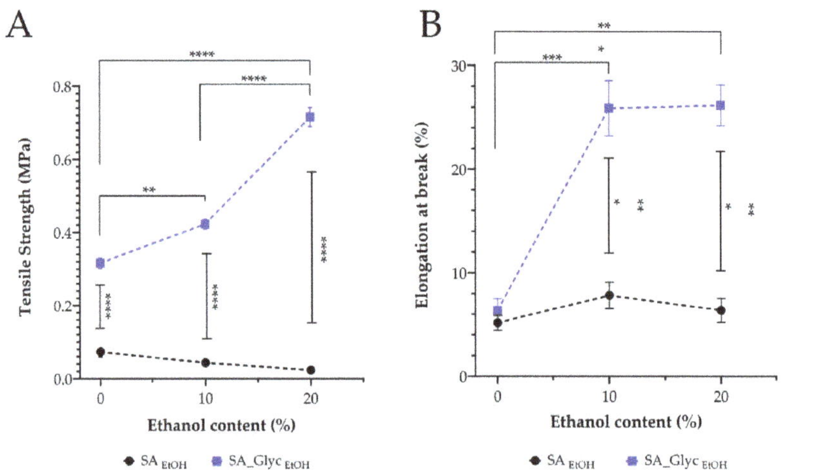

Figure 3. Mechanical properties of the films (n = 3). (**A**): Tensile strength. (**B**): Elongation at break. * $p < 0.05$, ** $p < 0.1$; *** $p < 0.01$; **** $p < 0.0001$.

3.5. Swelling Profile

Polymeric film swelling is important to understand films' water absorption capacity and obtain information about their water resistance [69]. The swelling profile of SA films, with and without glycerol treated with different ethanol concentrations, was recorded in Figure 4. The data obtained revealed the high-water absorption ability of the films in the first 30 s, stabilizing the swelling behavior over at least 300 s. This profile is described as suitable for buccal administration since polymers with high initial swelling rate could promote mucoadhesion [70]. The graphics also showed that after 240 s, the degradation of the film occurs for formulations without glycerol. In general, all glycerol-free films exhibit similar behavior with a maximum swelling percentage of 3578.7% ± 308.23.

In contrast, glycerol promoted a more controlled swelling profile in all formulations where the maximum swelling was 1441% ± 4.041. Adding a hydrophobic compound, such as glycerol, will impair the interaction with water molecules, decreasing the water absorption capacity. Another study reported that the increase in glycerol concentration reduced the swelling index of the fast oral dissolving films studied [71]. The swelling capacity of SA films is facilitated by carboxylic groups, which are strongly associated with water molecules [65]. In a drug delivery system, a moderate swelling profile is desirable, not compromising the system's stability [72]. Thus, based on the results, the SA_Glyc $_{EtOH10}$ formulation was selected to incorporate zein nanoparticles since it presented a swelling profile compatible to be applied as mucoadhesive drug delivery system for the buccal mucosa.

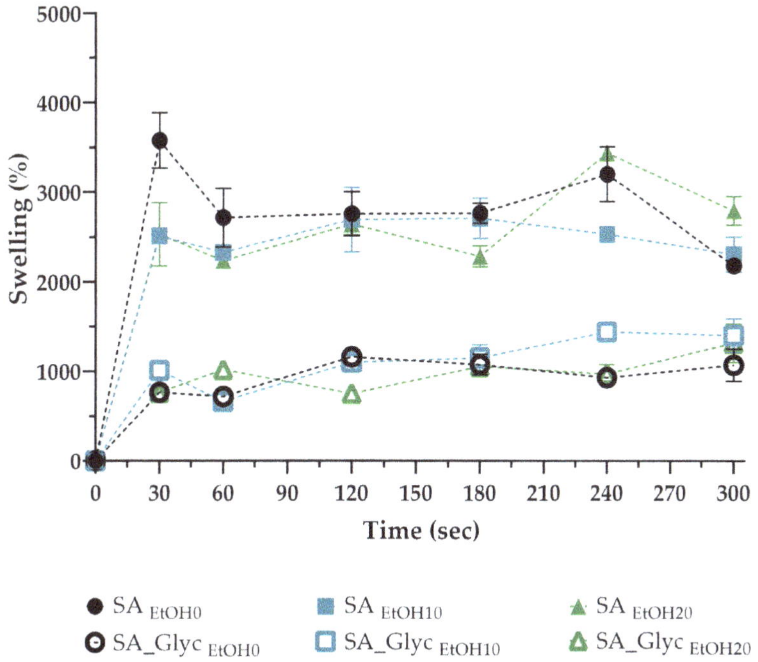

Figure 4. Swelling profile of the produced films (SA: Sodium alginate, EtOH: Ethanol, and Glyc: Glycerol).

3.6. Dissolution Time

The results obtained (Table 3) showed that the presence of ethanol induces an increase on dissolution time, which can be explained by the reduction of water molecule interactions and consequently delay the dissolution time [73]. In terms of the glycerol addition, the effects were just observed on formulations with 10% of ethanol, which increased the dissolution time [71].

Table 3. The dissolution time of oromucosal films ($n = 3$) is expressed as mean ± SEM (SA: Sodium alginate, EtOH: Ethanol, and Glyc: Glycerol).

Formulation	Dissolution Time (min)
SA $_{EtOH0}$	7.10 ± 0.41
SA_Glyc $_{EtOH0}$	6.27 ± 0.18
SA $_{EtOH10}$	8.88 ± 0.04
SA_Glyc $_{EtOH10}$	11.36 ± 0.68
SA $_{EtOH20}$	10.38 ± 0.05
SA_Glyc $_{EtOH20}$	9.00 ± 0.65

3.7. Characterization of Zein Nanoparticles

Nanoparticle drug carriers aim to achieve more efficient and sustained drug delivery. Their characteristics, such as particle size, charge, and hydrophobicity, are determinants of the permeability of the mucosal barrier [74]. The mean size of the zein nanoparticles without digoxin was 85.72 ± 0.360 nm, which increase when the digoxin concentration also augmented (Table 4). However, all produced nanoparticles displayed a mean diameter inferior to 200 nm, which is ideal for escaping recognition by the reticuloendothelial system and, consequently, prolong their half-life in the blood system [74]. Nevertheless, other authors described the particle size reduction of nanosuspensions as determinant for the increase in the surface area and enhancement in dissolution velocity of the drug [75,76]. In all cases, the PDI of the formulations remained under 0.4, indicating monodisperse nanosuspensions. In turn, the zeta potential indicates the surface charge of nanoparticles presenting values above 20 mV, considered as moderately stable [77–79]. Apart from the size of nanoparticles, their uptake is also dependent on charge density. The positive charge of zein nanoparticles and hydrophobic character of zein nanoparticles enables the ionic interaction with negatively charged groups available on the cell membrane surface and improves the epithelial endocytosis through the attachment of polymeric substances to the glycoproteins on epithelial surfaces, which allows for the increase of the mucoadhesion phenomenon [80–82]. This provides an intimate contact between drug formulation and mucosa tissue, increasing the drug absorption and residence time, resulting in improved drug therapeutic activity through high drug flux at absorptive mucosa [83]. Moreover, the mucoadhesive adhesion of zein nanoparticles on porcine buccal mucosa was already evaluated by other authors, who verified that the positively charged zein nanoparticles can anchor to the mucus layer by electrostatic interactions with negatively charged sialic acid residues in mucin, which is fundamental to prolong the residence time in the buccal mucosa [84].

Table 4. Characterization of the nanoparticles according to the digoxin concentration (n = 3), data are expressed as mean ± SEM (PDI: Polydispersity Index).

Formulation		Mean Size (nm)	PDI	Zeta Potential (mV)
Zein 2.5 mg/mL	Digoxin 0.00 mg/mL	85.72 ± 0.36	0.22 ± 0.00	24.23 ± 0.39
	Digoxin 0.25 mg/mL	87.20 ± 0.88	0.23 ± 0.00	21.23 ± 0.07
	Digoxin 0.50 mg/mL	92.16 ± 0.77	0.20 ± 0.01	23.40 ± 1.72
	Digoxin 1.00 mg/mL	123.20 ± 2.42	0.36 ± 0.01	22.30 ± 0.25

In addition, the stability of the aqueous nanoparticles suspension, stored at room temperature, was evaluated for 26 days (Figure 5). It was possible to verify that the zein nanoparticles incorporating 0.25 mg/mL of digoxin maintained their size for 12 days, with a PDI value of 0.23 ± 0.00, suggesting an ideal stability. In terms of zeta potential, no significant differences were observed between 6 and 20 days ($p > 0.999$) for this formulation. Thus, it can be concluded that this formulation is stable over at least 20 days and it was chosen to be incorporated into the film. Through this strategy, it is possible to combine the mucoadhesive behavior of zein, allowing the strong electrostatic interactions with mucin, as highlighted previously [84], and acting as novel platform for the buccal delivery of the poorly water-soluble digoxin.

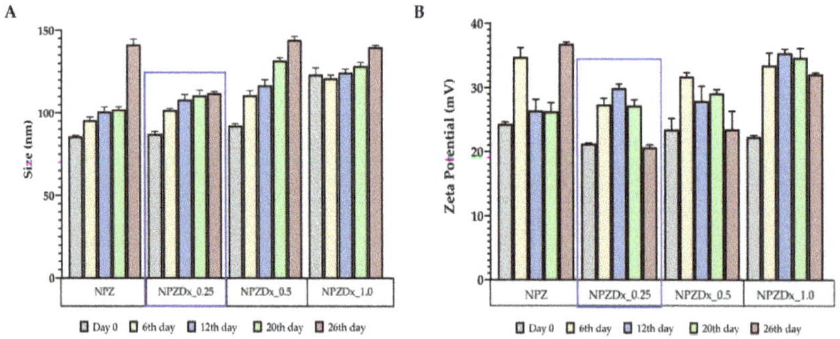

Figure 5. Stability of nanoparticles over time, n = 3 (NPZ: Zein nanoparticles, NPZDx: Zein-digoxin nanoparticles): (**A**): Particle size (nm). (**B**): Zeta potential (mV). The blue square evidence the nanoparticles formulation with more suitable morphological properties.

3.8. Digoxin Encapsulation Efficiency

The digoxin was incorporated into zein nanoparticles with a drug encapsulation efficiency of 91 ± 0.03%. This result is of utmost relevance since high drug encapsulation allows for lower concentrations of nanoparticles compared to other dosage forms, and the controlled delivery of drugs. To the best of our knowledge, this is the first work evaluating the performance of zein nanoparticles for digoxin delivery. In other studies it is only possible to find works reporting the production of zein nanoparticles incorporated with other biologically active compounds, achieving encapsulation efficiencies ranging between 47.80 and 92.60% [40,85–87]. One study reported the use of simple coacervates of zein to encapsulate gitoxin, a naturally occurring cardiac glycoside (such as digoxin) and proved the stability and maintenance of the biological activity of glycosides [88]. On the other hand, the incorporation of digoxin into other polymeric nanoparticles has been previously described, and the results showed high encapsulation efficiency and revealed that digoxin-loaded nanoparticles increased permeability across cell layers [89]. In addition, the digoxin incorporation into nanosystems affords different potentialities, as verified by Das et al., where the in vivo studies revealed an increase on digoxin bioavailability in solid lipid nanoparticles when compared with a digoxin solution after oral administration (0.25 mg) [90]. Taking this into account, we consider that the digoxin encapsulation into zein nanoparticles should not compromise its biological activity and represents a promising approach for the development of novel and safer formulations.

3.9. Characterization of SA Films Embedded with Zein-Digoxin Nanoparticles

Considering the optimal film formulation obtained, the nanoparticles suspension was embedded into the formulation by direct mixing with the SA_glycerol solution. The casting method with ethanol for film production followed the previous described approach. The results obtained for the characterization of films embedded with zein-digoxin (ZnDx) nanoparticles are summarized in Table 5. The addition of nanoparticles into the film did not change their thickness, with a mean value of 0.08 ± 0.90 mm. In turn, a significant decrease of EAB of the film (5.72 ± 0.58) was registered, while TS was not changed. Such can occur due to the addition of hydrophobic compounds, such as zein and digoxin, which prevent the interaction between the hydrophilic groups of SA and water [91].

Table 5. Characterization of the final formulation, data are expressed as mean ± SEM (SA: Sodium alginate, Glyc: Glycerol, EtOH: Ethanol, Zn: Zein, and Dx: Digoxin).

Formulation	Thickness (mm)	Tensile Strength (MPa)	Elongation at Break (%)	Dissolution Time (min)
SA_Glyc $_{EtOH10}$	0.09 ± 0.02	0.42 ± 0.01	27.85 ± 4.59	11.36 ± 0.68
SA_Glyc $_{EtOH10}$_ZnDx0.25	0.08 ± 0.90	0.40 ± 0.04	5.72 ± 0.58	13.75 ± 0.37

In terms of the swelling profile, there are no significant differences for both formulations (Figure 6). These formulations demonstrated an increase in the swelling capability after 30 s, suggesting a suitable film swelling, able to accelerate the release of the drug by diffusion and erosion [92]. Drug-loaded films dissolved significantly slower ($p = 0.02$) than the equivalent drug-free formulation (Table 5). This could be due to the poorly water-soluble character of digoxin. Besides, hydrophobic polymers (zein) do not allow for quick hydration upon contact with simulated saliva and, hence, delay the dissolution time of the films [93].

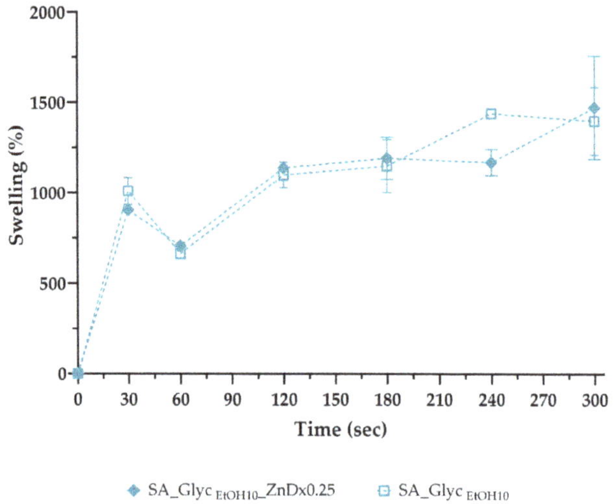

Figure 6. Swelling profile of the optimized film with zein-digoxin nanoparticles incorporated (SA: Sodium alginate, EtOH: Ethanol, Glyc: Glycerol, Zn: Zein, and Dx: Digoxin). Results are expressed as mean ± SEM.

4. Conclusions

In this study, a novel SA_Glyc $_{EtOH10}$ film containing ZnD × 0.25 nanoparticles was successfully prepared by incorporating drug nanosuspensions with mucoadhesive films mainly composed of SA, which provides a new route of transforming nanosuspensions of poorly water-soluble drugs (such as digoxin) into a solid dosage, which due to the bioadhesive behavior, reduced the number of administrations. SA films were successfully prepared by solution casting with different concentrations of ethanol. Then, the effect of the glycerol plasticizing agent on films' properties was also evaluated, where it was verified that the films containing glycerol presented a more controlled swelling profile. In addition, the zein nanoparticles incorporating digoxin were also successfully produced through the nanoprecipitation method, which displayed a size and surface charge stable for at least 12 days.

In this way, the mucoadhesive SA film incorporated with ZnD × 0.25 nanoparticles presented a swelling profile and mechanical properties compatible with the application as drug delivery system through the buccal mucosa. The development of this technological innovation becomes pertinent and necessary since it allows for the achievement of a more controlled drug release, greater therapeutic effect, reduction of side effects, and also to improve therapeutic compliance in patients with dysphagia.

In the near future, complementary assays, such as drug permeation, mucoadhesiveness, pharmacokinetic profile, and bioavailability, would allow for the successful scale-up of the new oromucosal film produced as alternative dosage form for digoxin and for drugs suffering from first-pass effect, especially those with a narrow therapeutic index.

Supplementary Materials: The following are available online at https://www.mdpi.com/article/10.3390/pharmaceutics13122030/s1, Figure S1: SEM micrographs of films morphology (SA: Sodium alginate, EtOH: Ethanol, and Glyc: Glycerol). A: SA $_{EtOH0}$. B: SA $_{EtOH10}$. C: SA_Glyc $_{EtOH0}$. D: SA_Glyc $_{EtOH10}$.

Author Contributions: Conceptualization, F.R. and P.C.; methodology, S.P.M., J.L., M.R. and P.C.; validation, J.L. and M.R.; formal analysis, D.A.R., S.P.M., F.R. and P.C.; investigation, D.A.R., S.P.M., F.R. and P.C.; resources, M.R.; data curation, D.A.R., S.P.M., J.L., F.R. and P.C.; writing—original draft preparation, D.A.R.; writing—review and editing, S.P.M., F.R. and P.C.; supervision, F.R. and P.C.;

project administration, F.R. and P.C.; funding acquisition, M.R., F.R. and P.C. All authors have read and agreed to the published version of the manuscript.

Funding: This work was developed within the scope of the CICS-UBI projects UIDB/00709/2020 and UIDP/00709/2020, financed by national funds through the Portuguese Foundation for Science and Technology/MCTES. This research was funded by the projects APIMedOlder [PTDC/MED-FAR/31598/2017] and ZAPGO [PTDC/NAN-MAT/28989/2017] funded by FEDER, through COMPETE2020—Programa Operacional Competitividade e Internacionalização (POCI-01-0145-FEDER-031598), and by national funds (OE), through the Portuguese Foundation for Science and Technology (FCT/MCTES), and project number 0633_BIOIMPACE_4_A co-financed by European Union/ERDF, ESF, European Regional Development Fund ERDF under the Interreg V A Spain-Portugal (POCTEP) 2014–2020 program.

Institutional Review Board Statement: Not applicable.

Informed Consent Statement: Not applicable.

Data Availability Statement: Not applicable.

Acknowledgments: Daniela A. Rodrigues acknowledges a fellowship from APIMedOlder project [PTDC/MEDFAR/31598/2017].

Conflicts of Interest: The authors declare no conflict of interest.

References

1. Groenewegen, A.; Rutten, F.H.; Mosterd, A.; Hoes, A.W. Epidemiology of heart failure. *Eur. J. Heart Fail.* **2020**, *22*, 1342–1356. [CrossRef]
2. Lippi, G.; Sanchis-Gomar, F. Global epidemiology and future trends of heart failure. *AME Med. J.* **2020**, *5*, 15. [CrossRef]
3. Gheorghiade, M.; Adams, K.F.; Colucci, W.S. Digoxin in the management of cardiovascular disorders. *Circulation* **2004**, *109*, 2959–2964. [CrossRef]
4. Cheng, J.W.M.; Rybak, I. Use of digoxin for heart failure and atrial fibrillation in elderly patients. *Am. J. Geriatr. Pharmacother.* **2010**, *8*, 419–427. [CrossRef] [PubMed]
5. Lloyd-Jones, D.; Adams, R.J.; Brown, T.M.; Carnethon, M.; Dai, S.; De Simone, G.; Ferguson, T.B.; Ford, E.; Furie, K.; Gillespie, C.; et al. Heart disease and stroke statistics—2010 update: A report from the American heart association. *Circulation* **2010**, *121*, e46–e215. [PubMed]
6. Angraal, S.; Nuti, S.V.; Masoudi, F.A.; Freeman, J.V.; Murugiah, K.; Shah, N.D.; Desai, N.R.; Ranasinghe, I.; Wang, Y.; Krumholz, H.M. Digoxin Use and Associated Adverse Events Among Older Adults. *Am. J. Med.* **2019**, *132*, 1191–1198. [CrossRef] [PubMed]
7. Ewy, G.A. Digoxin: The art and science. *Am. J. Med.* **2015**, *128*, 1272–1274. [CrossRef] [PubMed]
8. Renom-Guiteras, A.; Meyer, G.; Thürmann, P.A. The EU(7)-PIM list: A list of potentially inappropriate medications for older people consented by experts from seven European countries. *Eur. J. Clin. Pharmacol.* **2015**, *71*, 861–875. [CrossRef] [PubMed]
9. Idrees, H.; Zaidi, S.Z.J.; Sabir, A.; Khan, R.U.; Zhang, X.; Hassan, S.U. A review of biodegradable natural polymer-based nanoparticles for drug delivery applications. *Nanomaterials* **2020**, *10*, 1970. [CrossRef]
10. Campisi, G.; Paderni, C.; Saccone, R.; Fede, O.; Wolff, A.; Giannola, L. Human Buccal Mucosa as an Innovative Site of Drug Delivery. *Curr. Pharm. Des.* **2010**, *16*, 641–652. [CrossRef]
11. Kumar, A.; Naik, P.K.; Pradhan, D.; Ghosh, G.; Rath, G. Mucoadhesive formulations: Innovations, merits, drawbacks, and future outlook. *Pharm. Dev. Technol.* **2020**, *25*, 797–814. [CrossRef] [PubMed]
12. Shojaei, A.H. Buccal mucosa as a route for systemic drug delivery: A review. *J. Pharm. Pharm. Sci.* **1998**, *1*, 15–30.
13. Boddupalli, B.M.; Mohammed, Z.N.K.; Nath, A.R.; Banji, D. Mucoadhesive drug delivery system: An overview. *J. Adv. Pharm. Technol. Res.* **2010**, *1*, 381. [CrossRef] [PubMed]
14. Mansuri, S.; Kesharwani, P.; Jain, K.; Tekade, R.K.; Jain, N.K. Mucoadhesion: A promising approach in drug delivery system. *React. Funct. Polym.* **2016**, *100*, 151–172. [CrossRef]
15. Slavkova, M.; Breitkreutz, J. Orodispersible drug formulations for children and elderly. *Eur. J. Pharm. Sci.* **2015**, *75*, 2–9. [CrossRef] [PubMed]
16. Yir-Erong, B.; Bayor, M.T.; Ayensu, I.; Gbedema, S.Y.; Boateng, J.S. Oral thin films as a remedy for noncompliance in pediatric and geriatric patients. *Ther. Deliv.* **2019**, *10*, 443–464. [CrossRef] [PubMed]
17. Shaikh, R.; Singh, T.R.R.; Garland, M.J.; Woolfson, A.D.; Donnelly, R.F. Mucoadhesive drug delivery systems. *J. Pharm. Bioallied Sci.* **2011**, *3*, 89–100. [CrossRef] [PubMed]
18. Lau, E.T.L.; Steadman, K.J.; Cichero, J.A.Y.; Nissen, L.M. Dosage form modification and oral drug delivery in older people. *Adv. Drug Deliv. Rev.* **2018**, *135*, 75–84. [CrossRef]
19. Irfan, M.; Rabel, S.; Bukhtar, Q.; Qadir, M.I.; Jabeen, F.; Khan, A. Orally disintegrating films: A modern expansion in drug delivery system. *Saudi Pharm. J.* **2016**, *24*, 537–546. [CrossRef] [PubMed]

20. Arya, A.; Chandra, A.; Sharma, V.; Pathak, K. Fast dissolving oral films: An innovative drug delivery system and dosage form. *Int. J. ChemTech Res.* **2010**, *2*, 576–583.
21. Kadajji, V.G.; Betageri, G.V. Water soluble polymers for pharmaceutical applications. *Polymers* **2011**, *3*, 1972–2009. [CrossRef]
22. Sellimi, S.; Younes, I.; Ayed, H.B.; Maalej, H.; Montero, V.; Rinaudo, M.; Dahia, M.; Mechichi, T.; Hajji, M.; Nasri, M. Structural, physicochemical and antioxidant properties of sodium alginate isolated from a Tunisian brown seaweed. *Int. J. Biol. Macromol.* **2015**, *72*, 1358–1367. [CrossRef] [PubMed]
23. Castro, P.M.; Sousa, F.; Magalhães, R.; Ruiz-Henestrosa, V.M.P.; Pilosof, A.M.R.; Madureira, A.R.; Sarmento, B.; Pintado, M.E. Incorporation of beads into oral films for buccal and oral delivery of bioactive molecules. *Carbohydr. Polym.* **2018**, *194*, 411–421. [CrossRef] [PubMed]
24. Morales, J.O.; McConville, J.T. Manufacture and characterization of mucoadhesive buccal films. *Eur. J. Pharm. Biopharm.* **2011**, *77*, 187–199. [CrossRef]
25. Şen, F.; Uzunsoy, İ.; Baştürk, E.; Kahraman, M.V. Antimicrobial agent-free hybrid cationic starch/sodium alginate polyelectrolyte films for food packaging materials. *Carbohydr. Polym.* **2017**, *170*, 264–270. [CrossRef] [PubMed]
26. Puscaselu, R.; Gutt, G.; Amariei, S. The use of edible films based on sodium alginate in meat product packaging: An eco-friendly alternative to conventional plastic materials. *Coatings* **2020**, *10*, 166.
27. Jain, D.; Bar-Shalom, D. Alginate drug delivery systems: Application in context of pharmaceutical and biomedical research. *Drug Dev. Ind. Pharm.* **2014**, *40*, 1576–1584. [CrossRef]
28. Grottkau, B.; Cai, X.; Wang, J.; Yang, X.; Lin, Y. Polymeric Nanoparticles for a Drug Delivery System. *Curr. Drug Metab.* **2013**, *14*, 840–846. [CrossRef]
29. Wilczewska, A.Z.; Niemirowicz, K.; Markiewicz, K.H.; Car, H. Nanoparticles as drug delivery systems. *Pharmacol. Rep.* **2012**, *64*, 1020–1037. [CrossRef]
30. Argos, P.; Pedersen, K.; Marks, M.D.; Larkins, B.A. A structural model for maize zein proteins. *J. Biol. Chem.* **1982**, *257*, 9984–9990. [CrossRef]
31. Luo, Y.; Wang, Q. Zein-based micro- and nano-particles for drug and nutrient delivery: A review. *J. Appl. Polym. Sci.* **2014**, *131*, 16. [CrossRef]
32. Pascoli, M.; de Lima, R.; Fraceto, L.F. Zein nanoparticles and strategies to improve colloidal stability: A mini-review. *Front. Chem.* **2018**, *6*, 6. [CrossRef] [PubMed]
33. Paliwal, R.; Palakurthi, S. Zein in controlled drug delivery and tissue engineering. *J. Control. Release* **2014**, *189*, 108–122. [CrossRef] [PubMed]
34. Berardi, A.; Bisharat, L.; AlKhatib, H.S.; Cespi, M. Zein as a Pharmaceutical Excipient in Oral Solid Dosage Forms: State of the Art and Future Perspectives. *AAPS PharmSciTech* **2018**, *19*, 2009–2022. [CrossRef] [PubMed]
35. Tapia-Hernández, J.A.; Rodríguez-Felix, F.; Juárez-Onofre, J.E.; Ruiz-Cruz, S.; Robles-García, M.A.; Borboa-Flores, J.; Wong-Corral, F.J.; Cinco-Moroyoqui, F.J.; Castro-Enríquez, D.D.; Del-Toro-Sánchez, C.L. Zein-polysaccharide nanoparticles as matrices for antioxidant compounds: A strategy for prevention of chronic degenerative diseases. *Food Res. Int.* **2018**, *111*, 451–471. [CrossRef] [PubMed]
36. da Rosa, C.G.; de Oliveira Brisola Maciel, M.V.; de Carvalho, S.M.; de Melo, A.P.Z.; Jummes, B.; da Silva, T.; Martelli, S.M.; Villetti, M.A.; Bertoldi, F.C.; Barreto, P.L.M. Characterization and evaluation of physicochemical and antimicrobial properties of zein nanoparticles loaded with phenolics monoterpenes. *Colloids Surf. A Physicochem. Eng. Asp.* **2015**, *481*, 337–344. [CrossRef]
37. Alhakamy, N.A.; Ahmed, O.A.A.; Aldawsari, H.M.; Alfaifi, M.Y.; Eid, B.G.; Abdel-Naim, A.B.; Fahmy, U.A. Encapsulation of lovastatin in zein nanoparticles exhibits enhanced apoptotic activity in hepg2 cells. *Int. J. Mol. Sci.* **2019**, *20*, 5788. [CrossRef]
38. Boateng-Marfo, Y.; Dong, Y.; Ng, W.K.; Lin, H.S. Artemether-loaded zein nanoparticles: An innovative intravenous dosage form for the management of severe malaria. *Int. J. Mol. Sci.* **2021**, *22*, 1141. [CrossRef]
39. Cheng, W.; Wang, B.; Zhang, C.; Dong, Q.; Qian, J.; Zha, L.; Chen, W.; Hong, L. Preparation and preliminary pharmacokinetics study of GNA-loaded zein nanoparticles. *J. Pharm. Pharmacol.* **2019**, *71*, 1626–1634. [CrossRef]
40. Dong, F.; Dong, X.; Zhou, L.; Xiao, H.; Ho, P.Y.; Wong, M.S.; Wang, Y. Doxorubicin-loaded biodegradable self-assembly zein nanoparticle and its anti-cancer effect: Preparation, in vitro evaluation, and cellular uptake. *Colloids Surf. B Biointerfaces* **2016**, *140*, 324–331. [CrossRef]
41. Lai, L.F.; Guo, H.X. Preparation of new 5-fluorouracil-loaded zein nanoparticles for liver targeting. *Int. J. Pharm.* **2011**, *404*, 317–323. [CrossRef] [PubMed]
42. Lee, H.S.; Kang, N.W.; Kim, H.; Kim, D.H.; Chae, J.W.; Lee, W.; Song, G.Y.; Cho, C.W.; Kim, D.D.; Lee, J.Y. Chondroitin sulfate-hybridized zein nanoparticles for tumor-targeted delivery of docetaxel. *Carbohydr. Polym.* **2021**, *253*, 117187. [CrossRef] [PubMed]
43. Shinde, P.; Agraval, H.; Srivastav, A.K.; Yadav, U.C.S.; Kumar, U. Physico-chemical characterization of carvacrol loaded zein nanoparticles for enhanced anticancer activity and investigation of molecular interactions between them by molecular docking. *Int. J. Pharm.* **2020**, *588*, 119795. [CrossRef] [PubMed]
44. Yu, X.; Wu, H.; Hu, H.; Dong, Z.; Dang, Y.; Qi, Q.; Wang, Y.; Du, S.; Lu, Y. Zein nanoparticles as nontoxic delivery system for maytansine in the treatment of non-small cell lung cancer. *Drug Deliv.* **2020**, *27*, 100–109. [CrossRef] [PubMed]
45. Reboredo, C.; González-Navarro, C.J.; Martínez-Oharriz, C.; Martínez-López, A.L.; Irache, J.M. Preparation and evaluation of PEG-coated zein nanoparticles for oral drug delivery purposes. *Int. J. Pharm.* **2021**, *597*, 120287. [CrossRef] [PubMed]

46. Rao, J.P.; Geckeler, K.E. Polymer nanoparticles: Preparation techniques and size-control parameters. *Prog. Polym. Sci.* **2011**, *36*, 887–913. [CrossRef]
47. Gültekin, H.E.; Değim, Z. Biodegradable polymeric nanoparticles are effective systems for controlled drug delivery. *Fabad J. Pharm. Sci.* **2013**, *38*, 107–118.
48. Kamaly, N.; Yameen, B.; Wu, J.; Farokhzad, O.C. Degradable controlled-release polymers and polymeric nanoparticles: Mechanisms of controlling drug release. *Chem. Rev.* **2016**, *116*, 2602–2663. [CrossRef]
49. Sánchez, A.; Mejía, S.P.; Orozco, J. Recent advances in polymeric nanoparticle-encapsulated drugs against intracellular infections. *Molecules* **2020**, *25*, 3760. [CrossRef]
50. Bruschi, M.L.; De Freitas, O. Oral bioadhesive drug delivery systems. *Drug Dev. Ind. Pharm.* **2005**, *31*, 293–310. [CrossRef]
51. Li, J.; He, J.; Huang, Y.; Li, D.; Chen, X. Improving surface and mechanical properties of alginate films by using ethanol as a co-solvent during external gelation. *Carbohydr. Polym.* **2015**, *123*, 208–216. [CrossRef]
52. Alopaeus, J.F.; Hellfritzsch, M.; Gutowski, T.; Scherließ, R.; Almeida, A.; Sarmento, B.; Škalko-Basnet, N.; Tho, I. Mucoadhesive buccal films based on a graft co-polymer—A mucin-retentive hydrogel scaffold. *Eur. J. Pharm. Sci.* **2020**, *142*, 105142. [CrossRef] [PubMed]
53. Marques, M.R.C.; Loebenberg, R.; Almukainzi, M. Simulated biological fluids with possible application in dissolution testing. *Dissolution Technol.* **2011**, *18*, 15–28. [CrossRef]
54. Han, J.; Zhu, Z.; Qian, H.; Wohl, A.R.; Beaman, C.J.; Hoye, T.R.; Macosko, C.W. A simple confined impingement jets mixer for flash nanoprecipitation. *J. Pharm. Sci.* **2012**, *101*, 4018–4023. [CrossRef] [PubMed]
55. Milenković, M.Z.; Marinković, V.D.; Sibinović, P.S.; Palić, R.M.; Milenović, D.M. An HPLC method for the determination of digoxin in dissolution samples. *J. Serbian Chem. Soc.* **2010**, *75*, 1583–1594. [CrossRef]
56. Qin, Z.Y.; Jia, X.W.; Liu, Q.; Kong, B.H.; Wang, H. Fast dissolving oral films for drug delivery prepared from chitosan/pullulan electrospinning nanofibers. *Int. J. Biol. Macromol.* **2019**, *137*, 224–231. [CrossRef]
57. Shen, B.D.; Shen, C.Y.; Yuan, X.D.; Bai, J.X.; Lv, Q.Y.; Xu, H.; Dai, L.; Yu, C.; Han, J.; Yuan, H.L. Development and characterization of an orodispersible film containing drug nanoparticles. *Eur. J. Pharm. Biopharm.* **2013**, *85*, 1348–1356. [CrossRef]
58. Silva, T.A.; Stefano, J.S.; Janegitz, B.C. Sensing Materials: Nanomaterials Definition. In *Reference Module in Biomedical Sciences*; Elsevier: Amsterdam, The Netherlands, 2021.
59. Wasilewska, K.; Winnicka, K. How to assess orodispersible film quality? A review of applied methods and their modifications. *Acta Pharm.* **2019**, *69*, 155–176. [CrossRef]
60. Helmiyati; Aprilliza, M. Characterization and properties of sodium alginate from brown algae used as an ecofriendly superabsorbent. *IOP Conf. Series: Mater. Sci. Eng.* **2017**, *188*, 012019. [CrossRef]
61. Shen, W.; Hsieh, Y. Lo Biocompatible sodium alginate fibers by aqueous processing and physical crosslinking. *Carbohydr. Polym.* **2014**, *102*, 893–900. [CrossRef]
62. Gurikov, P.; Smirnova, I. Non-conventional methods for gelation of alginate. *Gels* **2018**, *4*, 14. [CrossRef]
63. Tkalec, G.; Knez, Ž.; Novak, Z. Formation of polysaccharide aerogels in ethanol. *RSC Adv.* **2015**, *5*, 77362–77371. [CrossRef]
64. Cerqueira, M.A.; Souza, B.W.S.; Teixeira, J.A.; Vicente, A.A. Effect of glycerol and corn oil on physicochemical properties of polysaccharide films—A comparative study. *Food Hydrocoll.* **2012**, *27*, 175–184. [CrossRef]
65. Lee, K.Y.; Mooney, D.J. Alginate: Properties and biomedical applications. *Prog. Polym. Sci.* **2012**, *37*, 106–126. [CrossRef] [PubMed]
66. Nair, A.B.; Kumria, R.; Harsha, S.; Attimarad, M.; Al-Dhubiab, B.E.; Alhaider, I.A. In vitro techniques to evaluate buccal films. *J. Control. Release* **2013**, *166*, 10–21. [CrossRef] [PubMed]
67. Dave, R.H.; Shah, D.A.; Patel, P.G. Development and Evaluation of High Loading Oral Dissolving Film of Aspirin and Acetaminophen. *J. Pharm. Sci. Pharmacol.* **2014**, *1*, 112–122. [CrossRef]
68. Bitencourt, C.M.; Fávaro-Trindade, C.S.; Sobral, P.J.A.; Carvalho, R.A. Gelatin-based films additivated with curcuma ethanol extract: Antioxidant activity and physical properties of films. *Food Hydrocoll.* **2014**, *40*, 145–152. [CrossRef]
69. Sevinç Özakar, R.; Özakar, E. Current overview of oral thin films. *Turkish J. Pharm. Sci.* **2021**, *18*, 111–121. [CrossRef]
70. Nafee, N.A.; Ismail, F.A.; Boraie, N.A.; Mortada, L.M. Mucoadhesive delivery systems. I. Evaluation of mucoadhesive polymers for buccal tablet formulation. *Drug Dev. Ind. Pharm.* **2004**, *30*, 985–993. [CrossRef]
71. Al-Mogherah, A.I.; Ibrahim, M.A.; Hassan, M.A. Optimization and evaluation of venlafaxine hydrochloride fast dissolving oral films. *Saudi Pharm. J.* **2020**, *28*, 1374–1382. [CrossRef]
72. Gilhotra, R.M.; Ikram, M.; Srivastava, S.; Gilhotra, N. A clinical perspective on mucoadhesive buccal drug delivery systems. *J. Biomed. Res.* **2014**, *28*, 81–97. [CrossRef] [PubMed]
73. Borges, A.F.; Silva, C.; Coelho, J.F.J.; Simões, S. Oral films: Current status and future perspectives: I-Galenical development and quality attributes. *J. Control. Release* **2015**, *206*, 1–19. [CrossRef] [PubMed]
74. Liu, J.; Leng, P.; Liu, Y. Oral drug delivery with nanoparticles into the gastrointestinal mucosa. *Fundam. Clin. Pharmacol.* **2021**, *35*, 86–96. [CrossRef] [PubMed]
75. Hong, J.; Li, Y.; Xiao, Y.; Li, Y.; Guo, Y.; Kuang, H.; Wang, X. Annonaceous acetogenins (ACGs) nanosuspensions based on a self-assembly stabilizer and the significantly improved anti-tumor efficacy. *Colloids Surf. B Biointerfaces* **2016**, *145*, 319–327. [CrossRef] [PubMed]
76. Pu, X.; Sun, J.; Wang, Y.; Wang, Y.; Liu, X.; Zhang, P.; Tang, X.; Pan, W.; Han, J.; He, Z. Development of a chemically stable 10-hydroxycamptothecin nanosuspensions. *Int. J. Pharm.* **2009**, *379*, 167–173. [CrossRef] [PubMed]

77. Bhattacharjee, S. DLS and zeta potential—What they are and what they are not? *J. Control. Release* **2016**, *235*, 337–351. [CrossRef] [PubMed]
78. Gagliardi, A.; Paolino, D.; Iannone, M.; Palma, E.; Fresta, M.; Cosco, D. Sodium deoxycholate-decorated zein nanoparticles for a stable colloidal drug delivery system. *Int. J. Nanomed.* **2018**, *13*, 601–614. [CrossRef] [PubMed]
79. Lakshmi, P.; Kumar, G.A. Nanosuspension technology: A review. *Int. J. Pharm. Pharm. Sci.* **2010**, *2*, 35–40.
80. Bennett, C.F.; Chiang, M.Y.; Chan, H.; Shoemaker, J.E.E.; Mirabelli, C.K. Cationic lipids enhance cellular uptake and activity of phosphorothioate antisense oligonucleotides. *Mol. Pharmacol.* **1992**, *41*, 1023–1033. [PubMed]
81. Sahoo, S.K.; Panyam, J.; Prabha, S.; Labhasetwar, V. Residual polyvinyl alcohol associated with poly (D,L-lactide-co-glycolide) nanoparticles affects their physical properties and cellular uptake. *J. Control. Release* **2002**, *82*, 105–114. [CrossRef]
82. Verma, A.; Stellacci, F. Effect of surface properties on nanoparticle-cell interactions. *Small* **2010**, *6*, 12–21. [CrossRef] [PubMed]
83. Punitha, S.; Girish, Y. Polymers in mucoadhesive buccal drug delivery system—A review. *Int. J. Res. Pharm. Sci.* **2010**, *1*, 2.
84. Esposito, D.; Conte, C.; d'Angelo, I.; Miro, A.; Ungaro, F.; Quaglia, F. Mucoadhesive zein/beta-cyclodextrin nanoparticles for the buccal delivery of curcumin. *Int. J. Pharm.* **2020**, *586*, 119587. [CrossRef] [PubMed]
85. Ghalei, S.; Asadi, H.; Ghalei, B. Zein nanoparticle-embedded electrospun PVA nanofibers as wound dressing for topical delivery of anti-inflammatory diclofenac. *J. Appl. Polym. Sci.* **2018**, *135*, 46643. [CrossRef]
86. Liu, Q.; Jing, Y.; Han, C.; Zhang, H.; Tian, Y. Encapsulation of curcumin in zein/ caseinate/sodium alginate nanoparticles with improved physicochemical and controlled release properties. *Food Hydrocoll.* **2019**, *93*, 432–442. [CrossRef]
87. Luo, Y.; Teng, Z.; Wang, Q. Development of zein nanoparticles coated with carboxymethyl chitosan for encapsulation and controlled release of vitamin D3. *J. Agric. Food Chem.* **2012**, *60*, 836–843. [CrossRef]
88. Muthuselvi, L.; Dhathathreyan, A. Simple coacervates of zein to encapsulate Gitoxin. *Colloids Surf. B Biointerfaces* **2006**, *51*, 39–43. [CrossRef]
89. Albekairi, N.A.; Al-Enazy, S.; Ali, S.; Rytting, E. Transport of digoxin-loaded polymeric nanoparticles across BeWo cells, an in vitro model of human placental trophoblast. *Ther. Deliv.* **2015**, *6*, 1325–1334. [CrossRef]
90. Das, S.; Chaudhury, A. Recent advances in lipid nanoparticle formulations with solid matrix for oral drug delivery. *AAPS PharmSciTech* **2011**, *12*, 62–76. [CrossRef]
91. Kuan, Y.L.; Navin Sivanasvaran, S.; Pui, L.P.; Yusof, Y.A.; Senphan, T. Physicochemical properties of sodium alginate edible film incorporated with mulberry (Morus australis) leaf extract. *Pertanika J. Trop. Agric. Sci.* **2020**, *43*, 359–376.
92. Mohamad, S.A.; Salem, H.; Yassin, H.A.; Mansour, H.F. Bucco-adhesive film as a pediatric proper dosage form for systemic delivery of propranolol hydrochloride: In-vitro and in-vivo evaluation. *Drug Des. Devel. Ther.* **2020**, *14*, 4277–4289. [CrossRef] [PubMed]
93. Irwan, A.W.; Berania, J.E.; Liu, X. A comparative study on the effects of amphiphilic and hydrophilic polymers on the release profiles of a poorly water-soluble drug. *Pharm. Dev. Technol.* **2016**, *21*, 231–238. [CrossRef] [PubMed]

pharmaceutics

MDPI

Article

The Impact of an Efflux Pump Inhibitor on the Activity of Free and Liposomal Antibiotics against *Pseudomonas aeruginosa*

Douweh Leyla Gbian and Abdelwahab Omri *

Department of Chemistry and Biochemistry, The Novel Drug and Vaccine Delivery Systems Facility, Laurentian University, Sudbury, ON P3E 2C6, Canada; Douweh@laurentian.ca
* Correspondence: aomri@laurentian.ca; Tel.: +1-705-675-1151-2190; Fax: +1-705-675-4844

Abstract: The eradication of *Pseudomonas aeruginosa* in cystic fibrosis patients has become continuously difficult due to its increased resistance to treatments. This study assessed the efficacy of free and liposomal gentamicin and erythromycin, combined with Phenylalanine arginine beta-naphthylamide (PABN), a broad-spectrum efflux pump inhibitor, against *P. aeruginosa* isolates. Liposomes were prepared and characterized for their sizes and encapsulation efficiencies. The antimicrobial activities of formulations were determined by the microbroth dilution method. Their activity on *P. aeruginosa* biofilms was assessed, and the effect of sub-inhibitory concentrations on bacterial virulence factors, quorum sensing (QS) signals and bacterial motility was also evaluated. The average diameters of liposomes were 562.67 ± 33.74 nm for gentamicin and 3086.35 ± 553.95 nm for erythromycin, with encapsulation efficiencies of 13.89 ± 1.54% and 51.58 ± 2.84%, respectively. Liposomes and PABN combinations potentiated antibiotics by reducing minimum inhibitory and bactericidal concentrations by 4–32 fold overall. The formulations significantly inhibited biofilm formation and differentially attenuated virulence factor production as well as motility. Unexpectedly, QS signal production was not affected by treatments. Taken together, the results indicate that PABN shows potential as an adjuvant of liposomal macrolides and aminoglycosides in the management of lung infections in cystic fibrosis patients.

Keywords: cystic fibrosis; *Pseudomonas aeruginosa*; liposomes; efflux pump inhibitor; PABN; aminoglycosides; macrolides

Citation: Gbian, D.L.; Omri, A. The Impact of an Efflux Pump Inhibitor on the Activity of Free and Liposomal Antibiotics against *Pseudomonas aeruginosa*. *Pharmaceutics* **2021**, *13*, 577. https://doi.org/10.3390/pharmaceutics13040577

Academic Editors: Ana Isabel Fernandes, Angela Faustino Jozala and Hwa-Jeong Lee

Received: 16 January 2021
Accepted: 15 April 2021
Published: 18 April 2021

1. Introduction

Pseudomonas aeruginosa is an opportunistic Gram-negative bacterium and the principal pathogen found in the lungs of cystic fibrosis (CF) patients [1,2]. Chronic and persistent pulmonary infections caused by *P. aeruginosa* lead to progressive lung damage, and eventually respiratory failure and death [3]. They are the leading cause of death in CF [4]. Aminoglycosides and macrolides are commonly prescribed for the management of *P. aeruginosa* infections in CF, as they inhibit protein synthesis in the bacteria [2,5–8]. Moreover, macrolides such as azithromycin are recommended for CF patients because they reduce pulmonary exacerbations over long periods [9,10]. However, due to the bacteria's increased resistance to clinically acceptable levels of antibiotics and the associated toxicity of macrolides and aminoglycosides at those high concentrations, it is crucial to develop new ways to revitalize those drugs [2,11–13]. Poor drug penetration is a major issue behind bacterial resistance to antibiotics. It can be attributable to reduced membrane permeability to antibiotics [14] and to the expression of efflux pumps which thwart the activity of antimicrobials by inducing their expulsion from the cell [15–18].

The main efflux systems with the highest clinical significance in *P. aeruginosa* are MexAB-OprM, MexCD-OprJ, MexEF-OprN, and MexXY-OprM pumps, which belong to the resistance nodulation cell division family and export metabolites, antibiotics and even quorum sensing (QS) molecules [15,19]. The MexAB-OprM pump transports beta-lactams, macrolides, tetracyclines [20], and 3-oxo-dodecanoyl homoserine lactone ($3OC_{12}$-HSL, QS signal) [21] among others, while the MexXY-OprM pump exports aminoglycosides, fluoroquinolones, tetracyclines and macrolides [22–24].

QS is used by bacteria to coordinate group behaviors at high cell density via the production of signaling molecules called autoinducers [25]. *P. aeruginosa* has three main interconnected QS systems organized hierarchically, namely the LasI/R system at the top, followed by the RhlI/R and the *Pseudomonas* Quinolone Signal (PQS) systems, respectively [26,27]. For QS to occur, autoinducers must be expressed extracellularly and detected by neighboring cells. N-butanoyl-homoserine lactone (C_4-HSL) signals produced by the Rhl system freely diffuse out of the cells, while $3OC_{12}$-HSL and PQS signals produced by Las and PQS, respectively, need to be exported by membrane transporters to cross the outer membrane [21,25]. *P. aeruginosa* upregulates virulence factors such as pyocyanin, proteases, motilities and forms robust biofilms through QS, causing destructive infections and inflammations [28–30]. Pyocyanin is a redox-active toxin that plays a crucial role in the establishment of *P. aeruginosa*'s infection, while proteases and lipases target and degrade the host's proteins and lipids to facilitate the bacterium's invasion [29]. Pyoverdine, on the other hand, is a siderophore used for scavenging iron, vital for bacterial growth and virulence [31]. A summary of *P. aeruginosa*'s main efflux pumps, QS systems and virulence factors along with their functions is provided in Table 1 below. Biofilms are communities of bacteria attached to a surface, protected by an exopolysaccharide matrix that can be 10–1000 times more resistant to antibiotics than planktonic bacteria [32]. Furthermore, recent studies have suggested a positive connection between biofilms and efflux pumps [33]. However, the exact mechanism behind this is not fully elucidated.

Table 1. Summary of *P. aeruginosa*'s main efflux pumps, quorum sensing (QS) systems and virulence factors.

Efflux Pumps	Substrates	QS Systems (Molecules)	Function	Virulence Factors	Function
MexAB-OprM	Beta-lactams, macrolides, tetracyclines [20], and 3-oxo-dodecanoyl homoserine lactone ($3OC_{12}$-HSL, QS signal) [21]	LasI/R ($3OC_{12}$-HSL)	Regulates elastase, protease, exotoxin A, biofilm formation and induces PQS and Rhl systems [34,35]	Protease	Immune invasion and host tissue damage [7,29]
MexXY-OprM	Aminoglycosides, fluoroquinolones, tetracyclines and macrolides [22–24]	RhlI/R (C_4-HSL)	Regulates the production of pyocyanin, rhamnolipids, elastase and hydrogen cyanide [36]	Pyocyanin	Induces oxidative stress, neutrophil apoptosis, inhibits ciliary beating in the airways, and causes cytotoxicity [37,38]
MexCD-OprJ	Macrolides, cephalosporins, fluoroquinolones, tetracyclines and organic solvents [39]	PQS [1] (PQS signal)	Regulates the expression of pyoverdine, pyocyanin, rhamnolipids and the RhlI/R system [35]	Pyoverdine	Iron scavenging, vital for pathogenesis. Sequestrates iron from host, which is used for biofilm formation [40]
MexEF-OprN	Chloramphenicol, tetracycline, fluoroquinolones, HHQ [2] (QS signal) [39]			Lipase	Degrades lipids in the host [29]

[1] *Pseudomonas* quinolone signal, [2] 4-hydroxy-2-heptylquinoline.

Combining efflux pump inhibitors with antibiotics could therefore represent a good strategy to bypass efflux resistance [41]. One such compound is Phenylalanine-Arginine Naphthylamide (PABN), a broad-spectrum competitive efflux pump inhibitor thought to behave as a substrate of efflux pumps by binding to their transporter domains [42]. PABN acts directly on efflux pumps without affecting the proton gradient and the electrical potential across the inner cell membrane [43]. It is reported to potentiate in vitro activity of various anti-pseudomonal drugs including fluoroquinolones, beta-lactams and aminoglycosides against multidrug resistant *P. aeruginosa* strains [44] and to even inhibit QS and virulence factors [43].

Antibiotics' encapsulation into liposomes can also be used to overcome poor drug penetration. Liposomes are spherical lipid vesicles of one or more lipid bilayers that serve as carriers for hydrophilic, lipophilic and amphiphilic compounds [45]. They protect drugs from undesired metabolic breakdown, increase their accumulation at the target site and reduce their toxicity, as less product is needed for therapeutic effect [46,47]. Arikayce® (Insmed), for instance, is a liposomal preparation of amikacin recently approved by the FDA (Food and Drug Administration, USA), used against *Mycobacterium avium* complex and *P. aeruginosa*, showing superior efficacy than its free counterpart [48,49]. Furthermore, previous work from our group demonstrated that liposomal antibiotics showed increased antimicrobial activities against resistant *P. aeruginosa* strains isolated from CF patients [47,50–52].

In the present study, we prepared liposomal gentamicin (GEN) and erythromycin (ERY), and their antimicrobial activity in combination with PABN was assessed against *P. aeruginosa* strains. Indeed, their impact on bacteria's biofilms, virulence factors and QS signal production as well as motilities was evaluated.

2. Materials and Methods

2.1. Chemicals and Media

Gentamicin, agarose, chloroform and casamino acids were obtained from Fisher Scientific (Ottawa, ON, Canada). Erythromycin was purchased from Caledon Laboratories LTD (Georgetown, WA, Canada). Phenylalanine-Arginine-β-Naphthylamide, cholesterol and Triton X-100 were purchased from Sigma Aldrich (Oakville, ON, Canada). The compound 2-Nitrophenyl-β-D-galactopyranoside was obtained from Thermo Fisher Scientific (Ottawa, ON, Canada). DPPC (1,2-Dipalmitoyl-*sn*-glycero-3-phosphocholine) was obtained from Avanti Polar Lipids Inc. (Alabaster, AL, USA). Mueller–Hinton broth (MHB) and Lysogeny broth (LB) and agar were purchased from Becton Dickinson (Francklin Lakes, NJ, USA) and Becton Dickinson Microbiology Systems (Oakville, ON, Canada), respectively. ABt medium and Z buffer were prepared as described previously [47,51].

2.2. Bacterial Strains

PA01 was a generous gift from Dr R.E.W Hancock (University of British Columbia, Vancouver, BC, Canada), and the clinical strain PA11 was obtained from the Memorial Hospital's Clinical Microbiology Laboratory (Sudbury, ON, Canada). *Staphylococcus aureus* (ATCC 29213) and *Bacillus subtilis* (ATCC 6633) strains purchased from PML Microbiologicals (Mississauga, ON, Canada) were used as indicator organisms for gentamicin and erythromycin, respectively [53]. All strains were stored at −80 °C in MHB supplemented with 10% glycerol (v/v) in a −86 °C ULT Freezer, Thermo Forma. The *Agrobacterium tumefaciens* strain A136 (pCF218)(pCF372) (Ti-) kindly donated by Dr Fuqua (Indiana University, Bloomington, IN, USA) was used as the biosensor strain and cultured in LB broth at 30 °C for the detection of acyl homoserine lactones (AHLs) [47].

2.3. Preparation of Liposomes

Gentamicin and erythromycin were encapsulated into liposomes composed of DPPC (0.11382 g/mL) and cholesterol (0.01 g/mL) at a molar ratio of 6:1 (DPPC to cholesterol), using the dehydration–rehydration vesicle (DRV) method as previously described [52]. Erythromycin was directly mixed with the lipids in the organic solvent for a final concentration of 20 mg/mL after rehydration. The lipid layer was rehydrated with a solution of 3 mg/mL of gentamicin or PBS (Phosphate-Buffered Saline) for erythromycin. Lipid suspensions were vortexed for 5 min and sonicated for 2 × 15 min (cycles of 45 s ON and 10 s OFF) in an ultrasonic dismembrator bath (FS20H; Fisher Scientific, Ottawa, ON, Canada) with an amplitude of 45 Hz (Model 500, Fisher Scientific). Lipid suspensions were divided into aliquots of 1 mL and frozen for 15 min, then placed overnight in a freeze-dry system (model 77540, Labanco Corporation, Kansas City, MO, USA). Powdered formulations obtained were stored in a freezer at 0 °C until use. Liposomes were rehydrated as previously described [52]. One hundred microliters of PBS was added to the powders and the mixtures were vortexed and incubated for 5 min at 40 °C. This step was repeated three times and a final volume of 700 µL of PBS was added. The unencapsulated drug was removed with three rounds of washing with PBS using a centrifuge (16,000 *g* for 15 min at 4 °C). The Submicron Nicomp particle sizer Model 270 (Nicomp, Santa Barbara, CA, USA) was used to measure the average particle size of liposomes and determine the polydispersity index as reported earlier [52].

2.4. *Microbiological Assay for the Measurement of Gentamicin and Erythromycin in Liposomes*

To measure the concentrations of antibiotics incorporated into liposomes, a microbiological agar diffusion assay with indicator strains was performed as previously reported [52]. The quantifiable limit for both antibiotics was 7.81×10^{-3} mg/mL. Standard curves linearity extended over 0.00781–4 mg/mL and gave correlation coefficients >0.99. Concentrations obtained were the means of three independent experiments performed in triplicate.

2.5. *Determination of Encapsulation Efficiency*

Encapsulation efficiencies (EE) of liposomal antibiotics were determined as the percentage of antibiotics entrapped in liposomes with respect to the initial amount used, with the following Equation (1) [53]:

$$\text{Encapsulation efficiency } (\%) = \frac{\text{Concentration of encapsulated drug } \times 100}{\text{Initial drug concentration}} \tag{1}$$

2.6. *Determination of Minimum Inhibitory Concentrations (MICs) and Minimum Bactericidal Concentrations (MBCs)*

MICs and MBCs of bacteria exposed to free and liposomal gentamicin and erythromycin with and without PABN (at 25 mg/L) were determined using the microbroth dilution technique as reported previously [50,54]. Results were taken from three separate experiments. Reductions of 2 fold or more with PABN were considered significant [44].

2.7. *Minimum Biofilm Eradication Concentration (MBEC)*

Biofilms of PA01 and PA11 adjusted to 0.5 McFarland standard (1.5×10^8 CFU/mL) were grown for 72–96 h in MHB, in an MBEC^{TM} plate (CBD-Innovotech, Edmonton, AB, Canada) as recommended [55]. After incubation, the peg lid with biofilms was rinsed in a fresh 96-well plate filled with PBS, transferred to another plate containing serial dilutions of antibiotics combined with PABN at 25 mg/L and incubated for 24 h, at 37 °C, 110 rpm in the shaking incubator. Control wells were filled with MHB instead. After incubation, the peg lid was rinsed with PBS for a few seconds and placed in a recovery plate, a fresh 96-well plate with 200 µL of MHB per well and biofilms were sonicated for 30 min in an ultrasonic dismembrator bath. The recovery plate was incubated for 24 h at 37 °C, 110 rpm and the MBEC was determined as the smallest concentration of antibiotics to eradicate biofilms. Reductions of 2 fold or more with PABN were considered significant [44].

2.8. *Effects of Sub-Inhibitory Concentrations of Free and Liposomal Gentamicin and Erythromycin on the Growth of P. aeruginosa*

Bacterial solutions of *P. aeruginosa* equivalent to 2 times 0.5 McFarland standard or optical density at λ = 600 nm (OD600), absorbance 0.26 in MHB were prepared, modified from previous reports [56] and exposed to equal volumes of antibiotics at 1/2 MIC, 1/4 MIC, 1/8 MIC, 1/16 MIC and 1/32 MIC (when necessary). The study was performed for 7 h as described earlier [57]. Results were taken from three separate experiments.

2.9. Virulence Factor Assays

PA01 and PA11 standardized to 0.5 McFarland standard in LB broth supplemented with an equal volume of sub-inhibitory concentrations of antibiotics combined with PABN were incubated for 24 h at 200 rpm, 37 °C in a shaking incubator [58]. PBS was used instead for positive controls. After incubation, samples were centrifuged at 12,000 rpm, 4 °C for 20 min and the supernatant was filter sterilized for further use.

2.9.1. Protease Assay

The assay was carried out with 1.25% (*v*/*v*) skimmed milk and filtered supernatants as previously described [59]. Protease activity = OD_{600} of skimmed milk − OD_{600} of each sample. Experiments were performed three times in triplicate.

2.9.2. Pyocyanin and Pyoverdine Assays

Pyocyanin was extracted from supernatants with chloroform (1:3 *v*/*v* chloroform to supernatant) and quantified spectrophotometrically at $\lambda = 520$ nm as described earlier [57,58]. Pyoverdine in the aqueous layer was removed and the absorbance measured at 405 nm. Experiments were performed three times for pyocyanin and three times in triplicate for pyoverdine.

2.9.3. Lipase Assay

The assay was performed as reported earlier [52]. A 0.6 mL aliquot of filtered supernatants of bacteria was mixed in a 15 mL centrifuge tube with 0.6 mL of Tween® 80 in Tris-buffered saline (10% *v*/*v*), 0.1 mL of $CaCl_2$ (1 M), and 1.2 mL of H_2O and incubated for 24 h, at 37 °C and 200 rpm (Innova 4000 Incubator Shaker, New Brunswick Scientific, NJ, USA). In the presence of lipase, Tween is broken down and binds to calcium, which precipitates and can be quantified spectrophotometrically at $\lambda = 400$ nm. Experiments were performed three times in triplicate.

2.10. Beta-Galactosidase Activity Assay

AHL production levels from *P. aeruginosa* exposed to free and liposomal antibiotics at sub-inhibitory concentrations with and without PABN were evaluated with the reporter strain *A. tumefaciens* (A136) as previously described [52]. Briefly, 4 mL of the reporter strain was mixed with 1 mL of supernatant and incubated at 30 °C in a water bath for 5 h. The bacterial cell densities of the samples at 600 nm were then measured before centrifugation. The supernatant was discarded, and the pellet was resuspended in an equal volume of Z buffer, as described previously. The cells were permeabilized with 200 µL of chloroform and 100 µL of 0.1% SDS, before the addition of *o*-nitro phenol-β-D-galactopyranoside (4 mg/mL in PBS). After the development of a deep yellow color, the reaction was stopped with 1 mL of 1 M Na_2CO_3 and the absorbances of the samples were measured at 420 and 550 nm. Miller units of β-galactosidase activity were calculated as follows: $1000 \times [A_{420} - (1.75 \times A_{550})]/(\text{time} \times \text{volume} \times A_{600})$ [60].

2.11. Motility Studies

Motility studies were slightly modified from other investigators [51,58]. Standardized bacteria grown overnight (2 µL) were inoculated onto agar plates containing sub-inhibitory concentrations of free or liposomal antibiotics with and without PABN. Twitching, swarming and swimming plates were prepared as described earlier [51]. Plates were incubated in a CO_2 incubator at 37 °C. After 18 h, swimming and swarming diameters were measured while twitching diameters were measured after 24 h. Experiments were performed three times in triplicate.

2.12. Data Analysis

Data are represented as mean ± SEM (standard error of the mean) of three independent experiments. Comparison between groups was achieved by one-way analysis of variance (ANOVA) with a Tukey–Kramer Multiple Comparisons test with GraphPad prism (Graph-

Pad Software Inc., San Diego, CA, USA, version 8.4.3). Probability values of * $p < 0.05$, ** $p < 0.01$, *** $p < 0.001$ and **** $p < 0.0001$ were considered statistically significant.

3. Results

3.1. Liposomal Antibiotics Characterisations

The encapsulation efficiency (EE) of liposomal GEN was 13.89 ± 1.545% and the concentration entrapped was 0.42 ± 0.046 mg/mL (Table 2). On the other hand, the EE of ERY was 51.58 ± 2.846% with an entrapped concentration of 10.32 ± 0.571 mg/mL. The average diameters of liposomal GEN and ERY were 562.67 ± 33.74 nm and 3086.35 ± 553.95 nm, respectively. The polydispersity index, which is a measure of size distribution, comprised between 0.0 (homogeneous) and 1.0 (heterogeneous) ranged from 0.6 ± 0.12 to 0.7 ± 0.11 for ERY and GEN, respectively.

Table 2. Characterization of liposomal gentamicin and erythromycin.

Liposomal Antibiotics	Size (nm)	Polydispersity Index	Encapsulation Efficiency (%)	Concentration (mg/mL)
Gentamicin	562.67 ± 33.74	0.7 ± 0.11	13.89 ± 1.545	0.42 ± 0.046
Erythromycin	3086.35 ± 553.95	0.6 ± 0.12	51.58 ± 2.846	10.32 ± 0.571

3.2. Determination of MICs, MBCs and MBECs

Liposomal antibiotics combined with PABN reduced MICs and MBCs in both strains by 4–32 fold as presented in Table 3. For instance, the MIC of PA11 was 256 mg/L for free GEN, 32 mg/L for liposomal GEN and 8 mg/L for liposomal GEN with PABN. Similar trends were observed for the MBCs. Liposomal formulations with PABN also eradicated biofilms and strongly reduced MBECs by 8–32 fold for GEN and 2–16 fold for ERY in both strains (Table 4). However, in PA11 no significant changes in MBEC were noticed after the addition of PABN to liposomal ERY. Additionally, the MIC values of PABN alone were 256 mg/L and 512 mg/L in PA01 and PA11, respectively, and the MBC in both strains was of 512 mg/L (not shown here). The MICs and MBCs for quality control laboratory strains were within the acceptable limits established by CLSI, Clinical and Laboratory Standards Institute (formerly NCCLS, National Committee for Clinical Laboratory Standards), as previously found in our group [61]. The liposomes containing PBS (control) had no antibacterial activity. Likewise, the combination of empty liposomes with free drug had no additive effect on the antibacterial activity of GEN and ERY.

Table 3. Free and liposomal antibiotics susceptibility of *P. aeruginosa* isolates.

Strains	MIC (mg/L) (MBC *(mg/L))				MIC (mg/L) (MBC * (mg/L))			
	Free GEN		Lipo GEN		Free ERY		Lipo ERY	
	−PABN	+PABN	−PABN	+PABN	−PABN	+PABN	−PABN	+PABN
PA 01	8 (32)	8 (16)	2 (4)	1 (2)	512 (512)	256 (256)	128 (128)	128 (128)
PA 11	256 (1024)	32 (128)	32 (128)	8 (32)	1024 (1024)	512 (512)	128 (256)	64(256)

* Minimum bactericidal concentrations are shown in parentheses.

Table 4. Efficacy of free and liposomal antibiotics against biofilms of *P. aeruginosa* isolates.

Strains	MBEC (mg/L)							
	Free GEN		Lipo GEN		Free ERY		Lipo ERY	
	−PABN	+PABN	−PABN	+PABN	−PABN	+PABN	−PABN	+PABN
PA 01	64	16	4	2	1024	1024	128	64
PA 11	1024	128	256	128	1024	512	512	512

3.3. Effects of Sub-Inhibitory Concentrations of Free and Liposomal Antibiotics on the Growth of P. aeruginosa Strains

Sub-inhibitory concentrations of 1/16 and 1/32 the MIC did not seem to significantly inhibit PA01 growth (Figure 1A–D). In PA11, 1/16 MIC for both free and liposomal antibiotic tests did not affect bacterial growth (Figure 1A′–D′). Concentrations of 1/16 and 1/32 the MIC were therefore chosen to study the effects of sub-inhibitory concentrations of antibiotics on virulence factors, motility and the production of QS molecules in both strains.

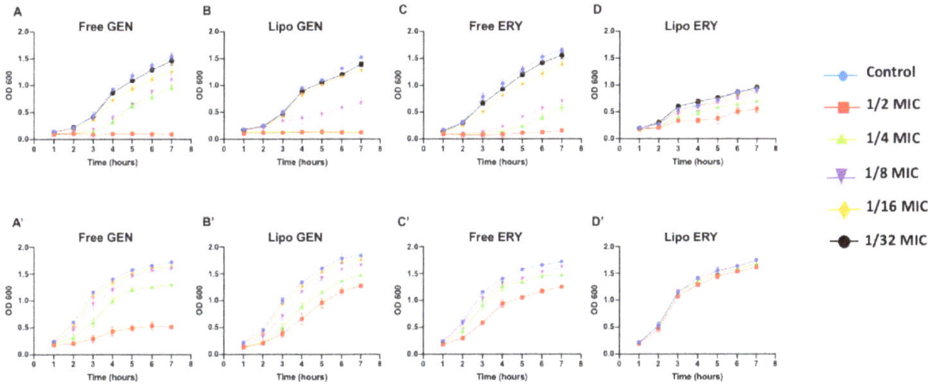

Figure 1. The effects of sub-inhibitory concentrations of free and liposomal gentamicin and erythromycin on the growth of PA01 and PA11 at 1/2, 1/4, 1/8, 1/16 and 1/32 the MIC. Shown are PA01 with free gentamicin (**A**), liposomal gentamicin (**B**), free erythromycin (**C**), liposomal erythromycin (**D**) and PA11 with free gentamicin (**A′**), liposomal gentamicin (**B′**), free erythromycin (**C′**) and liposomal erythromycin (**D′**).

3.4. Effect of Antibiotics and PABN on Bacterial Virulence Factors

Protease was significantly reduced by free erythromycin with and without PABN ($p < 0.001$) in both strains (Figure 2C,C′), liposomal erythromycin at 1/16 MIC with PABN in PA11 ($p < 0.01$) (Figure 2D′) and by PABN alone in PA01 ($p < 0.01$) (Figure 2E).

Only liposomal erythromycin combined with PABN seemed effective in significantly reducing pyocyanin production in PA01 ($p < 0.05$), as shown in Figure 3D. The reduction induced by free erythromycin (Figure 3C) seems considerable, but its significance appears to be prevented by variabilities in the control samples. Similarly, even though in Figure 3D the effects of 1/16 MIC and 1/16 MIC + P25 look identical, their respective values of 0.220 and 0.207 explain why the latter is significant while the other is not. No significant changes in the production of pyocyanin were noticed between the samples with and without PABN. It should be noted that the pyocyanin assay was only performed in PA01, as the strain PA11 did not appear to produce the compound.

Pyoverdine in PA01 was greatly reduced by free and liposomal erythromycin ($p < 0.001$) and free gentamicin ($p < 0.001$) with and without PABN and by PABN alone ($p < 0.001$) (Figure 4A,C–E). In PA11, pyoverdine was significantly lowered by free antibiotics with and without PABN ($p < 0.001$) (Figure 4A′,C′).

Finally, lipase production was significantly diminished by all our treatments in PA01 ($p < 0.05$, $p < 0.01$ and $p < 0.001$) (Figure 5A–E). In some instances, this effect was greater when PABN was added. Lipase production was also significantly reduced in PA11 by free and liposomal erythromycin ($p < 0.01$) and by free gentamicin ($p < 0.01$) in Figure 5A′,C′–E′. Furthermore, PABN alone was highly effective at reducing lipase in both strains ($p < 0.001$ in PA01 and $p < 0.05$ in PA11).

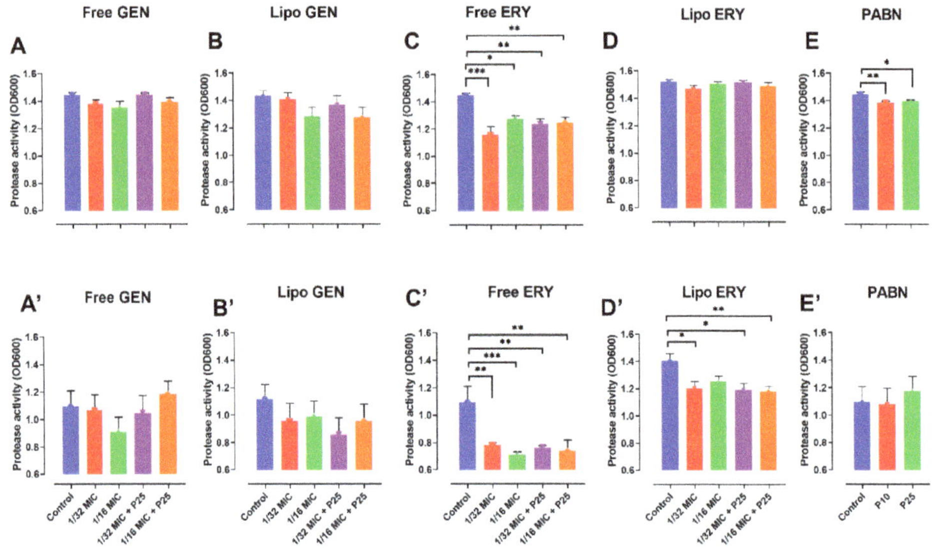

Figure 2. Effects of sub-inhibitory concentrations of free and liposomal gentamicin and erythromycin in the presence and absence of PABN on protease levels in PA01 and PA11. Shown are PA01 with free gentamicin (**A**), liposomal gentamicin (**B**), free erythromycin (**C**), liposomal erythromycin (**D**), PABN (**E**) and PA11 with free gentamicin (**A′**), liposomal gentamicin (**B′**), free erythromycin (**C′**), liposomal erythromycin (**D′**) and PABN (**E′**). The results represent the mean ± SEM of three independent experiments performed in triplicate. p values were considered significant when compared with the control and between groups: ***, $p < 0.001$; **, $p < 0.01$; *, $p < 0.05$. P10 and P25 correspond to PABN used at 10 and 25 mg/L, respectively.

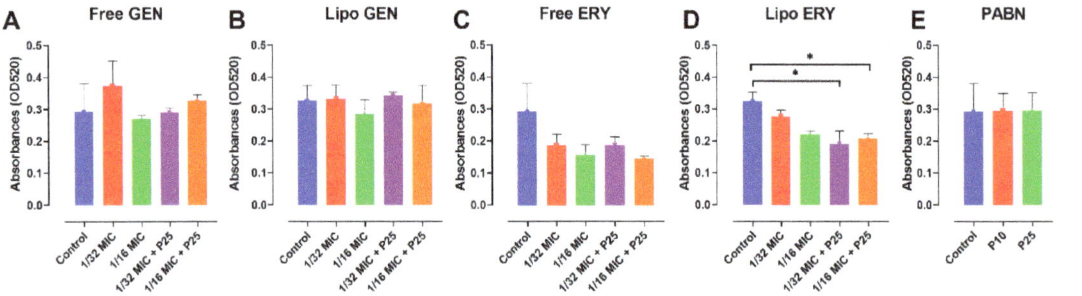

Figure 3. Effects of sub-inhibitory concentrations of free and liposomal gentamicin and erythromycin in the presence and absence of PABN on pyocyanin levels in PA01. Shown are PA01 with free gentamicin (**A**), liposomal gentamicin (**B**), free erythromycin (**C**), liposomal erythromycin (**D**) and PABN (**E**). The results represent the mean ± SEM of three independent experiments. p values were considered significant when compared with the control and between groups: *, $p < 0.05$. P10 and P25 correspond to PABN used at 10 and 25 mg/L, respectively.

3.5. Assessment of Quorum-Sensing Signal Production through a Beta-Galactosidase Assay

There were no statistically significant reductions observed in the levels of AHLs produced in both PA01 and PA11 from the β-galactosidase assay, as shown in Figure 6A–E′.

3.6. Effect of Antibiotics and PABN on Bacterial Motility

In PA01, twitching was significantly reduced at 1/16 MIC with PABN by liposomal gentamicin ($p < 0.01$) and liposomal erythromycin ($p < 0.001$) (Figure 7B,D). An example of the twitching motility is shown in Figure 8.

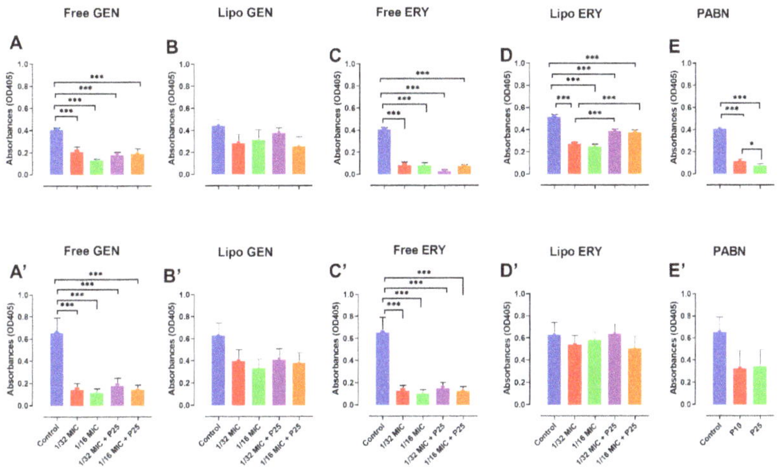

Figure 4. Effects of sub-inhibitory concentrations of free and liposomal gentamicin and erythromycin in the presence and absence of PABN on pyoverdine levels in PA01 and PA11. Shown are PA01 with free gentamicin (**A**), liposomal gentamicin (**B**), free erythromycin (**C**), liposomal erythromycin (**D**), PABN (**E**) and PA11 with free gentamicin (**A′**), liposomal gentamicin (**B′**), free erythromycin (**C′**), liposomal erythromycin (**D′**) and PABN (**E′**). The results represent the mean ± SEM of three independent experiments performed in triplicate. *p* values were considered significant when compared with the control and between groups: ***, $p < 0.001$; *, $p < 0.05$. P10 and P25 correspond to PABN used at 10 and 25 mg/L, respectively.

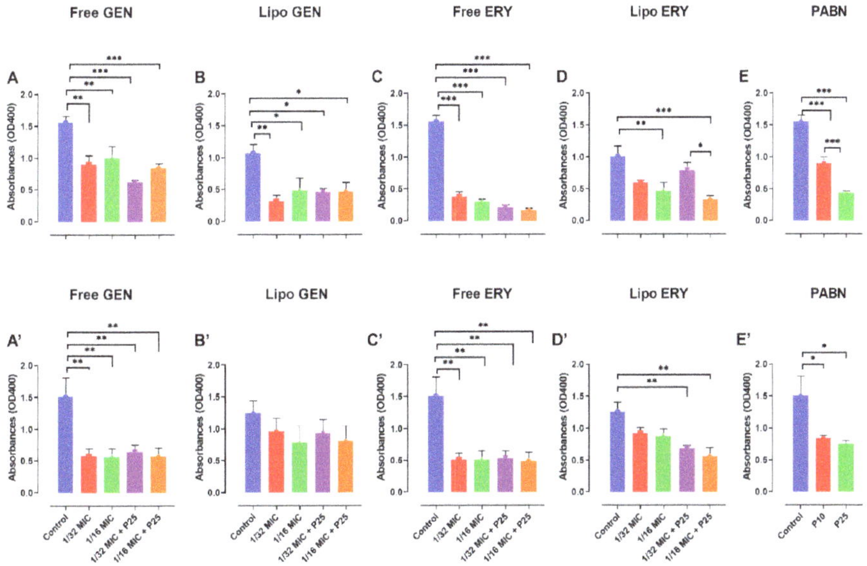

Figure 5. Effects of sub-inhibitory concentrations of free and liposomal gentamicin and erythromycin in the presence and absence of PABN on lipase levels in PA01 and PA11. Shown are PA01 with free gentamicin (**A**), liposomal gentamicin (**B**), free erythromycin (**C**), liposomal erythromycin (**D**), PABN (**E**) and PA11 with free gentamicin (**A′**), liposomal gentamicin (**B′**), free erythromycin (**C′**), liposomal erythromycin (**D′**) and PABN (**E′**). The results represent the mean ± SEM of three independent experiments performed in triplicate. *p* values were considered significant when compared with the control and between groups: ***, $p < 0.001$; **, $p < 0.01$; *, $p < 0.05$. P10 and P25 correspond to PABN used at 10 and 25 mg/L, respectively.

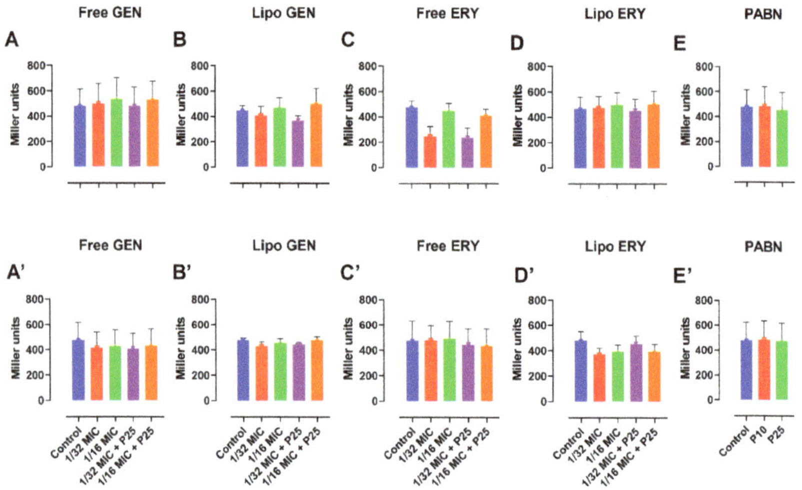

Figure 6. Effects of sub-inhibitory concentrations of free and liposomal gentamicin and erythromycin in the presence and absence of PABN on quorum sensing signals in PA01 and PA11. Shown are PA01 with free gentamicin (**A**), free erythromycin (**B**), liposomal gentamicin (**C**), liposomal erythromycin (**D**), PABN (**E**) and PA11 with free gentamicin (**A'**), free erythromycin (**B'**), liposomal gentamicin (**C'**), liposomal erythromycin (**D'**) and PABN (**E'**). The results represent the mean ± SEM of three independent experiments performed in triplicate. P10 and P25 correspond to PABN used at 10 and 25 mg/L, respectively.

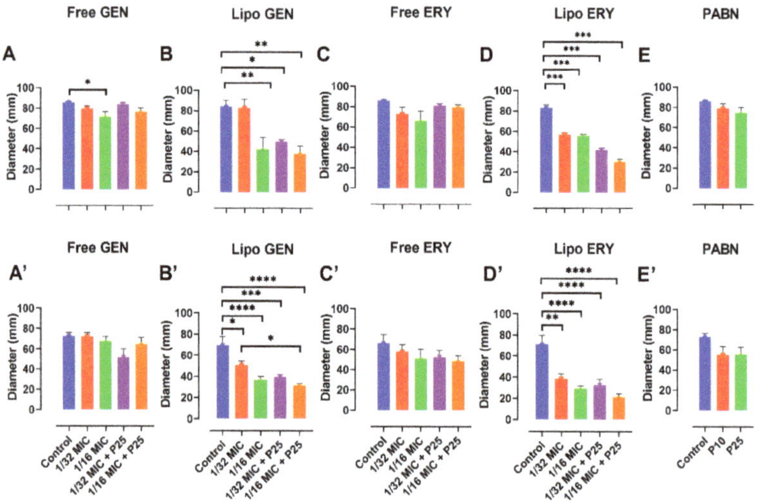

Figure 7. Impact of sub-inhibitory concentrations of free and liposomal gentamicin and erythromycin with PABN on PA01 and PA11 twitching motility. Twitching was examined with free and liposomal antibiotics at 1/16 and 1/32 the MIC in the presence and absence of PABN (10 and 25 mg/L). Shown are PA01 with free gentamicin (**A**), liposomal gentamicin (**B**), free erythromycin (**C**), liposomal erythromycin (**D**), PABN (**E**) and PA11 with free gentamicin (**A'**), liposomal gentamicin (**B'**), free erythromycin (**C'**), liposomal erythromycin (**D'**) and PABN (**E'**). The results are represented as the mean ± SEM of three independent experiments in triplicates. *p* values were considered significant compared with the control and between groups: ****, $p < 0.0001$; ***, $p < 0.001$; **, $p < 0.01$; *, $p < 0.05$. P10 and P25 correspond to PABN used at 10 and 25 mg/L, respectively.

Swarming and swimming were also considerably inhibited by all formulations ($p < 0.05$, $p < 0.01$ and $p < 0.001$) (Figure 9A–E and Figure 10A–E). In PA11, only liposomal gentamicin and erythromycin significantly inhibited twitching ($p < 0.0001$) at 1/16 MIC with and without PABN (Figure 7B',D'). Swarming was strongly inhibited by liposomal antibiotics at 1/16 MIC ($p < 0.0001$), free erythromycin with PABN ($p < 0.05$) and PABN alone ($p < 0.05$ and $p < 0.01$) (Figure 9B′–E′). Finally, swimming was significantly reduced by liposomal gentamicin and erythromycin with PABN ($p < 0.01$ and $p < 0.0001$, respectively) and by free erythromycin at 1/16 MIC ($p < 0.05$) (Figure 10B′–D′).

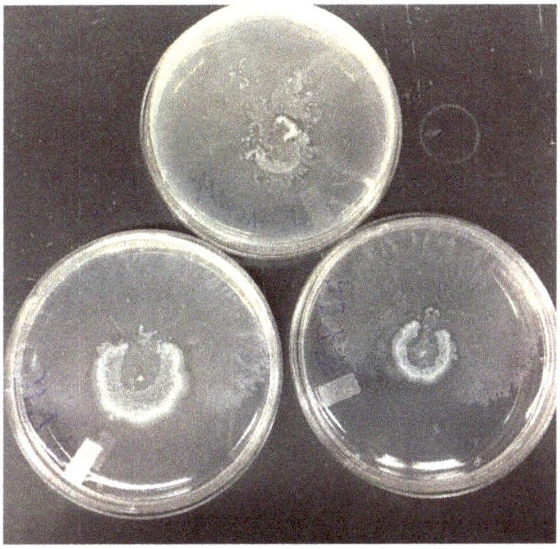

Figure 8. Twitching motility of PA11 with PABN at 10 and 25 mg/L. This picture shows an example of twitching motility observed with one of our strains. For consistency, the largest value for the diameters was used during the motility studies.

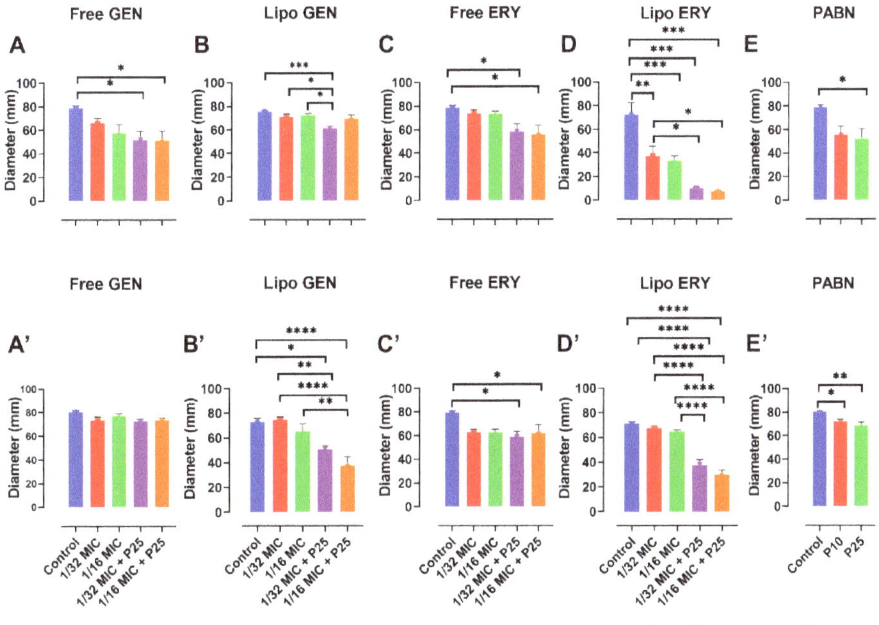

Figure 9. Impact of sub-inhibitory concentrations of free and liposomal gentamicin and erythromycin with PABN on PA01 and PA11 swarming motility. Swarming was examined with free and liposomal antibiotics at 1/16 and 1/32 the MIC in the presence and absence of PABN (10 and 25 mg/L). Shown are PA01 with free gentamicin (**A**), liposomal gentamicin (**B**), free erythromycin (**C**), liposomal erythromycin (**D**), PABN (**E**) and PA11 with free gentamicin (**A′**), liposomal gentamicin (**B′**), free

erythromycin (**C′**), liposomal erythromycin (**D′**) and PABN (**E′**). The results are represented as the mean ± SEM of three independent experiments in triplicates. *p* values were considered significant compared with the control and between groups: ****, $p < 0.0001$; ***, $p < 0.001$; **, $p < 0.01$; *, $p < 0.05$. P10 and P25 correspond to PABN used at 10 and 25 mg/L, respectively.

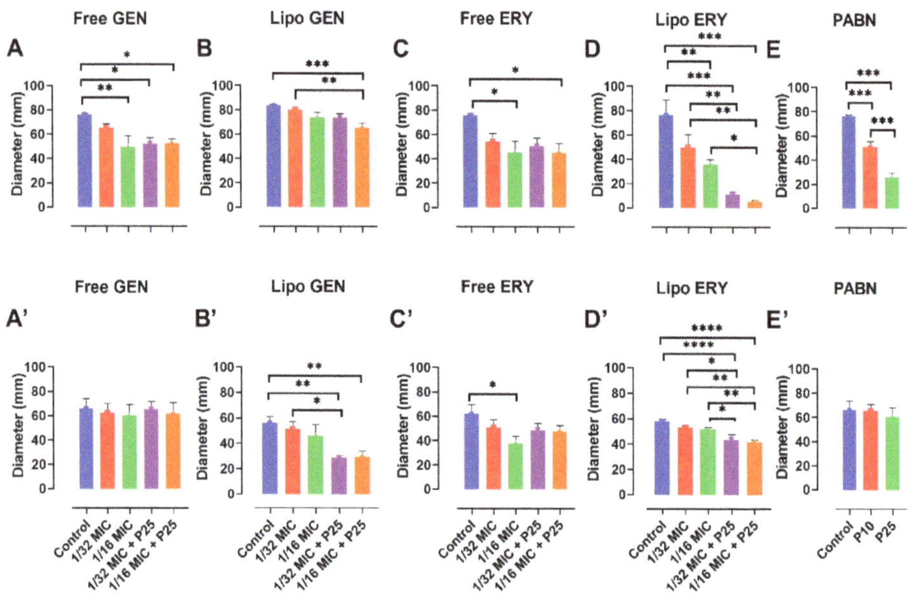

Figure 10. Impact of sub-inhibitory concentrations of free and liposomal gentamicin and erythromycin with PABN on PA01 and PA11 swimming motility. Swimming was examined with free and liposomal antibiotics at 1/16 and 1/32 the MIC in the presence and absence of PABN (10 and 25 mg/L). Shown are PA01 with free gentamicin (**A**), liposomal gentamicin (**B**), free erythromycin (**C**), liposomal erythromycin (**D**), PABN (**E**) and PA11 with free gentamicin (**A′**), liposomal gentamicin (**B′**), free erythromycin (**C′**), liposomal erythromycin (**D′**) and PABN (**E′**). The results are represented as the mean ± SEM of three independent experiments in triplicates. *p* values were considered significant compared with the control and between groups: ****, $p < 0.0001$; ***, $p < 0.001$; **, $p < 0.01$; *, $p < 0.05$. P10 and P25 correspond to PABN used at 10 and 25 mg/L, respectively.

4. Discussion

In the present study, liposomal gentamicin and erythromycin composed of DPPC-cholesterol were prepared by the DRV method in an attempt to increase their antimicrobial activity against resistant strains of *P. aeruginosa*. The polydispersity indexes indicate that our liposomal samples were fairly heterogeneous overall. Liposomal gentamicin showed superior EE than previous studies that reported values of 4.51% with DMPC-cholesterol and 1.8% with DPPC-cholesterol, respectively, for gentamicin [50,62]. Similarly, our EE for erythromycin was higher than earlier studies with erythromycin (32.06%) [53] and other macrolides such as azithromycin (23.08%) [52] and clarithromycin (15.96%) [51]. The direct dissolution of erythromycin in the organic solution with lipids due to its lipophilic nature, combined with an increased sonication time in our method (5 min vs. 30 min), might be behind these results. In fact, increased sonication time was shown to enhance drug EEs [63].

Liposomal formulations showed enhanced inhibitory and bactericidal activities against *P. aeruginosa* in comparison to free drugs. Indeed, bacteria went from resistant to intermediate or susceptible to treatments. Similar observations were reported by earlier studies with liposomal aminoglycosides and macrolides, showing that liposomes increased bacterial killing of free antibiotics [18,50,62,64,65]. Liposomes' increased activity was proposed to be the result of their fusion, disruption of the bacterial cell membrane and the subsequent intracellular uptake of their content [61,64]. When added, PABN further decreased

MICs and MBCs especially in PA11, suggesting that efflux pumps could be one of the main resistance mechanisms in this strain. The ability of PABN to inhibit efflux pumps in *P. aeruginosa* was evaluated by Lamers and coworkers as well through a fluorescence assay, with a fluorescent probe that is also an efflux substrate. The probe's fluorescence is only observed when it is bound to nucleic acids inside cells. PABN caused significant increases in fluorescence by 23–32% at 25 mg/L, indicating its significant inhibition of efflux in those strains [44]. We expect similar reductions in efflux activity in our strains treated with PABN, although further studies are needed to confirm this. Liposomes and PABN considerably reduced MBECs in both strains. Our results extend the findings of Ye et al. and Bandara et al., who found that tobramycin/clarithromycin proliposomes and liposomal ciprofloxacin, respectively, significantly eradicated *P. aeruginosa* biofilms when compared to free drugs [65,66]. Furthermore, Halwani et al. demonstrated that liposomal gentamicin co-encapsulated with gallium completely eradicated *P. aeruginosa* biofilms in vitro [54]. Similarly, Ferrer et al. reported that efflux pump inhibitors such as PABN combined with membrane permeabilizing peptides render *P. aeruginosa* strains that are overexpressing MexAB-OprM pumps more sensitive to antibiotics [42]. This strategy is interesting as it is believed to considerably reduce the associated toxicity of EPIs such as PABN. The minimum biofilm eradication concentration (MBIC) is the lowest concentration of an antimicrobial substance that induces no time dependent increase in the mean number of biofilm viable cells. It is commonly used to assess the inhibitory effects of formulations on biofilms [67]. It could be useful for future studies to determine the MBIC to fully and accurately determine the effects of our formulations on *P. aeruginosa* biofilms.

Virulence factors were reduced by most of our formulations to various extents, especially by free and liposomal erythromycin. This might account for the role of macrolides in the attenuation of *P. aeruginosa* inflammation at sub-inhibitory concentrations through the inhibition of virulence factors among other mechanisms [68,69]. Khan et al. also showed that free aminoglycosides including gentamicin significantly inhibited virulence factors such as pyoverdine, protease and pyocyanin in *P. aeruginosa* strains [7,70]. Earlier studies demonstrated an increased inhibitory activity of liposomal antibiotics on protease, elastase, lipase and chitinase production [47,51,52]. In contrast, our liposomal formulations did not appear to show superior activity overall against *P. aeruginosa* virulence factors. However, even in those instances liposomes are still of interest since studies have demonstrated their reduced toxicity and enhanced distribution in vivo [18]. Our results compare well with El-Shaer et al., who found that PABN alone reduced virulence factors in *P. aeruginosa* [43]. The results also extend the findings of Giordano et al., who indicated that PABN has a profound impact on *P. aeruginosa* transcriptome and affects virulence factors differentially [71].

Unexpectedly, none of our treatments showed significant reductions in the production of AHLs in both strains, even though virulence factors controlled by QS seemed to have been reduced. Similar studies report a reduction in QS signal levels in *P. aeruginosa* by sub-inhibitory concentrations of antibiotics or adjuvants [72–75]. El-Shaer et al., for example, reported a reduction in QS signals with PABN alone in *P. aeruginosa* strains isolated from urinary tract and wound infections [43]. However, this effect was not observed for all their strains, as C_4-HSL levels in wound isolates were unchanged and the level of reduction reported varied significantly between strains. This suggests a strain-dependant activity of PABN which might explain the differences in our results. It is also possible our treatments affected the detection (signal/receptor interaction) and/or the transport of autoinducers as well as reduced the expression of virulence genes. For instance, Khan et al. recently showed through an in silico docking analysis that aminoglycosides interact with *P. aeruginosa* QS receptor LasR. They proposed this to be a mechanism by which they inhibit QS associated virulence factors in the bacterium, as it prevents the binding of LasR receptor to $3OC_{12}$-HSL signals [7]. Furthermore, Burr et al. reported that sub-inhibitory concentrations of erythromycin strongly inhibited the expression of *P. aeruginosa* QS genes such as LasR and PqsA in non-CF bronchiectasis airways [69]. Similarly, El-Shaer and coworkers showed that PABN reduced the expression of QS genes such as LasI/R (with more specificity for

LasR), RhlI/R and PqsA/R as well as virulence genes, suggesting again an activity of PABN on *P. aeruginosa* transcription, beyond efflux inhibition [43]. Interestingly, Giordano et al. found that PABN enhanced the transcription of *qteE*, a gene coding for a protein that inhibits the activity of $3OC_{12}$-HSL receptor, LasR [71]. Numerous lines of evidence also demonstrated the involvement of efflux pumps in the transport of some autoinducers. Indeed, the MexAB-OprM pump is implicated in the efflux of $3OC_{12}$-HSL and QS-regulated factors are affected by its activity [21]. Furthermore, MexEF-OprN and MexGHI-OpmD pumps were shown to export precursors of the PQS signals, facilitate QS and bacterial growth and to promote virulence [76–78]. It is therefore possible that by inhibiting efflux pumps, PABN could have affected the transport of some autoinducers. This could result in less signals being transported and detected, and therefore lead to a reduced expression of QS related genes like virulence factors and motility [43].

In *P. aeruginosa*, twitching is modulated by type IV pili and is evident on solid surfaces [79], while swarming is a coordinated group movement on semi-solid surfaces that requires both flagella and type IV pili, and as such, it is regulated by QS [80]. Swimming, on the other hand, occurs in a liquid environment and also requires the use of flagella [79,81]. All those motilities play a determining role in bacterial attachment, colonization and their ability to cause widespread infections [7]. Motilities in bacteria were significantly reduced by our formulations to various extents. However, liposomal antibiotics proved to be more efficacious, especially in PA11. It was found that PABN alone inhibited motilities in *P. aeruginosa* [43]. Our results are also supported by previous studies which showed that erythromycin inhibited swarming in *P. aeruginosa* and that azithromycin and gentamicin inhibited twitching and swarming in PA01 [82,83]. The former study explained that macrolides inhibit flagellin expression in the bacteria, which is needed for the production of flagella, used in swarming and swimming.

5. Conclusions

Adjuvant therapy is an interesting strategy to revitalize the activity of old antibiotics. Indeed, liposomal gentamicin and erythromycin combined with PABN proved efficacious overall in inhibiting *P. aeruginosa* growth, eradicating biofilms and reducing the production of virulence factors and motility, even though the production of QS autoinducers did not appear to be affected. This suggests a possible impairment of the detection and/or transport of QS signals by our formulations, which should be confirmed through molecular studies. Furthermore, in vivo studies are needed to fully appreciate the impact of our treatments on the course of an infection in biological systems. Liposomal gentamicin and erythromycin with PABN therefore show potential in the management of *P. aeruginosa* infections in cystic fibrosis patients.

Author Contributions: Conceptualization, A.O. Writing—original draft preparation, D.L.G. Writing—review and editing, A.O. and D.L.G.; Supervision, A.O. Project administration, A.O.; Funding acquisition, A.O. Both authors have read and agreed to the published version of the manuscript.

Funding: This work was partially supported by the Laurentian University Research Fund (LURF).

Institutional Review Board Statement: Not applicable.

Informed Consent Statement: Not applicable.

Data Availability Statement: Not applicable.

Conflicts of Interest: The authors declare no conflict of interest.

References

1. Malhotra, S.; Hayes, D.; Wozniak, D.J. Mucoid Pseudomonas Aeruginosa and Regional Inflammation in the Cystic Fibrosis Lung. *J. Cyst. Fibros.* **2019**, *18*, 796–803. [CrossRef]
2. Abdelghany, S.M.; Quinn, D.J.; Ingram, R.J.; Gilmore, B.F.; Donnelly, R.F.; Taggart, C.C.; Scott, C.J. Gentamicin-Loaded Nanoparticles Show Improved Antimicrobial Effects towards Pseudomonas Aeruginosa Infection. *Int. J. Nanomed.* **2012**, *7*, 4053–4063. [CrossRef]

3. Magalhães, A.P.; Azevedo, N.F.; Pereira, M.O.; Lopes, S.P. The Cystic Fibrosis Microbiome in an Ecological Perspective and Its Impact in Antibiotic Therapy. *Appl. Microbiol. Biotechnol.* **2016**, *100*, 1163–1181. [CrossRef]
4. López-Causapé, C.; Rubio, R.; Cabot, G.; Oliver, A. Evolution of the Pseudomonas Aeruginosa Aminoglycoside Mutational Resistome In Vitro and in the Cystic Fibrosis Setting. *Antimicrob. Agents Chemother.* **2018**, *62*, e02583-17. [CrossRef] [PubMed]
5. Bassetti, M.; Castaldo, N.; Cattelan, A.; Mussini, C.; Righi, E.; Tascini, C.; Menichetti, F.; Mastroianni, C.M.; Tumbarello, M.; Grossi, P.; et al. Ceftolozane/Tazobactam for the Treatment of Serious Pseudomonas Aeruginosa Infections: A Multicentre Nationwide Clinical Experience. *Int. J. Antimicrob. Agents* **2019**, *53*, 408–415. [CrossRef] [PubMed]
6. Juhas, M.; Widlake, E.; Teo, J.; Huseby, D.L.; Tyrrell, J.M.; Polikanov, Y.S.; Ercan, O.; Petersson, A.; Cao, S.; Aboklaish, A.F.; et al. In Vitro Activity of Apramycin against Multidrug-, Carbapenem- and Aminoglycoside-Resistant Enterobacteriaceae and Acinetobacter Baumannii. *J. Antimicrob. Chemother.* **2019**, *74*, 944–952. [CrossRef] [PubMed]
7. Khan, F.; Lee, J.-W.; Javaid, A.; Park, S.-K.; Kim, Y.-M. Inhibition of Biofilm and Virulence Properties of Pseudomonas Aeruginosa by Sub-Inhibitory Concentrations of Aminoglycosides. *Microb. Pathog.* **2020**, *146*, 104249. [CrossRef]
8. Hoshino, K.; Imai, Y.; Mukai, K.; Hamauzu, R.; Ochi, K.; Hosaka, T. A Putative Mechanism Underlying Secondary Metabolite Overproduction by Streptomyces Strains with a 23S RRNA Mutation Conferring Erythromycin Resistance. *Appl. Microbiol. Biotechnol.* **2020**, *104*, 2193–2203. [CrossRef]
9. Chalmers, J.D.; Boersma, W.; Lonergan, M.; Jayaram, L.; Crichton, M.L.; Karalus, N.; Taylor, S.L.; Martin, M.L.; Burr, L.D.; Wong, C.; et al. Long-Term Macrolide Antibiotics for the Treatment of Bronchiectasis in Adults: An Individual Participant Data Meta-Analysis. *Lancet Respir. Med.* **2019**, *7*, 845–854. [CrossRef]
10. Mayer-Hamblett, N.; Retsch-Bogart, G.; Kloster, M.; Accurso, F.; Rosenfeld, M.; Albers, G.; Black, P.; Brown, P.; Cairns, A.; Davis, S.D.; et al. Azithromycin for Early Pseudomonas Infection in Cystic Fibrosis. The OPTIMIZE Randomized Trial. *Am. J. Respir. Crit. Care Med.* **2018**, *198*, 1177–1187. [CrossRef]
11. Lababidi, N.; Ofosu Kissi, E.; Elgaher, W.A.M.; Sigal, V.; Haupenthal, J.; Schwarz, B.C.; Hirsch, A.K.H.; Rades, T.; Schneider, M. Spray-Drying of Inhalable, Multifunctional Formulations for the Treatment of Biofilms Formed in Cystic Fibrosis. *J. Control. Release* **2019**, *314*, 62–71. [CrossRef] [PubMed]
12. Belotti, S.; Rossi, A.; Colombo, P.; Bettini, R.; Rekkas, D.; Politis, S.; Colombo, G.; Balducci, A.G.; Buttini, F. Spray Dried Amikacin Powder for Inhalation in Cystic Fibrosis Patients: A Quality by Design Approach for Product Construction. *Int. J. Pharm.* **2014**, *471*, 507–515. [CrossRef] [PubMed]
13. Kordes, A.; Preusse, M.; Willger, S.D.; Braubach, P.; Jonigk, D.; Haverich, A.; Warnecke, G.; Häussler, S. Genetically Diverse Pseudomonas Aeruginosa Populations Display Similar Transcriptomic Profiles in a Cystic Fibrosis Explanted Lung. *Nat. Commun.* **2019**, *10*, 1–10. [CrossRef]
14. Sonnleitner, E.; Pusic, P.; Wolfinger, M.T.; Bläsi, U. Distinctive Regulation of Carbapenem Susceptibility in Pseudomonas Aeruginosa by Hfq. *Front. Microbiol.* **2020**, *11*, 1001. [CrossRef]
15. Abbasi, F.; Yusefi, S.; Yavar, S.A. Minimum Inhibitory Concentration of Ciprofloxacin against Pseudomonas Aeruginosa in the Presence of the Efflux Inhibitor Phenylalanine-Arginine Beta-Naphthylamide. *Intern. Med. Med. Investig. J.* **2018**, *3*. [CrossRef]
16. Pu, Y.; Ke, Y.; Bai, F. Active Efflux in Dormant Bacterial Cells – New Insights into Antibiotic Persistence. *Drug Resist. Updat.* **2017**, *30*, 7–14. [CrossRef] [PubMed]
17. Pang, Z.; Raudonis, R.; Glick, B.R.; Lin, T.-J.; Cheng, Z. Antibiotic Resistance in Pseudomonas Aeruginosa: Mechanisms and Alternative Therapeutic Strategies. *Biotechnol. Adv.* **2019**, *37*, 177–192. [CrossRef] [PubMed]
18. Sans-Serramitjana, E.; Jorba, M.; Fusté, E.; Pedraz, J.L.; Vinuesa, T.; Viñas, M. Free and Nanoencapsulated Tobramycin: Effects on Planktonic and Biofilm Forms of Pseudomonas. *Microorganisms* **2017**, *5*, 35. [CrossRef] [PubMed]
19. Tetard, A.; Zedet, A.; Girard, C.; Plésiat, P.; Llanes, C. Cinnamaldehyde Induces Expression of Efflux Pumps and Multidrug Resistance in Pseudomonas Aeruginosa. *Antimicrob. Agents Chemother.* **2019**, *63*, e01081-19. [CrossRef]
20. Tafti, F.A.; Eslami, G.; Zandi, H.; Barzegar, K. Mutations in Nalc Gene of Mex AB-OprM Efflux Pump in Carbapenem Resistant Pseudomonas Aeruginosa Isolated from Burn Wounds in Yazd, Iran. *Iran J. Microbiol.* **2020**, *12*, 32–36.
21. Minagawa, S.; Inami, H.; Kato, T.; Sawada, S.; Yasuki, T.; Miyairi, S.; Horikawa, M.; Okuda, J.; Gotoh, N. RND Type Efflux Pump System MexAB-OprM of Pseudomonas Aeruginosa Selects Bacterial Languages, 3-Oxo-Acyl-Homoserine Lactones, for Cell-to-Cell Communication. *BMC Microbiol.* **2012**, *12*, 70. [CrossRef] [PubMed]
22. Singh, M.; Sykes, E.M.; Li, Y.; Kumar, A. MexXY RND Pump of Pseudomonas Aeruginosa PA7 Effluxes Bi-Anionic β-Lactams Carbenicillin and Sulbenicillin When It Partners with the Outer Membrane Factor OprA but Not with OprM. *Microbiology* **2020**, *166*, 1095–1106. [CrossRef]
23. Seupt, A.; Schniederjans, M.; Tomasch, J.; Häussler, S. Expression of the MexXY Aminoglycoside Efflux Pump and Presence of an Aminoglycoside-Modifying Enzyme in Clinical Pseudomonas Aeruginosa Isolates Are Highly Correlated. *Antimicrob. Agents Chemother.* **2020**, *65*, e01166-20. [CrossRef] [PubMed]
24. Puja, H.; Bolard, A.; Noguès, A.; Plésiat, P.; Jeannot, K. The Efflux Pump MexXY/OprM Contributes to the Tolerance and Acquired Resistance of Pseudomonas Aeruginosa to Colistin. *Antimicrob. Agents Chemother.* **2020**, *64*, e02033-19. [CrossRef]
25. Cruz, R.L.; Asfahl, K.L.; Van den Bossche, S.; Coenye, T.; Crabbé, A.; Dandekar, A.A. RhlR-Regulated Acyl-Homoserine Lactone Quorum Sensing in a Cystic Fibrosis Isolate of Pseudomonas Aeruginosa. *mBio* **2020**, *11*, e00532-20. [CrossRef]
26. Gökalsın, B.; Aksoydan, B.; Erman, B.; Sesal, N.C. Reducing Virulence and Biofilm of Pseudomonas Aeruginosa by Potential Quorum Sensing Inhibitor Carotenoid: Zeaxanthin. *Microb. Ecol.* **2017**, *74*, 466–473. [CrossRef]

27. Karthick Raja Namasivayam, S.; Angel, J.; Bharani, R.S.A.; Nachiyar, C.V. Terminalia Chebula and Ficus Racemosa Principles Mediated Repression of Novel Drug Target Las R—The Transcriptional Regulator and Its Controlled Virulence Factors Produced by Multiple Drug Resistant Pseudomonas Aeruginosa—Biocompatible Formulation against Drug Resistant Bacteria. *Microb. Pathog.* **2020**, *148*, 104412. [CrossRef]
28. Ahmed, T.; Pattnaik, S.; Khan, M.B.; Ampasala, D.R.; Busi, S.; Sarma, V.V. Inhibition of Quorum Sensing–Associated Virulence Factors and Biofilm Formation in Pseudomonas Aeruginosa PAO1 by Mycoleptodiscus Indicus PUTY1. *Braz. J. Microbiol.* **2020**, *51*, 467–487. [CrossRef]
29. Mishra, R.; Kushveer, J.S.; Khan, M.I.K.; Pagal, S.; Meena, C.K.; Murali, A.; Dhayalan, A.; Venkateswara Sarma, V. 2,4-Di-Tert-Butylphenol Isolated From an Endophytic Fungus, Daldinia Eschscholtzii, Reduces Virulence and Quorum Sensing in Pseudomonas Aeruginosa. *Front. Microbiol.* **2020**, *11*, 1668. [CrossRef]
30. Armijo, L.M.; Wawrzyniec, S.J.; Kopciuch, M.; Brandt, Y.I.; Rivera, A.C.; Withers, N.J.; Cook, N.C.; Huber, D.L.; Monson, T.C.; Smyth, H.D.C.; et al. Antibacterial Activity of Iron Oxide, Iron Nitride, and Tobramycin Conjugated Nanoparticles against Pseudomonas Aeruginosa Biofilms. *J. Nanobiotechnol.* **2020**, *18*, 1–27. [CrossRef]
31. Bonneau, A.; Roche, B.; Schalk, I.J. Iron Acquisition in Pseudomonas Aeruginosa by the Siderophore Pyoverdine: An Intricate Interacting Network Including Periplasmic and Membrane Proteins. *Sci. Rep.* **2020**, *10*, 1–11. [CrossRef]
32. Harrington, N.E.; Sweeney, E.; Harrison, F. Building a Better Biofilm - Formation of in Vivo-like Biofilm Structures by Pseudomonas Aeruginosa in a Porcine Model of Cystic Fibrosis Lung Infection. *Biofilm* **2020**, *2*, 100024. [CrossRef]
33. Rojo-Molinero, E.; Macià, M.D.; Oliver, A. Social Behavior of Antibiotic Resistant Mutants Within Pseudomonas Aeruginosa Biofilm Communities. *Front. Microbiol.* **2019**, *10*, 570. [CrossRef] [PubMed]
34. O'Loughlin, C.T.; Miller, L.C.; Siryaporn, A.; Drescher, K.; Semmelhack, M.F.; Bassler, B.L. A Quorum-Sensing Inhibitor Blocks Pseudomonas Aeruginosa Virulence and Biofilm Formation. *Proc. Natl. Acad. Sci. USA* **2013**, *110*, 17981–17986. [CrossRef]
35. Malgaonkar, A.; Nair, M. Quorum Sensing in Pseudomonas Aeruginosa Mediated by RhlR Is Regulated by a Small RNA PhrD. *Sci. Rep.* **2019**, *9*, 1–11. [CrossRef]
36. Sankar Ganesh, P.; Ravishankar Rai, V. Attenuation of Quorum-Sensing-Dependent Virulence Factors and Biofilm Formation by Medicinal Plants against Antibiotic Resistant Pseudomonas Aeruginosa. *J. Tradit. Complement. Med.* **2018**, *8*, 170–177. [CrossRef]
37. Caldwell, C.C.; Chen, Y.; Goetzmann, H.S.; Hao, Y.; Borchers, M.T.; Hassett, D.J.; Young, L.R.; Mavrodi, D.; Thomashow, L.; Lau, G.W. Pseudomonas Aeruginosa Exotoxin Pyocyanin Causes Cystic Fibrosis Airway Pathogenesis. *Am. J. Pathol.* **2009**, *175*, 2473–2488. [CrossRef] [PubMed]
38. Managò, A.; Becker, K.A.; Carpinteiro, A.; Wilker, B.; Soddemann, M.; Seitz, A.P.; Edwards, M.J.; Grassmé, H.; Szabò, I.; Gulbins, E. Pseudomonas Aeruginosa Pyocyanin Induces Neutrophil Death via Mitochondrial Reactive Oxygen Species and Mitochondrial Acid Sphingomyelinase. *Antioxid. Redox Signal.* **2015**, *22*, 1097–1110. [CrossRef]
39. Du, D.; Wang-Kan, X.; Neuberger, A.; Van Veen, H.W.; Pos, K.M.; Piddock, L.J.V.; Luisi, B.F. Multidrug Efflux Pumps: Structure, Function and Regulation. *Nat. Rev. Microbiol.* **2018**, *16*, 523–539. [CrossRef]
40. Kirienko, D.R.; Kang, D.; Kirienko, N.V. Novel Pyoverdine Inhibitors Mitigate Pseudomonas Aeruginosa Pathogenesis. *Front. Microbiol.* **2019**, *9*, 3317. [CrossRef]
41. Kishk, R.M.; Abdalla, M.O.; Hashish, A.A.; Nemr, N.A.; El Nahhas, N.; Alkahtani, S.; Abdel-Daim, M.M.; Kishk, S.M. Efflux MexAB-Mediated Resistance in P. Aeruginosa Isolated from Patients with Healthcare Associated Infections. *Pathogens* **2020**, *9*, 471. [CrossRef]
42. Ferrer-Espada, R.; Shahrour, H.; Pitts, B.; Stewart, P.S.; Sánchez-Gómez, S.; Martínez-de-Tejada, G. A Permeability-Increasing Drug Synergizes with Bacterial Efflux Pump Inhibitors and Restores Susceptibility to Antibiotics in Multi-Drug Resistant Pseudomonas Aeruginosa Strains. *Sci. Rep.* **2019**, *9*, 1–12. [CrossRef]
43. El-Shaer, S.; Shaaban, M.; Barwa, R.; Hassan, R. Control of Quorum Sensing and Virulence Factors of Pseudomonas Aeruginosa Using Phenylalanine Arginyl β-Naphthylamide. *J. Med. Microbiol.* **2016**, *65*, 1194–1204. [CrossRef]
44. Lamers, R.P.; Cavallari, J.F.; Burrows, L.L. The Efflux Inhibitor Phenylalanine-Arginine Beta-Naphthylamide (PAβN) Permeabilizes the Outer Membrane of Gram-Negative Bacteria. *PLoS ONE* **2013**, *8*, e60666. [CrossRef]
45. Jadhav, M.; Kalhapure, R.S.; Rambharose, S.; Mocktar, C.; Singh, S.; Kodama, T.; Govender, T. Novel Lipids with Three C18-Fatty Acid Chains and an Amino Acid Head Group for PH-Responsive and Sustained Antibiotic Delivery. *Chem. Phys. Lipids* **2018**, *212*, 12–25. [CrossRef]
46. Obuobi, S.; Julin, K.; Fredheim, E.G.A.; Johannessen, M.; Škalko-Basnet, N. Liposomal Delivery of Antibiotic Loaded Nucleic Acid Nanogels with Enhanced Drug Loading and Synergistic Anti-Inflammatory Activity against *S. aureus* Intracellular Infections. *J. Control. Release* **2020**, *324*, 620–632. [CrossRef]
47. Alhariri, M.; Omri, A. Efficacy of Liposomal Bismuth-Ethanedithiol-Loaded Tobramycin after Intratracheal Administration in Rats with Pulmonary Pseudomonas Aeruginosa Infection. *Antimicrob. Agents Chemother.* **2013**, *57*, 569–578. [CrossRef]
48. Zhang, J.; Leifer, F.; Rose, S.; Chun, D.Y.; Thaisz, J.; Herr, T.; Nashed, M.; Joseph, J.; Perkins, W.R.; DiPetrillo, K. Amikacin Liposome Inhalation Suspension (ALIS) Penetrates Non-Tuberculous Mycobacterial Biofilms and Enhances Amikacin Uptake Into Macrophages. *Front. Microbiol.* **2018**, *9*, 915. [CrossRef]
49. Cipolla, D.; Blanchard, J.; Gonda, I. Development of Liposomal Ciprofloxacin to Treat Lung Infections. *Pharmaceutics* **2016**, *8*, 6. [CrossRef]

50. Rukholm, G.; Mugabe, C.; Azghani, A.O.; Omri, A. Antibacterial Activity of Liposomal Gentamicin against Pseudomonas Aeruginosa: A Time–Kill Study. *Int. J. Pharm.* **2006**, *27*, 247–252. [CrossRef]
51. Alhajlan, M.; Alhariri, M.; Omri, A. Efficacy and Safety of Liposomal Clarithromycin and Its Effect on Pseudomonas Aeruginosa Virulence Factors. *Antimicrob. Agents Chemother.* **2013**, *57*, 2694–2704. [CrossRef]
52. Solleti, V.S.; Alhariri, M.; Halwani, M.; Omri, A. Antimicrobial Properties of Liposomal Azithromycin for Pseudomonas Infections in Cystic Fibrosis Patients. *J. Antimicrob. Chemother.* **2015**, *70*, 784–796. [CrossRef]
53. Mugabe, C.; Azghani, A.O.; Omri, A. Preparation and Characterization of Dehydration–Rehydration Vesicles Loaded with Aminoglycoside and Macrolide Antibiotics. *Int. J. Pharm.* **2006**, *307*, 244–250. [CrossRef] [PubMed]
54. Halwani, M.; Yebio, B.; Suntres, Z.E.; Alipour, M.; Azghani, A.O.; Omri, A. Co-Encapsulation of Gallium with Gentamicin in Liposomes Enhances Antimicrobial Activity of Gentamicin against Pseudomonas Aeruginosa. *J. Antimicrob. Chemother.* **2008**, *62*, 1291–1297. [CrossRef] [PubMed]
55. Innovotech MBEC Assay®. Available online: https://www.innovotech.ca/products/mbec-assays/ (accessed on 17 April 2021).
56. Alipour, M.; Omri, A.; Suntres, Z.E. Ginseng Aqueous Extract Attenuates the Production of Virulence Factors, Stimulates Twitching and Adhesion, and Eradicates Biofilms of Pseudomonas Aeruginosa. *Can. J. Physiol. Pharmacol.* **2011**, *89*, 419–427. [CrossRef] [PubMed]
57. Alipour, M.; Suntres, Z.E.; Lafrenie, R.M.; Omri, A. Attenuation of Pseudomonas Aeruginosa Virulence Factors and Biofilms by Co-Encapsulation of Bismuth–Ethanedithiol with Tobramycin in Liposomes. *J. Antimicrob. Chemother.* **2010**, *65*, 684–693. [CrossRef]
58. Vasavi, H.S.; Sudeep, H.V.; Lingaraju, H.B.; Shyam Prasad, K. Bioavailability-Enhanced Resveramax™ Modulates Quorum Sensing and Inhibits Biofilm Formation in Pseudomonas Aeruginosa PAO1. *Microb. Pathog.* **2017**, *104*, 64–71. [CrossRef]
59. El-Mowafy, S.A.; Abd El Galil, K.H.; El-Messery, S.M.; Shaaban, M.I. Aspirin Is an Efficient Inhibitor of Quorum Sensing, Virulence and Toxins in Pseudomonas Aeruginosa. *Microb. Pathog.* **2014**, *74*, 25–32. [CrossRef]
60. Miller, J.H.; Miller, J.B. *Experiments in Molecular Genetics*; Bacterial genetics-*E. coli*; Cold Spring Harbor Laboratory: New York, NY, USA, 1972; ISBN 978-0-87969-106-6.
61. Mugabe, C.; Halwani, M.; Azghani, A.O.; Lafrenie, R.M.; Omri, A. Mechanism of Enhanced Activity of Liposome-Entrapped Aminoglycosides against Resistant Strains of Pseudomonas Aeruginosa. *Antimicrob. Agents Chemother.* **2006**, *50*, 2016–2022. [CrossRef]
62. Alhariri, M.; Majrashi, M.A.; Bahkali, A.H.; Almajed, F.S.; Azghani, A.O.; Khiyami, M.A.; Alyamani, E.J.; Aljohani, S.M.; Halwani, M.A. Efficacy of Neutral and Negatively Charged Liposome-Loaded Gentamicin on Planktonic Bacteria and Biofilm Communities. *Int. J. Nanomed.* **2017**, *12*, 6949–6961. [CrossRef]
63. He, Y.; Luo, L.; Liang, S.; Long, M.; Xu, H. Influence of Probe-Sonication Process on Drug Entrapment Efficiency of Liposomes Loaded with a Hydrophobic Drug. *Int. J. Polym. Mater.* **2019**, *68*, 193–197. [CrossRef]
64. Jia, Y.; Joly, H.; Omri, A. Characterization of the Interaction between Liposomal Formulations and Pseudomonas Aeruginosa. *J. Liposome Res.* **2010**, *20*, 134–146. [CrossRef]
65. Ye, T.; Sun, S.; Sugianto, T.D.; Tang, P.; Parumasivam, T.; Chang, Y.K.; Astudillo, A.; Wang, S.; Chan, H.-K. Novel Combination Proliposomes Containing Tobramycin and Clarithromycin Effective against Pseudomonas Aeruginosa Biofilms. *Int. J. Pharm.* **2018**, *552*, 130–138. [CrossRef]
66. Bandara, H.M.H.N.; Herpin, M.J.; Kolacny, D.; Harb, A.; Romanovicz, D.; Smyth, H.D.C. Incorporation of Farnesol Significantly Increases the Efficacy of Liposomal Ciprofloxacin against Pseudomonas Aeruginosa Biofilms in Vitro. *Mol. Pharm.* **2016**, *13*, 2760–2770. [CrossRef] [PubMed]
67. Thieme, L.; Hartung, A.; Tramm, K.; Klinger-Strobel, M.; Jandt, K.D.; Makarewicz, O.; Pletz, M.W. MBEC versus MBIC: The Lack of Differentiation between Biofilm Reducing and Inhibitory Effects as a Current Problem in Biofilm Methodology. *Biol. Proced. Online* **2019**, *21*, 1–5. [CrossRef]
68. Sandri, A.; Ortombina, A.; Boschi, F.; Cremonini, E.; Boaretti, M.; Sorio, C.; Melotti, P.; Bergamini, G.; Lleo, M. Inhibition of Pseudomonas Aeruginosa Secreted Virulence Factors Reduces Lung Inflammation in CF Mice. *Virulence* **2018**, *9*, 1008–1018. [CrossRef]
69. Burr, L.D.; Rogers, G.B.; Chen, A.C.-H.; Hamilton, B.R.; Pool, G.F.; Taylor, S.L.; Venter, D.; Bowler, S.D.; Biga, S.; McGuckin, M.A. Macrolide Treatment Inhibits Pseudomonas Aeruginosa Quorum Sensing in Non–Cystic Fibrosis Bronchiectasis. An Analysis from the Bronchiectasis and Low-Dose Erythromycin Study Trial. *Ann. Am. Thorac. Soc.* **2016**, *13*, 1697–1703. [PubMed]
70. Khan, F.; Lee, J.-W.; Pham, D.T.N.; Lee, J.-H.; Kim, H.-W.; Kim, Y.-K.; Kim, Y.-M. Streptomycin Mediated Biofilm Inhibition and Suppression of Virulence Properties in Pseudomonas Aeruginosa PAO1. *Appl. Microbiol. Biotechnol.* **2020**, *104*, 799–816. [CrossRef]
71. Rampioni, G.; Pillai, C.R.; Longo, F.; Bondì, R.; Baldelli, V.; Messina, M.; Imperi, F.; Visca, P.; Leoni, L. Effect of Efflux Pump Inhibition on Pseudomonas Aeruginosa Transcriptome and Virulence. *Sci. Rep.* **2017**, *7*, 1–14. [CrossRef]
72. Gupta, P.; Chhibber, S.; Harjai, K. Subinhibitory Concentration of Ciprofloxacin Targets Quorum Sensing System of Pseudomonas Aeruginosa Causing Inhibition of Biofilm Formation & Reduction of Virulence. *Indian J. Med. Res.* **2016**, *143*, 643–651. [CrossRef]
73. Kiymaci, M.E.; Altanlar, N.; Gumustas, M.; Ozkan, S.A.; Akin, A. Quorum Sensing Signals and Related Virulence Inhibition of Pseudomonas Aeruginosa by a Potential Probiotic Strain's Organic Acid. *Microb. Pathog.* **2018**, *121*, 190–197. [CrossRef]
74. El-Mowafy, S.A.; Galil, K.H.A.E.; Habib, E.-S.E.; Shaaban, M.I. Quorum Sensing Inhibitory Activity of Sub-Inhibitory Concentrations of β-Lactams. *Afr. Health Sci.* **2017**, *17*, 199–207. [CrossRef]

75. Nalca, Y.; Jänsch, L.; Bredenbruch, F.; Geffers, R.; Buer, J.; Häussler, S. Quorum-Sensing Antagonistic Activities of Azithromycin in Pseudomonas Aeruginosa PAO1: A Global Approach. *Antimicrob. Agents Chemother.* **2006**, *50*, 1680–1688. [CrossRef]
76. Alcalde-Rico, M.; Olivares-Pacheco, J.; Alvarez-Ortega, C.; Cámara, M.; Martínez, J.L. Role of the Multidrug Resistance Efflux Pump MexCD-OprJ in the Pseudomonas Aeruginosa Quorum Sensing Response. *Front. Microbiol.* **2018**, *9*, 2757. [CrossRef] [PubMed]
77. Lamarche, M.G.; Déziel, E. MexEF-OprN Efflux Pump Exports the Pseudomonas Quinolone Signal (PQS) Precursor HHQ (4-Hydroxy-2-Heptylquinoline). *PLoS ONE* **2011**, *6*, e24310. [CrossRef] [PubMed]
78. Aendekerk, S.; Diggle, S.P.; Song, Z.; Høiby, N.; Cornelis, P.; Williams, P.; Cámara, M. The MexGHI-OpmD Multidrug Efflux Pump Controls Growth, Antibiotic Susceptibility and Virulence in Pseudomonas Aeruginosa via 4-Quinolone-Dependent Cell-to-Cell Communication. *Microbiology* **2005**, *151*, 1113–1125. [CrossRef] [PubMed]
79. Xu, A.; Zhang, M.; Du, W.; Wang, D.; Ma, L.Z. A Molecular Mechanism for How Sigma Factor AlgT and Transcriptional Regulator AmrZ Inhibit Twitching Motility in Pseudomonas Aeruginosa. *Environ. Microbiol.* **2020**, *23*, 572–587. [CrossRef] [PubMed]
80. Dave, A.; Samarth, A.; Karolia, R.; Sharma, S.; Karunakaran, E.; Partridge, L.; MacNeil, S.; Monk, P.N.; Garg, P.; Roy, S. Characterization of Ocular Clinical Isolates of Pseudomonas Aeruginosa from Non-Contact Lens Related Keratitis Patients from South India. *Microorganisms* **2020**, *8*, 260. [CrossRef]
81. Lakshmanan, D.; Harikrishnan, A.; Jyoti, K.; Ali, M.I.; Jeevaratnam, K. A Compound Isolated from Alpinia Officinarum Hance. Inhibits Swarming Motility of Pseudomonas Aeruginosa and down Regulates Virulence Genes. *J. Appl. Microbiol.* **2020**, *128*, 1355–1365. [CrossRef]
82. Molinari, G.; Paglia, P.; Schito, G.C. Inhibition of Motility of Pseudomonas Aeruginosa and Proteus Mirabilis by Subinhibitory Concentrations of Azithromycin. *Eur. J. Clin. Microbiol. Infect. Dis.* **1992**, *11*, 469–471. [CrossRef]
83. Bahari, S.; Zeighami, H.; Mirshahabi, H.; Roudashti, S.; Haghi, F. Inhibition of Pseudomonas Aeruginosa Quorum Sensing by Subinhibitory Concentrations of Curcumin with Gentamicin and Azithromycin. *J. Glob. Antimicrob. Resist.* **2017**, *10*, 21–28. [CrossRef] [PubMed]

pharmaceutics MDPI

Review

Recent Advances in Hydrogel-Mediated Nitric Oxide Delivery Systems Targeted for Wound Healing Applications

Gina Tavares, Patrícia Alves * and Pedro Simões *

University of Coimbra, Chemical Process Engineering and Forest Products Research Centre, Department of Chemical Engineering, Rua Sílvio Lima, 3030-790 Coimbra, Portugal; ginatavares@eq.uc.pt
* Correspondence: palves@eq.uc.pt (P.A.); pnsim@eq.uc.pt (P.S.)

Abstract: Despite the noticeable evolution in wound treatment over the centuries, a functional material that promotes correct and swift wound healing is important, considering the relative weight of chronic wounds in healthcare. Difficult to heal in a fashionable time, chronic wounds are more prone to infections and complications thereof. Nitric oxide (NO) has been explored for wound healing applications due to its appealing properties, which in the wound healing context include vasodilation, angiogenesis promotion, cell proliferation, and antimicrobial activity. NO delivery is facilitated by molecules that release NO when prompted, whose stability is ensured using carriers. Hydrogels, popular materials for wound dressings, have been studied as scaffolds for NO storage and delivery, showing promising results such as enhanced wound healing, controlled and sustained NO release, and bactericidal properties. Systems reported so far regarding NO delivery by hydrogels are reviewed.

Keywords: Nitric oxide; hydrogel; wound dressing; chronic wounds

Citation: Tavares, G.; Alves, P.; Simões, P. Recent Advances in Hydrogel-Mediated Nitric Oxide Delivery Systems Targeted for Wound Healing Applications. *Pharmaceutics* **2022**, *14*, 1377. https://doi.org/10.3390/pharmaceutics14071377

Academic Editor: César Viseras

Received: 27 May 2022
Accepted: 27 June 2022
Published: 29 June 2022

1. Introduction—How Wound Care Is Still Relevant Nowadays

Wounds are ruptured and therefore structurally and physiologically compromised skin, caused by either trauma or physiological conditions. Depending on the time required to heal, wounds are typically categorized into acute or chronic [1]. Acute wounds tend to heal relatively fast, while chronic wounds take longer to properly heal. The latter most often arise from complications of specific diseases, with ulcers being the most common type of long-term wounds. Unfortunately, reoccurrence is a major issue in disease-caused chronic wounds, and it can only be avoided by the cure or management of the underlying disease [2]. Due to their high propensity to reappear, chronic wounds burden the healthcare system, and most importantly, negatively impact the quality of life of patients [3,4].

Chronic wounds (i.e., venous, arterial, pressure, and diabetic ulcers) have distinct causes but some characteristics in common, namely, infection, prolonged inflammatory phase, and biofilm formation. Cell abnormalities are also observed in chronic wounds, such as decreased growth factor receptors and reduced mitogenic potential, which impair cells from reacting to environmental signals [5]. These long-term wounds are more susceptible to infection, which further delays wound healing [6], and if left untreated, can cause impaired mobility, limb amputation, and eventually lead to death [7]. A study on the incidence of healthcare-associated infections in European Union countries, including Iceland, Norway, and the United Kingdom, during the period 2016–2017, showed that these infections easily exceeded 8 million per year, and over 3 million patients attained such infections each year at acute care hospitals [8]. Antimicrobial-resistant infections are responsible for large numbers of deaths (ca., 30,000 Europeans in 2020), and have been overshadowed by the still active coronavirus disease pandemic [9]. For further information regarding chronic wounds, we recommend reviews on this subject [4,5,7].

Wound healing is an elaborate cascade-like process that has four complex and overlapping phases (i.e., hemostasis, inflammation, proliferation, and remodeling [10]) that begin immediately after injury and last until re-epithelialization of the skin is completed [6,7] (Figure 1). Hemostasis starts immediately after injury and lasts between a few minutes to an hour. During this stage, platelets arrive to the wound bed, adhere to the extracellular matrix (ECM), and secrete proteins that initiate fibrin production and deposition, thus creating a clot that interrupts the bleeding. Throughout the process, these platelets also produce growth factors that attract neutrophils, macrophages, and fibroblasts to the wound bed. The next phase, inflammation, lasts for ca. 3 days, during which inflammation mediators increase the permeability of blood vessels and facilitate the arrival of neutrophils to the site. Neutrophils digest pathogens, foreign material, damaged cells, and ECM through phagocytosis. Once monocytes arrive and differentiate to macrophages, these instigate the proliferation of fibroblasts, smooth-muscle cells, and endothelial cells, hence beginning the proliferation stage. Starting around 48 h after injury, this phase consists of fibroblast proliferation, collagen and other ECM components production and deposition, and angiogenesis. The last phase, remodeling, starts 2–3 weeks after injury and can take several months to be completed. The ECM produced during the proliferation stage is remodeled by enzymes produced by fibroblasts, and lastly, macrophages and fibroblasts depart the wound site, ceasing the inflammation and proliferation stages [1,7].

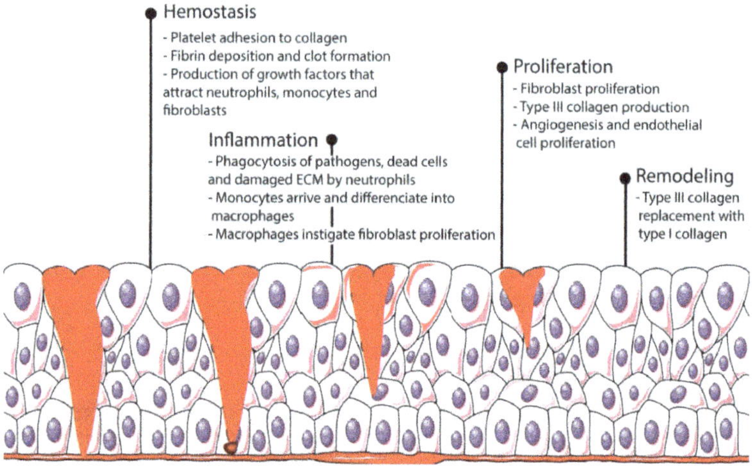

Figure 1. Schematic representation of the wound healing process.

Any imbalance in the process leads to impaired healing and chronic wound development. For instance, bacteria propagation enhances the inflammatory response and deeply compromises angiogenesis, thus impacting the amount of oxygen and nutrients capable of reaching the wound bed [10]. The evolution to chronic wounds can be prevented though a simple wound care regiment. Wound care is essentially performed in two steps: debridement and wound coverage. Debridement is the cleaning of the wound through removal of tissue debris that would otherwise be fuel for microbial proliferation and allows the exposure of healthy tissue to facilitate its proliferation [4,11]. The next step is the physical protection of the wound through the application of wound dressings.

Wound dressings are materials designed to cover damaged skin and are primarily meant to promote the wound healing process by acting as a pathogen penetration barrier while keeping the wound site moist through the absorption of excess exudate [12–14]. Moisture retention contributes to a proper and swift wound closure process as it aids the migration of new skin cells [4,15]. Deficient or excess exudate absorption is detrimental for proper wound healing as it leads to a microbial-friendly environment or dry wound site, respectively. Exudate levels differ during the healing stages, with high levels for the first 48 h [16]; thus, the main guideline is that wound dressings should ideally only absorb excess exudate without compromising the healing process [4]. Comparatively to normal skin, water loss is higher in wounds, reaching up to 5000 $g \cdot m^{-2}d^{-1}$, around 20-fold the water loss of normal skin when at 35 °C. It has been disclosed that wound healing benefits from water vapor transmission values of around 2000–2500 $g \cdot m^{-2}d^{-1}$ [17].

Since traditional wound dressings implicate constant reapplication and complementary methods to keep the wound aseptic, the development of wound dressings with attributes relevant for wound healing has been encouraged. Most research focuses on infection prevention, but besides antimicrobial properties, wound dressings can also be complemented with drugs or other components that accelerate the healing process, such as growth factors [18], anti-inflammatory drugs, and cytokines [19]. Growth factors, which are at low levels in chronic wounds, contribute to wound healing through the performance of several functions, including chemoattraction of macrophages, fibroblasts, and other cells; angiogenesis; and proliferation of fibroblasts and endothelial cells [18]. Cytokines have a role in wound healing and are responsible for inducing the migration of immune system cells to the wound site. Studies on the delivery of growth factors and cytokines showed increased wound closure [19].

For the past few decades, efforts have been made to confer antimicrobial properties to wound dressing supports such as foams, sponges, hydrogels, and gauzes. The simplest route is to load antimicrobial agents (e.g., silver [4], antibiotics, quaternary ammonium, and metallic nanoparticles [3]) into porous materials, but the materials can display antibacterial activity on their own (e.g., chitosan has been proven to have antibacterial activity [20]). Performance limitations of textile wound dressings (e.g., cotton or wool) have also fueled the search for different materials. Although soft in texture [3], textile wound dressings are devoid of the flexibility required for wounds located in mobility-related body parts such as joints [21]. When applied to burns, textile wound dressings adhere to the wound site in an uncontrollable manner, making its removal painful as the superficial layer of the wound bed is stripped in the process [1,22]. The ultimate wound dressings should be flexible [13], have antibacterial or at least bacteriostatic activity [21], exhibit adequate exudate absorption and gas permeability [13], allow a pain-free removal for the greater comfort possible, and be biocompatible [22–25]. The biocompatibility of a material is ascertained after an extensive array of tests that study the physical, chemical, and mechanical properties of the material as well as the potential adverse effects (i.e., allergenic, mutagenic, and cytotoxic) that may occur from its use, being crucial that the material does not elicit substantial damages or toxic effects to the body [26]. Research has shown that effective wound dressings exhibit porosity between 50% and 60%; these high values allow the transfer of oxygen and nutrients to the wound bed cells in contact with the dressing [17,23]. Pore size is also important since small pores physically hinder bacteria from reaching the wound site [11]. The interest is set on novel materials that intrinsically have a considerable number of desired properties (e.g., inherent antimicrobial activity and biocompatibility) and can perform well in wound environments. NO is a promising component regarding the design of ideal wound dressings. Due to its diminutive dimensions, this radical easily penetrates porous materials to reach the wound bed and triggers death cell mechanisms once it reaches bacterial membranes [27]. However, as a bioactive agent, NO demands storage and delivery vehicles. Therefore, it is theorized that hydrogels as vectors for the delivery of NO can be designed to fit the requirements of an excellent wound dressing. Polymers can form an assortment of materials that can accommodate the requirements of ideal wound dressings (e.g., foams, sponges, fibers and hydrogels), and due to a matrix similar to the extracellular matrix, nanofibers and hydrogels are the most explored polymeric materials for wound healing purposes [28]. The differentiating factor of NO-releasing hydrogels for wound healing is the functionality of NO. Antibacterial wound dressings on the market have an antimicrobial agent whose functionality is limited to preventing infections. NO, however, is unique because it participates in multiple aspects with regard to the evolution of the healing process besides infection prevention.

2. Hydrogels

Hydrogels are highly hydrated cross-linked polymers arranged in a matrix-like fashion that allow significant water retention (over 90% of their dry weight) in their three-dimensional network [29]. The most common natural polymers used for hydrogel formulation include collagen, alginate, hyaluronic acid [20], gelatin [30], cellulose [31], and chitosan [32]. Since most natural polymers already display biocompatibility and biodegradability [26], their high bioavailability further consolidates the proportion of interest in biopolymers over the past few decades [6]. However, biomedical applications are not exclusively reliant on natural polymers since many synthetic polymers are well-established biocompatible polymers (e.g., Poly(ethylene glycol) (PEG) [33] and Pluronic F-127 [34]) and are widely used for biomedical applications. Unlike natural polymers, synthetic polymers allow a greater degree of control over their composition. Biopolymers, however, require purification, and homogeneity is sometimes difficult to achieve due to different sources.

The structure and properties of hydrogels make them promising materials for the design of transdermal or injectable drug delivery systems, wound dressings, and adhesives [30,35]. Hydrogels are materials of great interest for wound healing due to their flexibility, adhesion, stability, and biodegradability, in addition to the capability of maintaining the wounded site moist, which helps to accelerate the healing rate [20,21,31,36]. Their porous extracellular matrix-like structure is also an important aspect to consider as it can facilitate the absorption of exudate from the wound bed [21,37] (Figure 2). Hydrogels can be modified to improve desired properties. For instance, knowing that hydrogel-tissue adhesion is limited in extreme wet conditions (e.g., bleeding), authors developed hemostatic hydrogels with enhanced tissue adhesion by grafting molecules that mimic adhesive components found in nature, namely methacrylate and dopamine [38].

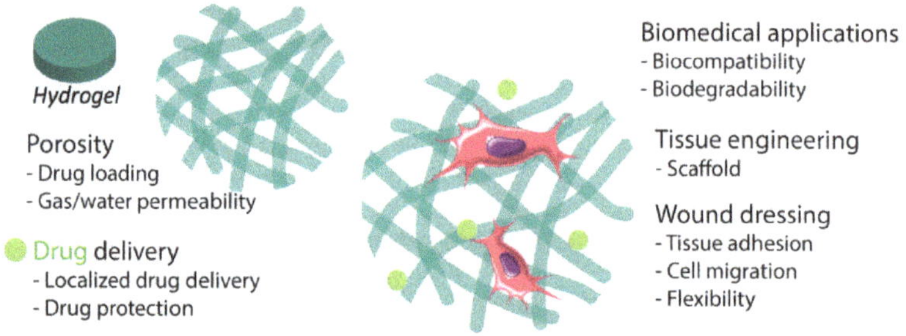

Figure 2. Hydrogel characteristics for wound healing, drug delivery, and tissue engineering.

Due to the characteristics mentioned above, hydrogels offer the possibility to simultaneously perform two functions, namely as a drug (or any bioactive agent relevant to wound closure) delivery system, and as a wound dressing [21]. In addition, hydrogels can be implemented as film/membranes [39], as a powder [40] (particles that gel in contact with liquid), or even be formed in situ (injectable [10,41–43]), making this class of materials highly convenient. For instance, hydrogel-forming powders better adapt to irregular wounds, and injectable hydrogels are excellent candidates for wounds located in mobility-related places [40,44]. In addition, powdering hydrogels has been reported as a route to patch and/or recycle mechanically damaged hydrogels. Powdered self-healing hydrogels regained their initial mechanical properties upon hydration [45].

3. Nitric Oxide and Its Donors

3.1. The Tiniest Antimicrobial Agent

Nitric oxide (NO) is a known bactericidal agent that has been explored for wound healing. It is effective towards a large range of bacteria, as well as fungi, parasites, and viruses [46–48]. NO stimulates the activity of immune cells at low concentrations (10^{-12}–10^{-9} M) and promotes inhibition and death of pathogens at higher concentrations

(10^{-6}–10^{-3} M) [49–51]. NO reacts with superoxide to form peroxynitrite (NO_3^-), a very reactive oxidant responsible for membrane disruption via lipid peroxidation, and inactivation of enzymes via protein oxidation and nitration [52], phenomena that ultimately lead to bacteria death (Figure 3) [46]. Moreover, it has been reported that the concentration of NO considered lethal to bacteria (ca., 200 ppm of gaseous NO) is tolerable and non-toxic to human fibroblasts, which further validates the use of NO in the context of wound healing [47]. A study determined that gaseous NO at pressures above 200 ppm decreased cell viability and immune cell proliferation in mouse lymphocytes [51]. Furthermore, NO is a much safer alternative to typical antibiotics, as the overuse of antibiotics can trigger the development of resistance mechanisms in bacteria. Multidrug-resistant bacteria strains, as indicated by the term, are resistant to a variety of antibiotics [6], rendering these ineffective in the fight against bacteria proliferation. Recent studies report that NO alone is effective against a wide range of bacteria without the creation of resistance, and most importantly, in a clinical set, the susceptibility of drug-resistant bacteria to antibiotics is enhanced when the latter are complemented with NO [53]. In general, antimicrobial agents tend to have higher cytotoxicity than desired while antibiotics require higher concentrations to be effective [16]. Hence, NO's adequacy for efficient antibacterial activity is supported by its synergetic antibacterial activity when allied to antibiotics, and although its cytotoxicity needs to be extensively studied, NO has inherent lower cytotoxicity compared to typical antimicrobial agents since NO is endogenously present in cells.

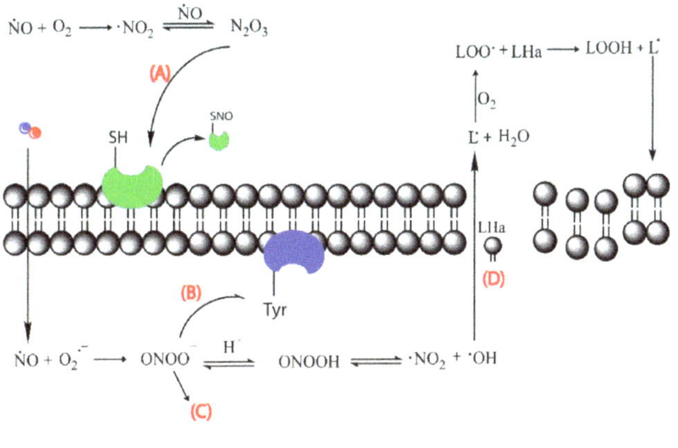

Figure 3. NO acting mechanism on bacteria cell membrane. Nitric oxide leads to thiol nitrosation (**A**), tyrosine nitration (**B**), DNA cleavage (**C**), and lipid peroxidation (**D**). Lipid (L) and allylic proton (Ha). Adapted with permission from ref. [27]. Copyright 2021 American Chemical Society and Adapted with permission from Ref. [54]. Copyright 2008 American Chemical Society.

The efficacy of an antibacterial agent differs from the conditions in which it is tested, namely against biofilm-inserted or planktonic bacteria. Bacteria can generate an extracellular matrix in which the diffusion of antibiotics is hindered, which complicates the fight against infections. More than the presence of planktonic bacteria, biofilm formation actually dictates if an acute wound becomes chronic [16] since biofilms are predominant in at least 60% of chronic wounds [55]. Biofilms allow gene transfer between bacteria, which could lead to the dissemination of genes associated with antibiotic resistance. Studies have shown that due to its size, NO diffusion is not hampered, and, most importantly, can disperse these films by restoring biofilm-incorporated bacteria to its planktonic state. NO-dispersed bacteria exhibit higher susceptibility to antibiotics [56]. Bacteria are more vulnerable in the free form, and most antibiotics are conceived to perform activity on planktonic bacteria [57]. Additionally, in respect to planktonic bacteria, biofilms require 2–10-fold NO and 1000–10,000-fold antibiotics to be destroyed. The ability to scatter biofilms makes NO a striking alternative to be considered in infection treatment and prevention. Moreover, NO directly kills biofilm-incorporated bacteria when the biofilm is exposed to high concentrations of NO [58].

Antibacterial activity is assessed by a variety of methods, through in vitro (inhibition zone on agar plates or inoculated broth in contact with the material), in vivo (i.e., mice), and ex vivo (excised animal skin) tests [59]. Anti-biofilm activity, as the ability of a material to destroy biofilms, is studied by allowing contact between a biofilm and the material being tested, followed by biofilm biomass determination through a staining protocol (e.g., crystal violet [60]) and determination of the viability of biofilm-embedded bacteria after exposure to the biocide (e.g., colony forming units count [61]). Depending on the method, additional information can be gathered; for example, by using a layered biofilm support, wound healing conditions can be mimicked and used to determine biocide efficacy (e.g., tetrazolium reduction used to assess cell viability) as well as its penetrability [62].

The most common bacteria detected in infected wounds are *Pseudomonas aeruginosa*, *Staphylococcus aureus*, *Klebsiella pneumoniae*, *Enterococcus faecalis*, *Acinetobacter baumannii* [55], and *Escherichia coli* [59]. Often, wounds are polymicrobial, and therefore, single-species biofilms might be inadequate to study the impact of antibacterial agents against typical in vivo infections. Some authors have reported the study of antibacterial efficacy in pluribacterial systems designed to better represent the bacterial composition and/or biocide susceptibility observed in of chronic wounds (i.e., *P. aeruginosa* and *S. aureus* biofilms) [59]. Although its use in wound healing is majorly due to its antimicrobial activity, NO has other properties that align with and further improve wound closure, such as promotion of angiogenesis, vasodilation, and fibroblast proliferation, among others [63]. Previous studies have shown that NO causes erythema when delivered topically owing to its vasodilator property. These tend to disappear a few minutes after NO delivery is interrupted [64]. NO has proven to direct endothelial differentiation of embryonic stem cells without growth factors by down-regulating pluripotent genes and up-regulating the expression of endothelial genes [65]. NO also accelerates endothelium proliferation, as demonstrated in a study with arterial grafts. Although no significant difference was observed after 3 months, NO-releasing arterial grafts exhibited greater endothelium coverage than the non-NO-releasing graft after the first month [66]. For further information about NO's role in cell proliferation, the interested reader is referred to reference [67].

3.2. Nitric Oxide Donors

Owing to its gaseous nature and subsequent difficulty to effectively be stored and administered, NO is exogenously delivered to tissues, most commonly through NO donors. NO donors are any molecule or complex capable of releasing NO (e.g., organic nitrates and nitrites, metal–NO complexes, N-diazeniumdiolates, and S-nitrosothiols). Several factors must be weighted in the selection of an ideal NO donor for biomedical applications, the most relevant being the release mechanism and rate, and toxicity of the by-products following NO donation. Different applications demand distinct profiles, and concerning NO release rate, short-burst and prolonged releases are valuable for localized immediate effects and long-lasting effects in which NO is supposed to be continuously delivered, respectively [48]. It has been reported that wound healing benefits from a mixed release profile, i.e., a spontaneous short release followed by a continuous release. Higher NO concentrations at an early stage are important to hasten inflammation, which occurs in the first few hours, whereas the sustained delivery of NO throughout the ensuing stages of wound healing is beneficial for endothelial differentiation, which is characteristic of the last stage of wound closure [68,69].

With the ability to donate two or one NO molecule(s) per each parent molecule, *N*-diazeniumdiolates and *S*-nitrosothiols (RSNO) are the most attractive NO donors for biomedical applications [49]. Any aminated or thiolated molecules, such as polymers and peptides, can be converted to RSNO or *N*-diazenium-based donors through nitrosation, which greatly expands the range of possibilities for NO donor materials.

S-nitrosothiols are a group of molecules in which a nitroso group is bonded to a sulfur atom (RS-N=O), and are formed by the reaction of thiols with NO derivatives (e.g., NO_2, N_2O_4, N_2O_3, and NO_2^-) [70,71]. *S*-nitrosoglutathione (GSNO) and *S*-nitrosocysteine (CySNO) are some of the most studied *S*-nitrosothiols with low molecular weight (Table 1). *S*-nitrosothiols are intermediates in biological processes, and thus stable in physiological conditions, namely at 37 °C and pH 7.4. However, the majority of RSNOs are easily decomposed at room temperature to form disulfides and NO, which limits their use [72]. These molecules release NO upon decomposition induced by enzymatic catalysis, light, and metal ions (i.e., Cu^{2+}, Fe^{2+}, Hg^{2+} and Ag^+). NO release is accompanied by the formation of a disulfide, which is formed by the reaction between two thiyl radicals (RS•) [73]. The molecular structure of *S*-nitrosothiols influences the decomposition rate. Primary and secondary RSNOs are less stable, and thus exhibit a higher NO release rate. Moreover, these molecules can transfer the NO moiety to thiols without releasing NO, in a reaction termed trans-nitrosation [74,75], which in turn translates into a decreased possibility of generating peroxynitrite [48,75]. Due to this property, RSNOs have been linked to greater antibacterial activity as the result of nitrosylation of thiolated proteins [58].

Table 1. Chemical structure of the most used S-nitrosothiols.

S-Nitrosothiol	Chemical Structure
GSNO *S*-nitrosogluthathione	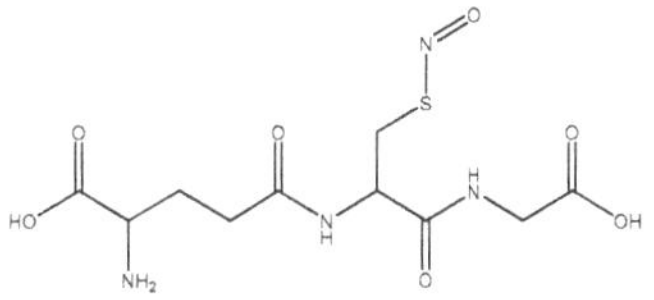
SNAC *S*-nitroso-*N*-acetylcysteine	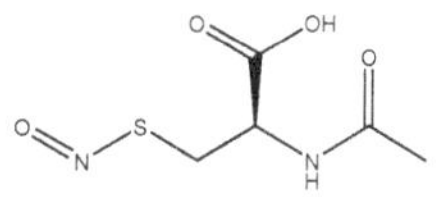
SNAP *S*-nitroso-*N*-acetylpenicillamine	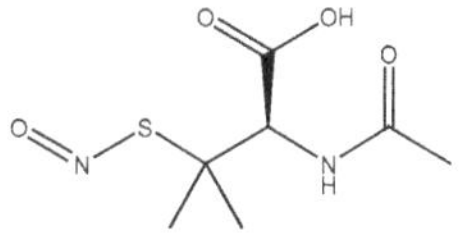
SNMSA *S*-nitroso-mercaptosuccinic acid	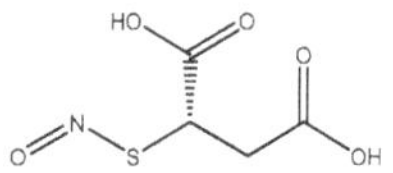

N-diazeniumdiolates are a class of compounds generally termed NONOates due to the functional group $[N(O)NO]^-$. *N*-diazeniumdiolates are stable molecules obtained by the reaction of secondary amines, present in both simple molecules and polymers, with NO at high pressures. Less common and less stable are NONOates formed with primary amines or amides, which in turn rely on protonated amines in the vicinity to achieve greater stability through hydrogen bonding formation [76,77]. NONOates undergo protonation to decompose into the parent amine and two molecules of NO, making NO release a pH-dependent process. These molecules are stable in basic media but undergo protonation at low pH to release NO. In other words, NO release is constrained in alkali media and triggered in acidic environments. The rate at which NO is released is entirely dependent on the donor structure (Table 2), and therefore subject to alterations. Diazeniumdiolates can be chemically modified at the second oxygen of the functional group, further contributing to the lengthening of NO release as it requires prior removal of the protecting moiety [47,78,79]. The potential of NONOates to form carcinogenic nitrosamines (R_2-N-N=O) is the main shortcoming of the use of these molecules in biomedical devices [47]. An approach to counteract the formation of these undesired molecules has been explored and lies on the chemical attachment of diazeniumdiolates to a larger molecule (i.e., polymer). Under these conditions, some authors also hypothesize that the half-life of NONOates is altered and possibly prolonged [80].

Table 2. Chemical structure and approximate half-life values, $t_{1/2}$, of NONOates at 37 °C and pH 7.4. Adapted from [81].

N-Diazeniumdiolate	Chemical Structure	$t_{1/2}$
PROLI/NO 1-[-2-(-carboxylate)pyrrolidine-1-yl] NONOate	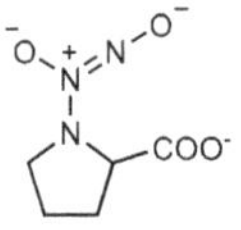	2 s
MAHMA/NO Methylamine hexamethylene methylamine NONOate	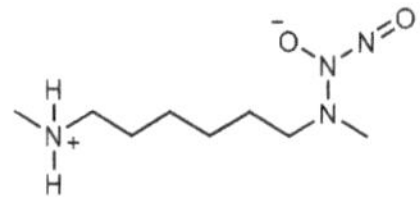	1 min
DEA/NO Diethylamine NONOate	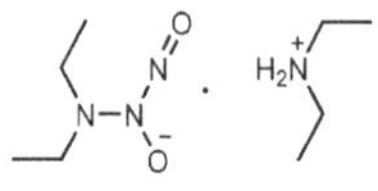	2 min
SPER/NO Spermine NONOate	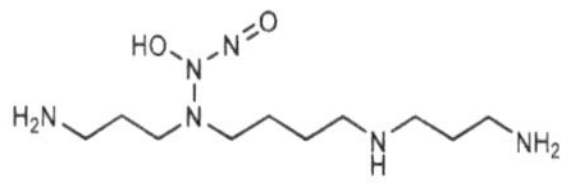	6 min
PAPA/NO Propylamine propylamine NONOate	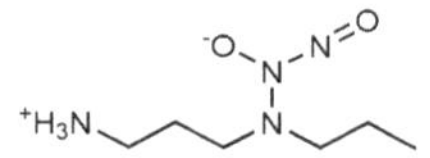	15 min
DPTA/NO Dipropylentriamine NONOate	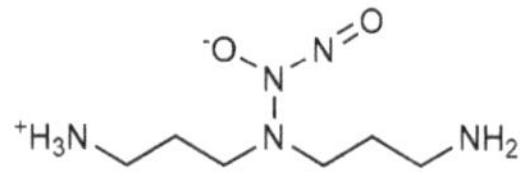	3 h

Generally, NO donors are subject to burst releases and short half-lives. As previously mentioned, environmental manipulation (e.g., pH, temperature, light, and enzymatic degradation) and chemical modification can be used to tune the NO release rate. However, the physical protection of NO donors from external stimuli by vesicles or matrices is an option that has been extensively explored, as well. Polymer-based and lipid-based vesicles such as dendrimers, micelles, and liposomes are among the most common carriers for NO donors meant to extend NO release [49]. Matrices such as hydrogels and fibers can also be used to store and protect NO donors [69,82,83]. For instance, inserting *S*-nitrosothiols in hydrogels improves the stability of these molecules and prolongs NO release [84,85]. Moreover, some studies suggest that polymers with poor water solubility better protect NO donors that decompose in solution by limiting the interaction between water and the NO donor [86].

Besides NO-extended release, polymer-mediated NO delivery has been reported for enhanced antimicrobial activity. For instance, a synthetic antimicrobial copolymer modified with NO donating groups showed synergistic biofilm dispersal and antibacterial activity against *P. aeruginosa* [87]. Inspired by peptides with antimicrobial activity, antimicrobial polymers have been created to mimic its structure and properties—ideally, with cationic and hydrophobic segments [88]. These amphiphilic molecules adhere to and accumulate in bacteria cell membranes, disrupting cell integrity and leading to death [89].

4. NO-Releasing Hydrogel-Based Systems

4.1. Physically Adsorbed NO Donors

NO-delivering materials require protective measures to prevent precocious NO release (due to unwanted NO donor decomposition) prior to application. Hydrogels, matrices of excellence for wound healing, besides being adequate to store and protect NO donors, offer the possibility to be devoid of moisture for storage purposes, and can regain their structure upon hydration, relevant behavior when NO donors with hydrolytic NO release are used.

The incorporation of bioactive compounds into hydrogels can be achieved through a variety of methods and can be grouped according to hydrogel–drug interactions, namely chemical modification and physical adsorption [29,47,51]. NO release systems formed by NO donors or precursors covalently and non-covalently bound to a hydrogel matrix are summarized in Tables 3 and 4. Most NO-releasing hydrogels were designed and tested for wound healing purposes, but due to the many properties of NO, other applications (i.e., antibacterial activity [41,90–92], vasodilation [39,93,94], biomedical applications or tissue engineering [65,92,95], anticancer activity [90,96,97]) were also targeted. NO is used in anticancer therapeutics as a way to make tumorous cells more susceptible to chemotherapeutic drugs. Poorly vascularized tumor masses produce HIF-1a (hypoxia-inducible factor), triggering cell resistance to death mechanisms (i.e., DNA damage, autophagy, and apoptosis) incited by radio or chemotherapy. Due to its angiogenic properties, NO normalizes tumor vasculature, thus ensuring the delivery of systemically administered drugs [98,99]. Oddly, NO plays a role in both encouraging and confining the proliferation of cancerous cells. Angiogenesis and proliferation facilitate cancer metastasis, whereas DNA damage leads to apoptosis [99]. As for tissue engineering applications, NO is advantageous because it can inhibit platelet adhesion and aggregation [100] on implanted materials, thus preventing blockages and subsequent cardiovascular complications. In other words, NO is implemented for its antimicrobial, angiogenic, and vasodilation properties, all important for the wound healing process.

Table 3. NO-releasing hydrogels based on physically adsorbed NO donors.

Hydrogel	NO Donor	NO Release Features	References
pHEMA	Manganese nitrosyl	Light-activated	[82]
Methacrylate-modified gelatin /hyaluronic acid graft dopamine	*N,N′*-di–sec–butyl–*N,N′*-dinitroso-1,4-phenylenediamine (BNN6)		[101]
Gelatin methacrylate and oxide dextran	BNN6	Near-infrared release	[42]
Gelatin	Sodium nitrite		[83]
Gelatin methacrylate	SNAP (S-nitroso-N-acetylpenicillamine)		[102]
Gelatin and sodium alginate	SNAP	Burst release in first 4 h, sustained up to 120 h	[68]
F-127/PAA	GSNO	~200 min constant ~5 days	[103]
Pluronic F-127	GSNO	——	[34,104–107]
Pluronic F-127	GSNO SNAC (*S*-nitroso-*N*-acetylcysteine)	Thermal or photochemical release	[84,108,109]
Pluronic F-127	GSNO		[85]
Pluronic F-127 and alginate	GSNO		[110]
Pluronic F-127 Pluronic P-123	Nitroso-derivative of 4-amino-7-nitrobenzofurazan	Photochemical release	[111]
Alginate, pectin and PEG	GSNO	Release for at least 18 h of GSNO	[40]

Table 3. *Cont.*

Hydrogel	NO Donor	NO Release Features	References
Alginate	S-nitroso-mercaptosuccinic acid	Burst release in first 5 h, sustained in following hours (tested up to 18 h)	[112]
Chitosan	Isosorbide mononitrate (ISMN)		[113]
Chitosan	GSNO	Sustained for over 48 h	[46]
Chitosan, PEG, sugar	Sodium nitrite	Sustained for at least 24 h	[44]
Chitosan, PVP, PEG	Nitrite	Burst release for 120 min followed by sustained up to 8 h	[93]
Chitosan, PVA	SNAP	Continuous release for at least 120 h	[114]
Chitosan and Poly(vinyl alcohol)	Ruthenium nitrosyl	NIR-induced release	[90]
PEG, fibrinogen	SNAP	Photolytic and thermal activation	[43]
Fmoc-FF	SNAP	Burst release in the first 12 h, sustained over 7 days	[115]
Poly(β-cyclodextrin) and modified dextran	Nitro compound	Photochemical	[91,97,116,117]

Physically adsorbed NO donors are mainly based on small molecular weight RSNOs, GSNO being the most explored so far (Table 3). Even though a predilection is observed for natural polymers (e.g., gelatin, chitosan, and alginate), mostly due to the inherent biocompatibility and high bioavailability, the most explored polymer is Pluronic F-127, an amphiphilic poly(propylene oxide) and poly(ethylene oxide) co-polymer that easily forms micelles in solution [27]. A hydrogel system containing a metal–NO donor was tested for wound healing and promising results were obtained [82]. The light-activated NO release system was complemented with a coating for leaching prevention, thus allowing NO diffusion instead of the NO donor itself. Nitrite and organic nitrate-containing hydrogels meant to release NO were tested with special focus on the antibacterial activity of the systems, although the NO release profile of the systems was not explored in depth [83,113]. NO donors based on nitrosamines were also reported. A hydrogel with BNN6 exhibited excellent properties, namely NO release, antibacterial activity, mechanical properties, and, most important, biocompatibility, since the donor is a nitrosamine [101]. Some studies on nitrosamine-containing hydrogels are focused on the properties of the donor molecule and its potential use for antimicrobial activity, lacking further studies regarding cytotoxicity.

Biocompatible hydrogels are believed to make the overall system appropriate for topical delivery [111]. Since adverse responses are undesirable for wound healing, biocompatibility is a must for any material meant for this specific application. The repercussions of NO use and overuse on humans are yet to be uncovered. Most studies rely on in vitro tests, and the few in vivo tests are performed on mice. Mice wounds heal differently from human wounds, instead of re-epithelization, healing is made by wound edge closure. However, wound healing in pigs is made by re-epithelization and displays similar responses to growth factors. The different mechanisms might produce incongruent results when translating in vivo studies in rats to humans. Literature has shown that studies in pigs had a 78% concordance with human studies, higher than the 57% and 53% of in vitro and in vivo studies in rats, respectively [51]. Even if cytotoxic effects against mammalian cells are investigated in vitro and in vivo, complete studies of NO toxicity are needed [118].

Few systems exhibited the profile deemed best suited for wound healing, namely an initial uncontrolled release followed by a slow and constant release [68,93,112,115]. Sustained NO delivery has been reported using an antioxidant in parallel with a NONOate-based NO donor. Aiming to lessen the indiscriminate destructive power of peroxynitrite—a product of the reaction between NO and superoxide—an antioxidant was included in the formulation. The system exhibited a sustained NO release that lasted at least 12 h when complemented with the antioxidant curcumin. However, the formulation reduced collagen deposition, a process that occurs at the latter steps of wound closure [119]. Since peroxynitrite is responsible for the antimicrobial activity of NO, this system is not the most appropriate for wound healing materials. Basically, the material should remain compatible with its intended application whenever a component is added to counteract the perceived shortcomings of another component. Systems based on the addition of reducing agents (e.g., glucose, ascorbic acid) have also been reported. Ascorbic acid catalyzed a sustained NO release for the tested 36 h when used to complement a keratin-based RSNO electrospun with poly(urethane) and gelatin [63]. The higher release rate in the presence of ascorbic acid has been assigned to the reduction of Cu^{2+} to Cu^{+}, as the latter enhances NO release from RSNOs [73]. The role of copper ions in solution has been postulated to increase NO release by disrupting *N*-diazeniumdiolate and amine H-bonding [27].

Kinetic studies showed that water absorption by the hydrogel controlled NO release from GSNO-loaded Pluronic F-127 and PAA hydrogels [103]. The same NO donor, incorporated in Pluronic F-127/Chitosan hydrogels and Pluronic F-127-embedded chitosan nanoparticles, followed Higuchi with Fickian diffusion kinetics [34,85], and Korsmeyer-Peppas with Fickian diffusion kinetics when incorporated in chitosan hydrogels [46]. For the NO donor *S*-nitroso-mercaptosuccinic acid in alginate hydrogels, NO release best fitted the Higuchi model with Fickian diffusion [112]. Drug release in function of time can be predicted by mathematical models. The release rate of drugs from matrix systems is described by both Higuchi and Korsmeyer-Peppas equations, the latter being a semi-empirical model used for polymeric matrices such as hydrogels. Fickian diffusion means that the drug, in this case, NO, is released by diffusion instead of swelling or polymer relaxation [120].

Although some hydrogel formulations of physically absorbed donors have been reported to exhibit no leaching [117], the possibility of leaching is higher in the case of a donor incorporated by physical adsorption. The premature and unspecific release of the NO donor from the hydrogel matrix is extremely undesired and can be avoided by coating (e.g., poly(urethane) shells) or chemical attachment of NO donors to hydrogels [85].

4.2. Chemically Attached NO Donors

Chemically modified NO-releasing hydrogels are based on a wide array of polymers, such as chitosan, peptides, Pluronic F-127, PVA, and gelatin (see Table 4), with chitosan as the most studied polymer to date. This polymer, as the result of deacetylated chitin, a marine polysaccharide, has a heterogeneous chemical structure composed of *N*-acetyl-glucosamine and *N*-glucosamine units. Only second to chitosan hydrogels, peptide hydrogels are composed of macromolecules that confer biocompatibility and degradability which are great for biomedical applications such as wound healing [121]. Although less common, fibrin and fibrinogen-based hydrogels have been linked to augmented wound healing. Fibrinogen hydrogels facilitate cell adhesion, angiogenesis, and cell proliferation [43], while fibrin hydrogels allow cell proliferation and can be degraded by cells intervenient in wound healing to remodel the ECM [92].

Regarding NO donors, the diversity is limited, as it consists primarily of NONOates and RSNOs, apart from a metal-NO complex [122]. *S*-nitrosothiols and *N*-diazeniumdiolates are great NO donors for these specific systems, as functional groups such as thiols and amines can react to store NO, forming RSNOs and NONOates, respectively (Figure 4). Contrary to hydrogels with physically adsorbed NO donors, leaching is absent in hydrogels with chemically attached NO donors.

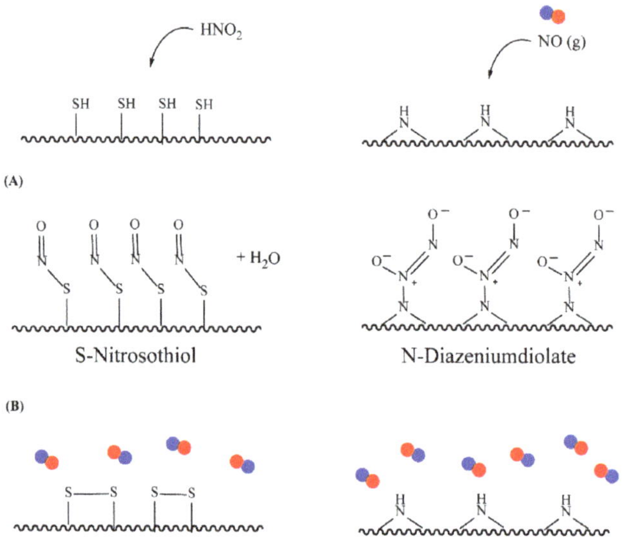

Figure 4. Nitric oxide capture (**A**) and release (**B**) by thiols (left) and amines (right) to originate *S*-nitrosothiols and *N*-diazeniumdiolates, respectively. Adapted from ref. [39].

Table 4. NO-releasing hydrogels based on covalently bound NO donors.

Hydrogel	**NO Donor**	**NO Release Features**	**Reference**
Poly(vinyl alcohol)	*N*-Diazeniumdiolate	~48 h	[123]
Poly(vinyl alcohol)	RSNO	Photochemical release	[39]
Pluronic F-127	RSNO		[124]
Pluronic F-127 and branched PEI	*N*-Diazeniumdiolate	Burst release in first hours, sustained up to 50 h	[77,125]
Chitosan	*N*-Diazeniumdiolate	Enzymatic deprotection by glycosidase	[126,127]
NapFFGEE peptide	*N*-Diazeniumdiolate	Enzymatic deprotection by glutathione/glutathione *S*-transferase	[96]
Naphthalene-terminated FFGGG peptide	*N*-Diazeniumdiolate	Enzymatic deprotection	[94]
Fmoc-Pexiganan and Pexiganan	*N*-Diazeniumdiolate	~400 h	[128]
Gelatin	SNAP	Burst release in first 2 h, sustained up to 72 h	[95]
Chitosan and hyaluronic acid	SNAC	Burst release in first 2 h, sustained up to 48 h	[41]
Chitosan	*N*-Diazeniumdiolate	~48 h Enzymatic deprotection	[65]
Fibrin	SNAP	Light exposure	[92]
Laponite-poly(pentaethylenehexamine) composite	*N*-diazeniumdiolate	Burst release	[129]

Table 4. *Cont.*

Hydrogel	NO Donor	NO Release Features	Reference
Alginate modified with DETA	*N*-Diazeniumdiolate	~4 days	[80]
PEG	*S*-nitrocysteine	~24 h	[130]
Poly(caprolactone)/Poly(sulfhydrylated polyester)	RSNO		[64]
Nap-FFKEGG	*N*-Diazeniumdiolate	No burst release	[131]
Alginate and branched PEI	*N*-Diazeniumdiolate	Addition of Cu (II) increases NO release rate	[27]
Chitosan, PEG, and glucose	Nitrite SNAC		[132]
Poly(ε-lysine)	*N*-Diazeniumdiolate	~15 h	[76]
Poly(2-hydroxyethyl methacrylate)	Ruthenium nitrosyl	Photochemical release	[122]

Swift and spontaneous NO donation is observed in NONOate-modified Laponite-poly(amine) composite hydrogels, though NO release is dependent on the laponite-to-polymer ratio, further attributed to tri-dimensional disposition. NO donors intercalated between Laponite disks are less susceptible to decomposition, as interaction with the medium is delayed, therefore extending NO release [129]. A mixed release profile is reported for few systems [41,77,95,125]. Controlled and paced NO release has been reported for the systems reliant on enzymatic catalysis [65,96,126,127]. Enzymatic sensitivity allows greater control over NO delivery and release rate, as the latter is dictated by enzyme kinetics. Briefly, a NO donor is either connected to a polymer backbone and a specific enzymatic substrate, or simply to a polymeric chain. NO release occurs after the protecting molecule (e.g., galactose) is modified by the enzyme (i.e., glycosidase enzyme for galactose substrate), deprotecting the NO donor, which then decomposes. Complex and specific molecules can also donate NO upon direct modification by enzymes [96]. Moreover, enzyme-responsive delivery systems hold their cargo in the absence of enzyme independently of the medium, therefore eliminating spontaneous release.

A unique approach in which a metal-NO complex is covalently bound to the polymeric chain through polymerization in the presence of 4-vinylpyridine attached do the metal-NO complex has been reported. The resulting polymer forms a highly stable hydrogel that promptly releases NO upon UV irradiation (Figure 5). Results indicate that the photoproduct remains retained within the hydrogel structure following irradiation and NO release, further supporting the suitability of the system for biomedical applications [122].

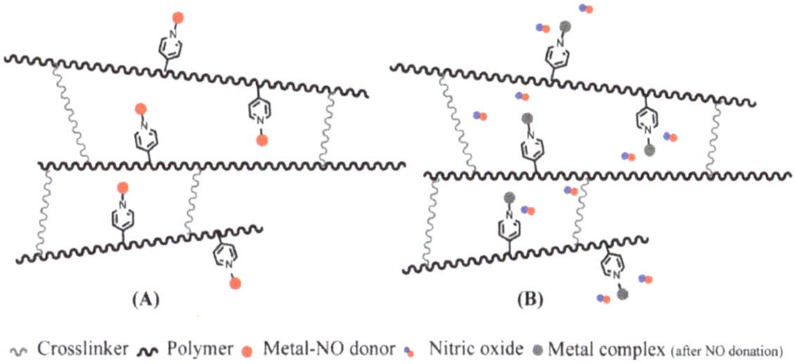

Figure 5. NO-releasing hydrogel with NO donor covalently linked to a pyridine derivate inserted in the polymeric chain. Before (**A**) and after (**B**) irradiation. Adapted from ref. [122].

A dual system based on a SNO-modified PVA film coupled with a GSNO-containing Pluronic F-127 hydrogel was tested for wound healing in rats (Figure 6). The film alone displayed spontaneous and fast NO release for the first couple hours, whereas the hydrogel itself showed sustained NO release. This dual phase dressing was designed to modulate NO delivery on the hypothesis that NO released from both PVA film and GSNO dispersed in the hydrogel would accumulate on the poly(propylene oxide) core of the micellar Pluronic F-127 hydrogel and be slowly released. In other words, even if NO is spontaneously released by PVA films, it will be retained in the hydrogel and slowly diffuse to the wound. Results showed that NO release occurs steadily for a period of at least 24 h when both layers are used. Moreover, the study demonstrated enhanced wound closure and a shortened inflammation phase [133].

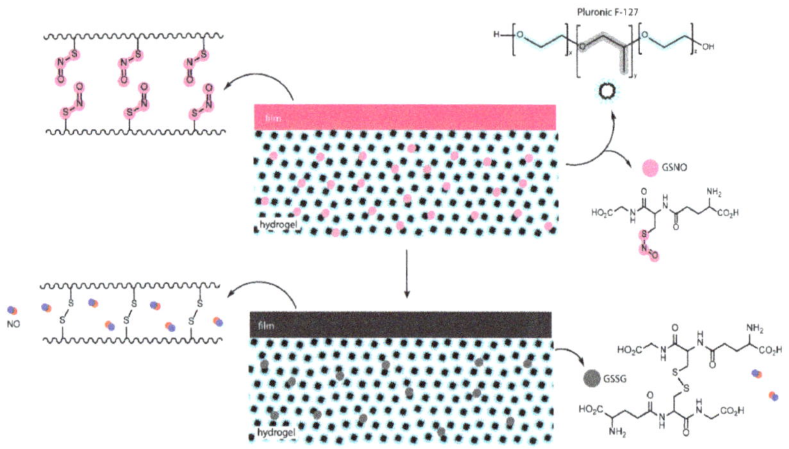

Figure 6. Poly(vinyl alcohol) films modified with SNO groups and GSNO-containing Pluronic F-127 hydrogels. Adapted from ref. [133].

Nitric oxide delivery would benefit from standardized results. NO is detected and measured through a variety of techniques (i.e., Griess assay, fluorescence, chemiluminescence, and electrochemical methods [50]), and independently of the technique used to detect and quantify NO release, the release profile can be easily observed with cumulative release plots. However, results remain difficult to compare because some authors report the percentage or molar concentration of released NO while others report molar concentrations of NO per mass or per area of the hydrogel. Although the total amount of NO present and released in the tested sample should always be presented, calculating partial release until NO release halts guarantees that the method and units used in NO quantification are normalized. Studies performed so far have shown that NO can indeed be stored in hydrogel matrices until release is desired and/or triggered. Since the performance of the system as a wound dressing capable of releasing NO depends on several factors (e.g., hydrogel composition, NO donor class, NO release mechanism, etc.), there is room for further studies since there are numerous formulations to choose from. Table 5 summarizes the advantages and disadvantages of the incorporation of NO donors in hydrogels and the type of mechanism behind NO release.

Table 5. Summary of advantages and disadvantages of NO donor incorporation in hydrogels and NO release mechanisms.

	Advantages	Limitations
Mechanism	NO Donor Incorporation	
Physical adsorption	Simple, no reactions or modifications required Any NO donor can be incorporated	Possible leaching Storage, stability, and release depend on hydrogel–donor interactions
Chemical attachment	No leaching Ease to create RSNOs and NONOates	Requires complex reactions
	NO release	
Hydrolysis	Uncomplicated release triggers	Undesired release in water containing environments
Enzymatic catalysis	Not subject to uncontrolled release due to specific triggers	Release rate depends on enzyme kinetics
Photocatalysis		Limited application, requires direct irradiation

4.3. Antibacterial Activity and Wound Healing of NO-Releasing Hydrogels

Nitric oxide is an efficient antibacterial agent, and NO-releasing hydrogels have shown bactericidal efficiency against Gram-positive *Staphilococcus aureus*, *Staphilococcus epidermis*, and *Streptococcus mutans*, and against Gram-negative *Escherichia coli* and *Pseudomonas aeruginosa* (Table 6). Bacteria are characterized as Gram-positive bacteria when they have a thick peptidoglycan layer, and Gram-negative when their thin peptidoglycan is followed by an outer membrane that unfortunately better protects the bacteria [58,134]. The antibacterial activity of NO against planktonic and biofilm-embedded *P. aeruginosa* was tested with the use of a chemically modified antimicrobial polymer (ethylene glycol, ethylhexyl, and cationic primary amine units). In addition to great bactericidal efficacy, the NO-releasing polymer induced biofilm dispersal [87].

Table 6. Antibacterial activity of NO-releasing hydrogels against Gram-positive and Gram-negative bacteria, with a focus on the systems with enhanced wound healing tested in vivo. Methicillin-resistant *S. aureus* (MRSA) and multidrug-resistant *P. aeruginosa* (MRPA).

Gram +	Gram −	Effect	NO Donor/Hydrogel	References
Antibacterial activity assessed in vitro				
S. aureus	*E. coli*	Bactericidal	Metal-NO complex/Chitosan, PVA	[90]
	E. coli	Bactericidal	Nitro compound/Poly(cyclodextrin)	[91]
S. epidermis	*E. coli*	Bactericidal	NONOate/Chitosan, Hyaluronic acid	[41]
S. mutans *S. aureus*	*E. coli*	Bactericidal	RSNO/Alginate	[112]
	P. aeruginosa	Bactericidal	GSNO/Chitosan, Pluronic F-127	[34]
S. aureus	*P. aeruginosa*	Bactericidal	NONOate/Alginate, PEI	[27]
	P. aeruginosa	Bactericidal Biofilm dispersal	NONOate/antimicrobial polymer	[87]
With enhanced wound healing tested in vivo				
S. aureus	*E. coli*	Bactericidal	BNN6/GelMA	[42]
S. aureus	*P. aeruginosa*	Bactericidal	GSNO/Chitosan	[46]
MRSA	*P. aeruginosa*	Bactericidal	GSNO/Alginate, Pectin, PEG	[40]
MRSA	MRPA	Bactericidal	GSNO/Alginate	[110]

As for wound healing, in vivo tests performed on rats showed that NO-releasing hydrogels enhanced wound closure. A combined effect of chitosan and NO was observed as chitosan hydrogels alone accelerated wound closure and GSNO-loaded chitosan hydrogels showed superior wound healing in rats [46]. Promising results were also obtained with alginate-based hydrogels loaded with GSNO, namely accelerated wound healing and bactericidal activity against drug-resistant Gram-positive and Gram-negative bacteria such as MRSA and MRPA [40,111]. These results support the suitability of NO for wound healing purposes.

5. Conclusions

The interest in functional materials has been rising in recent decades. Even though quality of life has improved enormously due to the advancements in healthcare and pharmaceutics, there is room for improved materials capable of promoting wound healing. NO has garnered increased interest over the past few years due to its antimicrobial properties and has proven to be efficient on its own, by enhancing the antibacterial efficiency of antibiotics and by decreasing resistance developed by bacteria strains, which is very important nowadays since multidrug resistant bacteria strains are difficult to eradicate. NO further aids wound healing by fastening inflammation, inducing angiogenesis and facilitating cell proliferation, making it an excellent bioactive compound for wound closure. Since NO is a gas, its delivery is made through molecules or systems capable of donating NO. Multiple classes of NO donors have been explored, with *N*-diazeniumdiolates and *S*-nitrosothiols being the most prevalent due to their higher stability relative to other classes of compounds capable of donating NO. Nonetheless, vesicles or matrices are generally used to extend NO donor stability and consequent shelf-life. Besides being popular polymeric matrices suitable for NO donor storage and protection, hydrogels are also a promising class of material for wound healing purposes since these structures can physically protect the wound bed from external factors.

Two approaches are observed in the preparation of hydrogels for NO delivery: NO donors incorporated in or chemically attached to hydrogel platforms. Hydrogels with chemically bound NO donors are devoid of NO donor leaching, contrary to some hydrogels with physically adsorbed NO donors. The profile of NO delivery is influenced by the class of donor, mechanism of decomposition into NO, and hydrogel loading method. The release profile itself can be modulated to a certain point, from abrupt to continuous, or even mixed. The latter is deemed more beneficial for wound healing. Photochemical or enzymatic responsiveness provides NO deliveries with ultimate control where the release is initiated upon stimulation instead of instantaneously.

The antibacterial activity of hydrogel-delivered NO has been tested against Gram-positive and Gram-negative bacteria, normal and drug-resistant strains, with promising results. In the future, antibacterial activity should include biofilm dispersal and eradication besides the typical planktonic bacteria eradication. The performance of NO-loaded hydrogels in wound healing tested in vivo is encouraging, with fastened wound healing. Although the cytotoxicity of NO against mammal cells is studied and disclosed on almost every report, further studies should be performed to determine the long-term effects of NO exposure in humans. In sum, NO-releasing hydrogels are proven to be excellent materials for wound healing purposes. According to the results reported, the interest in NO donors is far from ending since their role in wound dressings goes beyond antibacterial activity.

6. Future Perspective

The studies carried out to date prove the potential of both NO as a therapeutic agent for chronic wounds and hydrogels as protectors and vectors for the delivery of bioactive agents. Although the characteristics of each type of wound make it difficult or even impossible to formulate a one-size-fits-all wound dressing, it is viable to develop an optimized system for each type of wound only by modifying the properties of the hydrogel itself (adhesion, exudate absorption, water vapor, and gas permeability). An extensive characterization of the physicochemical properties of wound dressings, NO's release profile over time, as well as the impact of NO's toxicity given prolonged and/or recurrent exposure is essential. It is also necessary to explore the toxicity of the system and by-products after NO donation.

Funding: Gina Tavares acknowledges the PhD grant (ref: UI/BD/150855/2021) funded by Fundação para a Ciência e a Tecnologia (FCT), Portugal. Authors would like to thank the Strategic Research Center (CIEPQPF) Project UIDB/EQU/00102/2020 and UIDP/EQU/00102/2020, funded by FCT.

Conflicts of Interest: The authors declare no conflict of interest.

References

1. Ambekar, R.S.; Kandasubramanian, B. Advancements in nanofibers for wound dressing: A review. *Eur. Polym. J.* **2019**, *117*, 304–336. [CrossRef]
2. Wang, W.; Lu, K.J.; Yu, C.H.; Huang, Q.L.; Du, Y.Z. Nano-drug delivery systems in wound treatment and skin regeneration. *J. Nanobiotechnol.* **2019**, *17*, 82. [CrossRef] [PubMed]
3. Xiang, J.; Zhu, R.; Lang, S.; Yan, H.; Liu, G.; Peng, B. Mussel-inspired immobilization of zwitterionic silver nanoparticles toward antibacterial cotton gauze for promoting wound healing. *Chem. Eng. J.* **2021**, *409*, 128291. [CrossRef]
4. Han, G.; Ceilley, R. Chronic Wound Healing: A Review of Current Management and Treatments. *Adv. Ther.* **2017**, *34*, 599–610. [CrossRef] [PubMed]
5. Demidova-Rice, T.N.; Hamblin, M.R.; Herman, I.M. Acute and impaired wound healing: Pathophysiology and current methods for drug delivery, part 1: Normal and chronic wounds: Biology, causes, and approaches to care. *Adv. Skin Wound Care* **2012**, *25*, 304–314. [CrossRef]
6. El-Aassar, M.R.; Ibrahim, O.M.; Fouda, M.M.G.; Fakhry, H.; Ajarem, J.; Maodaa, S.N.; Allam, A.A.; Hafez, E.E. Wound dressing of chitosan-based-crosslinked gelatin/ polyvinyl pyrrolidone embedded silver nanoparticles, for targeting multidrug resistance microbes. *Carbohydr. Polym.* **2021**, *255*, 117484. [CrossRef]
7. Saghazadeh, S.; Rinoldi, C.; Schot, M.; Kashaf, S.S.; Sharifi, F.; Jalilian, E.; Nuutila, K.; Giatsidis, G.; Mostafalu, P.; Derakhshandeh, H.; et al. Drug delivery systems and materials for wound healing applications. *Adv. Drug Deliv. Rev.* **2018**, *127*, 138–166. [CrossRef]
8. Suetens, C.; Latour, K.; Kärki, T.; Ricchizzi, E.; Kinross, P.; Moro, M.L.; Jans, B.; Hopkins, S.; Hansen, S.; Lyytikäinen, O.; et al. Prevalence of healthcare-associated infections, estimated incidence and composite antimicrobial resistance index in acute care hospitals and long-term care facilities: Results from two European point prevalence surveys, 2016 to 2017. *Eurosurveillance* **2018**, *23*, 1800516. [CrossRef]
9. Monnet, D.L.; Harbarth, S. Will coronavirus disease (COVID-19) have an impact on antimicrobial resistance? *Eurosurveillance* **2020**, *25*, 2001886. [CrossRef]
10. Cheng, W.; Wang, M.; Chen, M.; Niu, W.; Li, Y.; Wang, Y.; Luo, M.; Xie, C.; Leng, T.; Lei, B. Injectable antibacterial antiinflammatory molecular hybrid hydrogel dressing for rapid MDRB-infected wound repair and therapy. *Chem. Eng. J.* **2021**, *409*, 128140. [CrossRef]
11. Ketabchi, N.; Dinarvand, R.; Adabi, M.; Gholami, M.; Firoozi, S.; Amanzadi, B.; Faridi-Majidi, R. Study of Third-Degree Burn Wounds Debridement and Treatment by Actinidin Enzyme Immobilized on Electrospun Chitosan/PEO Nanofibers in Rats. *Biointerface Res. Appl. Chem.* **2021**, *11*, 10358–10370. [CrossRef]
12. Matsliah, L.; Goder, D.; Giladi, S.; Zilberman, M. In vitro characterization of novel multidrug-eluting soy protein wound dressings. *J. Biomater. Appl.* **2021**, *35*, 978–993. [CrossRef]
13. Karakaya, P.S.; Oktay, A.; Seventekin, N.; Yesil-Celiktas, O. Design of a new generation wound dressing with pine bark extract. *J. Ind. Text.* **2021**, *50*, 1193–1204. [CrossRef]
14. Khan, T.A.; Peh, K.K.; Ch'ng, H.S. Mechanical, bioadhesive strength and biological evaluations of chitosan films for wound dressing. *J. Pharm. Pharm. Sci.* **2000**, *3*, 303–311.
15. Hajikhani, M.; Emam-Djomeh, Z.; Askari, G. Fabrication and characterization of mucoadhesive bioplastic patch via coaxial polylactic acid (PLA) based electrospun nanofibers with antimicrobial and wound healing application. *Int. J. Biol. Macromol.* **2021**, *172*, 143–153. [CrossRef]
16. Eriksson, E.; Liu, P.Y.; Schultz, G.S.; Martins-Green, M.M.; Tanaka, R.; Weir, D.; Gould, L.J.; Armstrong, D.G.; Gibbons, G.W.; Wolcott, R.; et al. Chronic wounds: Treatment consensus. *Wound Repair Regen.* **2022**, *30*, 156–171. [CrossRef]
17. Pan, H.; Fan, D.; Cao, W.; Zhu, C.; Duan, Z.; Fu, R.; Li, X.; Ma, X. Preparation and Characterization of Breathable Hemostatic Hydrogel Dressings and Determination of Their Effects on Full-Thickness Defects. *Polymers* **2017**, *9*, 727. [CrossRef]
18. Park, J.W.; Hwang, S.R.; Yoon, I.-S. Advanced Growth Factor Delivery Systems in Wound Management and Skin Regeneration. *Molecules* **2017**, *22*, 1259. [CrossRef]
19. Jimi, S.; Jaguparov, A.; Nurkesh, A.; Sultankulov, B.; Saparov, A. Sequential Delivery of Cryogel Released Growth Factors and Cytokines Accelerates Wound Healing and Improves Tissue Regeneration. *Front. Bioeng. Biotechnol.* **2020**, *8*, 345. [CrossRef]
20. Moeini, A.; Pedram, P.; Makvandi, P.; Malinconico, M.; Gomez d'Ayala, G. Wound healing and antimicrobial effect of active secondary metabolites in chitosan-based wound dressings: A review. *Carbohydr. Polym.* **2020**, *233*, 115839. [CrossRef]

21. Qu, J.; Zhao, X.; Liang, Y.; Zhang, T.; Ma, P.X.; Guo, B. Antibacterial adhesive injectable hydrogels with rapid self-healing, extensibility and compressibility as wound dressing for joints skin wound healing. *Biomaterials* **2018**, *183*, 185–199. [CrossRef] [PubMed]
22. Montaser, A.S.; Rehan, M.; El-Senousy, W.M.; Zaghloul, S. Designing strategy for coating cotton gauze fabrics and its application in wound healing. *Carbohydr. Polym.* **2020**, *244*, 116479. [CrossRef] [PubMed]
23. Mirmajidi, T.; Chogan, F.; Rezayan, A.H.; Sharifi, A.M. In vitro and in vivo evaluation of a nanofiber wound dressing loaded with melatonin. *Int. J. Pharm.* **2021**, *596*, 120213. [CrossRef] [PubMed]
24. Anjum, S.; Arora, A.; Alam, M.S.; Gupta, B. Development of antimicrobial and scar preventive chitosan hydrogel wound dressings. *Int. J. Pharm.* **2016**, *508*, 92–101. [CrossRef] [PubMed]
25. Zhang, M.; Yang, M.; Woo, M.W.; Li, Y.; Han, W.; Dang, X. High-mechanical strength carboxymethyl chitosan-based hydrogel film for antibacterial wound dressing. *Carbohydr. Polym.* **2021**, *256*, 117590. [CrossRef]
26. Porto, I.C.C.M. Polymer Biocompatibility. In *Polymerization*; Gomes, A.S., Ed.; IntechOpen: London, UK, 2012. [CrossRef]
27. Jeong, H.; Kim, T.; Earmme, T.; Hong, J. Acceleration of Nitric Oxide Release in Multilayer Nanofilms through Cu(II) Ion Intercalation for Antibacterial Applications. *Biomacromolecules* **2021**, *22*, 1312–1322. [CrossRef]
28. Contardi, M.; Kossyvaki, D.; Picone, P.; Summa, M.; Guo, X.; Heredia-Guerrero, J.A.; Giacomazza, D.; Carzino, R.; Goldoni, L.; Scoponi, G.; et al. Electrospun polyvinylpyrrolidone (PVP) hydrogels containing hydroxycinnamic acid derivatives as potential wound dressings. *Chem. Eng. J.* **2021**, *409*, 128144. [CrossRef]
29. Champeau, M.; Seabra, A.B.; de Oliveira, M.G. Hydrogels for Topical Nitric Oxide Delivery. In *Nitric Oxide Donors: Novel Biomedical Applications and Perspectives*; Seabra, A.B., Ed.; Elsevier: London, UK, 2017; pp. 313–330. [CrossRef]
30. Pal, A.; Bajpai, J.; Bajpai, A.K. Poly (acrylic acid) grafted gelatin nanocarriers as swelling controlled drug delivery system for optimized release of paclitaxel from modified gelatin. *J. Drug Deliv. Sci. Technol.* **2018**, *45*, 323–333. [CrossRef]
31. Gupta, A.; Briffa, S.M.; Swingler, S.; Gibson, H.; Kannappan, V.; Adamus, G.; Kowalczuk, M.; Martin, C.; Radecka, I. Synthesis of Silver Nanoparticles Using Curcumin-Cyclodextrins Loaded into Bacterial Cellulose-Based Hydrogels for Wound Dressing Applications. *Biomacromolecules* **2020**, *21*, 1802–1811. [CrossRef]
32. Ling, Z.; Chen, Z.; Deng, J.; Wang, Y.; Yuan, B.; Yang, X.; Lin, H.; Cao, J.; Zhu, X.; Zhang, X. A novel self-healing polydopamine-functionalized chitosan-arginine hydrogel with enhanced angiogenic and antibacterial activities for accelerating skin wound healing. *Chem. Eng. J.* **2021**, *420*, 130302. [CrossRef]
33. Hoang Thi, T.T.; Pilkington, E.H.; Nguyen, D.H.; Lee, J.S.; Park, K.D.; Truong, N.P. The Importance of Poly(ethylene glycol) Alternatives for Overcoming PEG Immunogenicity in Drug Delivery and Bioconjugation. *Polymers* **2020**, *12*, 298. [CrossRef]
34. Pelegrino, M.T.; Lima, B.D.; do Nascimento, M.H.M.; Lombello, C.B.; Brocchi, M.; Seabra, A.B. Biocompatible and Antibacterial Nitric Oxide-Releasing Pluronic F-127/Chitosan Hydrogel for Topical Applications. *Polymers* **2018**, *10*, 452. [CrossRef]
35. Wei, Q.Y.; Xu, Y.M.; Lau, A.T.Y. Recent progress of nanocarrier-based therapy for solid malignancies. *Cancers* **2020**, *12*, 2783. [CrossRef]
36. Zheng, Z.; Bian, S.; Li, Z.; Zhang, Z.; Liu, Y.; Zhai, X.; Pan, H.; Zhao, X. Catechol modified quaternized chitosan enhanced wet adhesive and antibacterial properties of injectable thermo-sensitive hydrogel for wound healing. *Carbohydr. Polym.* **2020**, *249*, 116826. [CrossRef]
37. Drury, J.L.; Mooney, D.J. Hydrogels for tissue engineering: Scaffold design variables and applications. *Biomaterials* **2003**, *24*, 4337–4351. [CrossRef]
38. Han, W.; Zhou, B.; Yang, K.; Xiong, X.; Luan, S.; Wang, Y.; Xu, Z.; Lei, P.; Luo, Z.; Gao, J.; et al. Biofilm-inspired adhesive and antibacterial hydrogel with tough tissue integration performance for sealing hemostasis and wound healing. *Bioact. Mater.* **2020**, *5*, 768–778. [CrossRef]
39. Lourenco, S.D.; de Oliveira, M.G. Topical photochemical nitric oxide release from porous poly(vinyl alcohol) membrane for visible light modulation of dermal vasodilation. *J. Photochem. Photobiol. A Chem.* **2017**, *346*, 548–558. [CrossRef]
40. Lee, J.; Hlaing, S.P.; Cao, J.F.; Hasan, N.; Ahn, H.J.; Song, K.W.; Yoo, J.W. In Situ Hydrogel-Forming/Nitric Oxide-Releasing Wound Dressing for Enhanced Antibacterial Activity and Healing in Mice with Infected Wounds. *Pharmaceutics* **2019**, *11*, 496. [CrossRef]
41. Yang, Y.; Zhou, Y.T.; Li, Y.L.; Guo, L.Y.; Zhou, J.; Chen, J.H. Injectable and self-healing hydrogel containing nitric oxide donor for enhanced antibacterial activity. *React. Funct. Polym.* **2021**, *166*, 10. [CrossRef]
42. Liu, H.L.; Zhu, X.L.; Guo, H.M.; Huang, H.L.; Huang, S.H.; Huang, S.S.; Xue, W.; Zhu, P.; Guo, R. Nitric oxide released injectable hydrogel combined with synergistic photothermal therapy for antibacterial and accelerated wound healing. *Appl. Mater. Today* **2020**, *20*, 12. [CrossRef]
43. Joseph, C.A.; McCarthy, C.W.; Tyo, A.G.; Hubbard, K.R.; Fisher, H.C.; Altscheffel, J.A.; He, W.L.; Pinnaratip, R.; Liu, Y.; Lee, B.P.; et al. Development of an Injectable Nitric Oxide Releasing Poly(ethylene) Glycol-Fibrin Adhesive Hydrogel. *ACS Biomater. Sci. Eng.* **2019**, *5*, 959–969. [CrossRef]
44. Friedman, A.J.; Han, G.; Navati, M.S.; Chacko, M.; Gunther, L.; Alfieri, A.; Friedman, J.M. Sustained release nitric oxide releasing nanoparticles: Characterization of a novel delivery platform based on nitrite containing hydrogel/glass composites. *Nitric Oxide* **2008**, *19*, 12–20. [CrossRef]
45. Miao, H.; Hao, W.; Liu, H.; Liu, Y.; Fu, X.; Huang, H.; Ge, M.; Qian, Y. Highly Flexibility, Powder Self-Healing, and Recyclable Natural Polymer Hydrogels. *Gels* **2022**, *8*, 89. [CrossRef]

46. Kim, J.O.; Noh, J.K.; Thapa, R.K.; Hasan, N.; Choi, M.; Kim, J.H.; Lee, J.H.; Ku, S.K.; Yoo, J.W. Nitric oxide-releasing chitosan film for enhanced antibacterial and in vivo wound-healing efficacy. *Int. J. Biol. Macromol.* **2015**, *79*, 217–225. [CrossRef]
47. Wo, Y.; Brisbois, E.J.; Bartlett, R.H.; Meyerhoff, M.E. Recent advances in thromboresistant and antimicrobial polymers for biomedical applications: Just say yes to nitric oxide (NO). *Biomater. Sci.* **2016**, *4*, 1161–1183. [CrossRef]
48. Fontana, K.; Mutus, B. Nitric Oxide-Donating Devices for Topical Applications. In *Nitric Oxide Donors: Novel Biomedical Applications and Perspectives*; Seabra, A.B., Ed.; Elsevier: London, UK, 2017; pp. 55–74. [CrossRef]
49. Yang, C.; Jeong, S.; Ku, S.; Lee, K.; Park, M.H. Use of gasotransmitters for the controlled release of polymer-based nitric oxide carriers in medical applications. *J. Control. Release* **2018**, *279*, 157–170. [CrossRef]
50. Rong, F.; Tang, Y.; Wang, T.; Feng, T.; Song, J.; Li, P.; Huang, W. Nitric oxide-releasing polymeric materials for antimicrobial applications: A review. *Antioxidants* **2019**, *8*, 556. [CrossRef]
51. Malone-Povolny, M.J.; Maloney, S.E.; Schoenfisch, M.H. Nitric Oxide Therapy for Diabetic Wound Healing. *Adv. Healthc. Mater.* **2019**, *8*, e1801210. [CrossRef]
52. Zaja-Milatovic, S.; Gupta, R.C. *Handbook of Toxicology of Chemical Warfare Agents*, 2nd ed.; Academic Press: Cambridge, MA, USA, 2015. [CrossRef]
53. Rouillard, K.R.; Novak, O.P.; Pistiolis, A.M.; Yang, L.; Ahonen, M.J.R.; McDonald, R.A.; Schoenfisch, M.H. Exogenous Nitric Oxide Improves Antibiotic Susceptibility in Resistant Bacteria. *ACS Infect. Dis.* **2021**, *7*, 23–33. [CrossRef]
54. Hetrick, E.M.; Shin, J.H.; Stasko, N.A.; Johnson, C.B.; Wespe, D.A.; Holmuhamedov, E.; Schoenfisch, M.H. Bactericidal Efficacy of Nitric Oxide-Releasing Silica Nanoparticles. *ACS Nano* **2008**, *2*, 235–246. [CrossRef]
55. Puca, V.; Marulli, R.Z.; Grande, R.; Vitale, I.; Niro, A.; Molinaro, G.; Prezioso, S.; Muraro, R.; Di Giovanni, P. Microbial Species Isolated from Infected Wounds and Antimicrobial Resistance Analysis: Data Emerging from a Three-Years Retrospective Study. *Antibiotics* **2021**, *10*, 1162. [CrossRef] [PubMed]
56. Nguyen, T.-K.; Selvanayagam, R.; Ho, K.K.K.; Chen, R.; Kutty, S.K.; Rice, S.A.; Kumar, N.; Barraud, N.; Duong, H.T.T.; Boyer, C. Co-delivery of nitric oxide and antibiotic using polymeric nanoparticles. *Chem. Sci.* **2016**, *7*, 1016–1027. [CrossRef] [PubMed]
57. Ravikumar, G.; Chakrapani, H. Synergistic activities of Nitric Oxide and Various Drugs. In *Nitric Oxide Donors: Novel Biomedical Applications and Perspectives*; Seabra, A.B., Ed.; Elseivier: London, UK, 2017; pp. 293–312. [CrossRef]
58. Yang, L.; Feura, E.S.; Ahonen, M.J.R.; Schoenfisch, M.H. Nitric Oxide–Releasing Macromolecular Scaffolds for Antibacterial Applications. *Adv. Healthc. Mater.* **2018**, *7*, 1800155. [CrossRef] [PubMed]
59. Maillard, J.-Y.; Kampf, G.; Cooper, R. Antimicrobial stewardship of antiseptics that are pertinent to wounds: The need for a united approach. *JAC-Antimicrob. Resist.* **2021**, *3*, dlab027. [CrossRef]
60. Castro, J.; Lima, Â.; Sousa, L.G.V.; Rosca, A.S.; Muzny, C.A.; Cerca, N. Crystal Violet Staining Alone Is Not Adequate to Assess Synergism or Antagonism in Multi-Species Biofilms of Bacteria Associated With Bacterial Vaginosis. *Front. Cell. Infect. Microbiol.* **2022**, *11*, 1375. [CrossRef]
61. Vazquez, N.M.; Mariani, F.; Torres, P.S.; Moreno, S.; Galván, E.M. Cell death and biomass reduction in biofilms of multidrug resistant extended spectrum β-lactamase-producing uropathogenic Escherichia coli isolates by 1,8-cineole. *PLoS ONE* **2020**, *15*, e0241978. [CrossRef]
62. Junka, A.F.; Żywicka, A.; Szymczyk, P.; Dziadas, M.; Bartoszewicz, M.; Fijałkowski, K. A.D.A.M. test (Antibiofilm Dressing's Activity Measurement)—Simple method for evaluating anti-biofilm activity of drug-saturated dressings against wound pathogens. *J. Microbiol. Methods* **2017**, *143*, 6–12. [CrossRef]
63. Wan, X.Z.; Liu, S.; Xin, X.X.; Li, P.F.; Dou, J.; Han, X.; Kang, I.K.; Yuan, J.; Chi, B.; Shen, J. S-nitrosated keratin composite mats with NO release capacity for wound healing. *Chem. Eng. J.* **2020**, *400*, 10. [CrossRef]
64. Baldim, V.; de Oliveira, M.G. Poly-epsilon-caprolactone/polysulfhydrylated polyester blend: A platform for topical and degradable nitric oxide-releasing materials. *Eur. Polym. J.* **2018**, *109*, 143–152. [CrossRef]
65. Nie, Y.; Zhang, K.; Zhang, S.Q.; Wang, D.; Han, Z.; Che, Y.; Kong, D.; Zhao, Q.; Han, Z.; He, Z.-X.; et al. Nitric oxide releasing hydrogel promotes endothelial differentiation of mouse embryonic stem cells. *Acta Biomater.* **2017**, *63*, 190–199. [CrossRef]
66. Yang, S.; Zheng, X.; Qian, M.; Wang, H.; Wang, F.; Wei, Y.; Midgley, A.C.; He, J.; Tian, H.; Zhao, Q. Nitrate-Functionalized poly(ε-Caprolactone) Small-Diameter Vascular Grafts Enhance Vascular Regeneration via Sustained Release of Nitric Oxide. *Front. Bioeng. Biotechnol.* **2021**, *9*, 770121. [CrossRef]
67. Napoli, C.; Paolisso, G.; Casamassimi, A.; Al-Omran, M.; Barbieri, M.; Sommese, L.; Infante, T.; Ignarro, L.J. Effects of Nitric Oxide on Cell Proliferation: Novel Insights. *J. Am. Coll. Cardiol.* **2013**, *62*, 89–95. [CrossRef]
68. Wu, Y.; Liang, T.Z.; Hu, Y.; Jiang, S.A.; Luo, Y.S.; Liu, C.; Wang, G.; Zhang, J.; Xu, T.; Zhu, L. 3D bioprinting of integral ADSCs-NO hydrogel scaffolds to promote severe burn wound healing. *Regen. Biomater.* **2021**, *8*, rbab014. [CrossRef]
69. Ramadass, S.K.; Nazir, L.S.; Thangam, R.; Perumal, R.K.; Manjubala, I.; Madhan, B.; Seetharaman, S. Type I collagen peptides and nitric oxide releasing electrospun silk fibroin scaffold: A multifunctional approach for the treatment of ischemic chronic wounds. *Colloids Surf. B Biointerfaces* **2019**, *175*, 636–643. [CrossRef]
70. Frost, M.C. Improving the Performance of Implantable Sensors with Nitric Oxide Release. In *Nitric Oxide Donors: Novel Biomedical Applications and Perspectives*; Seabra, A.B., Ed.; Elseivier: London, UK, 2017; pp. 191–220. [CrossRef]
71. Zhang, C.; Biggs, T.D.; Devarie-Baez, N.O.; Shuang, S.; Dong, C.; Xian, M. S-Nitrosothiols: Chemistry and reactions. *Chem. Commun.* **2017**, *53*, 11266–11277. [CrossRef]

72. Marazzi, M.; López-Delgado, A.; Fernández-González, M.A.; Castaño, O.; Frutos, L.M.; Temprado, M. Modulating nitric oxide release by S-nitrosothiol photocleavage: Mechanism and substituent effects. *J. Phys. Chem. A* **2012**, *116*, 7039–7049. [CrossRef]
73. Singh, R.J.; Hogg, N.; Joseph, J.; Kalyanaraman, B. Mechanism of nitric oxide release from S-nitrosothiols. *J. Biol. Chem.* **1996**, *271*, 18596–18603. [CrossRef]
74. de Oliveira, M.G. S-Nitrosothiols as Platforms for Topical Nitric Oxide Delivery. *Basic Clin. Pharmacol. Toxicol.* **2016**, *119*, 49–56. [CrossRef]
75. Gur, S.; Chen, A.L.; Kadowitz, P.J. Nitric Oxide Donors and Penile Erectile Function. In *Nitric Oxide Donors: Novel Biomedical Applications and Perspectives*; Seabra, A.B., Ed.; Elseivier: London, UK, 2017; pp. 121–140. [CrossRef]
76. Aveyard, J.; Deller, R.C.; Lace, R.; Williams, R.L.; Kaye, S.B.; Kolegraff, K.N.; Curran, J.M.; D'Sa, R.A. Antimicrobial Nitric Oxide Releasing Contact Lens Gels for the Treatment of Microbial Keratitis. *ACS Appl. Mater. Interfaces* **2019**, *11*, 37491–37501. [CrossRef]
77. Kim, J.; Lee, Y.; Singha, K.; Kim, H.W.; Shin, J.H.; Jo, S.; Han, D.K.; Kim, W.J. NONOates-Polyethylenimine Hydrogel for Controlled Nitric Oxide Release and Cell Proliferation Modulation. *Bioconjugate Chem.* **2011**, *22*, 1031–1038. [CrossRef]
78. Kashfi, K.; Duvalsaint, P.L. Nitric Oxide Donors and Therapeutic Applications in Cancer. In *Nitric Oxide Donors: Novel Biomedical Applications and Perspectives*; Seabra, A.B., Ed.; Elseivier: London, UK, 2017; pp. 75–120. [CrossRef]
79. Fu, J.; Han, J.; Meng, T.; Hu, J.; Yin, J. Novel α-ketoamide based diazeniumdiolates as hydrogen peroxide responsive nitric oxide donors with anti-lung cancer activity. *Chem. Commun.* **2019**, *55*, 12904–12907. [CrossRef]
80. Hasan, N.; Lee, J.; Kwak, D.; Kim, H.; Saparbayeva, A.; Ahn, H.J.; Yoon, I.S.; Kim, M.S.; Jung, Y.; Yoo, J.W. Diethylenetriamine/NONOate-doped alginate hydrogel with sustained nitric oxide release and minimal toxicity to accelerate healing of MRSA-infected wounds. *Carbohydr. Polym.* **2021**, *270*, 118387. [CrossRef]
81. Keefer, L.K. Nitric oxide (NO)- and nitroxyl (HNO)-generating diazeniumdiolates (NONOates): Emerging commercial opportunities. *Curr. Top. Med. Chem.* **2005**, *5*, 625–636. [CrossRef]
82. Halpenny, G.M.; Steinhardt, R.C.; Okialda, K.A.; Mascharak, P.K. Characterization of pHEMA-based hydrogels that exhibit light-induced bactericidal effect via release of NO. *J. Mater. Sci.-Mater. Med.* **2009**, *20*, 2353–2360. [CrossRef]
83. Dave, R.N.; Joshi, H.M.; Venugopalan, V.P. Biomedical evaluation of a novel nitrogen oxides releasing wound dressing. *J. Mater. Sci.-Mater. Med.* **2012**, *23*, 3097–3106. [CrossRef]
84. Shishido, S.M.; Seabra, A.B.; Loh, W.; De Oliveira, M.G. Thermal and photochemical nitric oxide release from S-nitrosothiols incorporated in Pluronic F127 gel: Potential uses for local and controlled nitric oxide release. *Biomaterials* **2003**, *24*, 3543–3553. [CrossRef]
85. Pelegrino, M.T.; de Araújo, D.R.; Seabra, A.B. S-nitrosoglutathione-containing chitosan nanoparticles dispersed in Pluronic F-127 hydrogel: Potential uses in topical applications. *J. Drug Deliv. Sci. Technol.* **2018**, *43*, 211–220. [CrossRef]
86. Wo, Y.; Li, Z.; Colletta, A.; Wu, J.; Xi, C.; Matzger, A.J.; Brisbois, E.J.; Bartlett, R.H.; Meyerhoff, M.E. Study of crystal formation and nitric oxide (NO) release mechanism from S-nitroso-N-acetylpenicillamine (SNAP)-doped CarboSil polymer composites for potential antimicrobial applications. *Compos. Part B Eng.* **2017**, *121*, 23–33. [CrossRef]
87. Namivandi-Zangeneh, R.; Sadrearhami, Z.; Bagheri, A.; Sauvage-Nguyen, M.; Ho, K.K.K.; Kumar, N.; Wong, E.H.H.; Boyer, C. Nitric Oxide-Loaded Antimicrobial Polymer for the Synergistic Eradication of Bacterial Biofilm. *ACS Macro Lett.* **2018**, *7*, 592–597. [CrossRef]
88. Kamaruzzaman, N.F.; Tan, L.P.; Hamdan, R.H.; Choong, S.S.; Wong, W.K.; Gibson, A.J.; Chivu, A.; Pina, M.d.F. Antimicrobial Polymers: The Potential Replacement of Existing Antibiotics? *Int. J. Mol. Sci.* **2019**, *20*, 2747. [CrossRef]
89. Nguyen, T.-K.; Lam, S.J.; Ho, K.K.K.; Kumar, N.; Qiao, G.G.; Egan, S.; Boyer, C.; Wong, E.H.H. Rational Design of Single-Chain Polymeric Nanoparticles That Kill Planktonic and Biofilm Bacteria. *ACS Infect. Dis.* **2017**, *3*, 237–248. [CrossRef]
90. Yu, Y.T.; Shi, S.W.; Wang, Y.; Zhang, Q.L.; Gao, S.H.; Yang, S.P.; Liu, J.G. A Ruthenium Nitrosyl-Functionalized Magnetic Nanoplatform with Near-Infrared Light-Controlled Nitric Oxide Delivery and Photothermal Effect for Enhanced Antitumor and Antibacterial Therapy. *ACS Appl. Mater. Interfaces* **2020**, *12*, 312–321. [CrossRef]
91. Kandoth, N.; Mosinger, J.; Gref, R.; Sortino, S. A NO photoreleasing supramolecular hydrogel with bactericidal action. *J. Mater. Chem. B* **2013**, *1*, 3458–3463. [CrossRef]
92. VanWagner, M.; Rhadigan, J.; Lancina, M.; Lebovsky, A.; Romanowicz, G.; Holmes, H.; Brunette, M.A.; Snyder, K.L.; Bostwick, M.; Lee, B.P.; et al. S-Nitroso-N-acetylpenicillamine (SNAP) Derivatization of Peptide Primary Amines to Create Inducible Nitric Oxide Donor Biomaterials. *ACS Appl. Mater. Interfaces* **2013**, *5*, 8430–8439. [CrossRef]
93. Mohamed, N.A.; Ahmetaj-Shala, B.; Duluc, L.; Mackenzie, L.S.; Kirkby, N.S.; Reed, D.M.; Lickiss, P.D.; Davies, R.P.; Freeman, G.R.; Wojciak-Stothard, B.; et al. A New NO-Releasing Nanoformulation for the Treatment of Pulmonary Arterial Hypertension. *J. Cardiovasc. Transl. Res.* **2016**, *9*, 162–164. [CrossRef]
94. Yao, X.P.; Liu, Y.; Gao, J.; Yang, L.; Mao, D.; Stefanitsch, C.; Li, Y.; Zhang, J.; Ou, L.L.; Kong, D.L.; et al. Nitric oxide releasing hydrogel enhances the therapeutic efficacy of mesenchymal stem cells for myocardial infarction. *Biomaterials* **2015**, *60*, 130–140. [CrossRef]
95. Xing, Q.; Yates, K.; Bailey, A.; Vogt, C.; He, W.L.; Frost, M.C.; Zhao, F. Effects of local nitric oxide release on human mesenchymal stem cell attachment and proliferation on gelatin hydrogel surface. *Surf. Innov.* **2013**, *1*, 224–232. [CrossRef]
96. Zhang, J.M.; Deng, M.G.; Shi, X.G.; Zhang, C.N.; Qu, X.W.; Hu, X.L.; Wang, W.W.; Kong, D.L.; Huang, P.S. Cascaded amplification of intracellular oxidative stress and reversion of multidrug resistance by nitric oxide prodrug based-supramolecular hydrogel for synergistic cancer chemotherapy. *Bioact. Mater.* **2021**, *6*, 3300–3313. [CrossRef]

97. Kandoth, N.; Malanga, M.; Fraix, A.; Jicsinszky, L.; Fenyvesi, É.; Parisi, T.; Colao, I.; Sciortino, M.T.; Sortino, S. A host-guest supramolecular complex with photoregulated delivery of nitric oxide and fluorescence imaging capacity in cancer cells. *Chem.-Asian J.* **2012**, *7*, 2888–2894. [CrossRef]
98. Sung, Y.-C.; Jin, P.-R.; Chu, L.-A.; Hsu, F.-F.; Wang, M.-R.; Chang, C.-C.; Chiou, S.-J.; Qiu, J.T.; Gao, D.-Y.; Lin, C.-C.; et al. Delivery of nitric oxide with a nanocarrier promotes tumour vessel normalization and potentiates anti-cancer therapies. *Nat. Nanotechnol.* **2019**, *14*, 1160–1169. [CrossRef]
99. Mintz, J.; Vedenko, A.; Rosete, O.; Shah, K.; Goldstein, G.; Hare, J.M.; Ramasamy, R.; Arora, H. Current Advances of Nitric Oxide in Cancer and Anticancer Therapeutics. *Vaccines* **2021**, *9*, 94. [CrossRef]
100. Holmes, A.J. The Role of L-Ascorbic Acid in S-Nitrosothiol Decomposition and Aspects of the Nitrosation of Thiones. Ph.D. Thesis, Durham University, Durham, UK, 2000.
101. Huang, S.S.; Liu, H.L.; Liao, K.D.; Hu, Q.Q.; Guo, R.; Deng, K.X. Functionalized GO Nanovehicles with Nitric Oxide Release and Photothermal Activity-Based Hydrogels for Bacteria-Infected Wound Healing. *ACS Appl. Mater. Interfaces* **2020**, *12*, 28952–28964. [CrossRef]
102. Zahid, A.A.; Augustine, R.; Dalvi, Y.B.; Reshma, K.; Ahmed, R.; Rehman, S.R.U.; Marei, H.E.; Alfkey, R.; Hasan, A. Development of nitric oxide releasing visible light crosslinked gelatin methacrylate hydrogel for rapid closure of diabetic wounds. *Biomed. Pharmacother.* **2021**, *140*, 111747. [CrossRef]
103. Champeau, M.; Povoa, V.; Militao, L.; Cabrini, F.M.; Picheth, G.F.; Meneau, F.; Jara, C.P.; de Araujo, E.P.; de Oliveira, M.G. Supramolecular poly(acrylic acid)/F127 hydrogel with hydration-controlled nitric oxide release for enhancing wound healing. *Acta Biomater.* **2018**, *74*, 312–325. [CrossRef]
104. Vercelino, R.; Cunha, T.M.; Ferreira, E.S.; Cunha, F.Q.; Ferreira, S.H.; de Oliveira, M.G. Skin vasodilation and analgesic effect of a topical nitric oxide-releasing hydrogel. *J. Mater. Sci.-Mater. Med.* **2013**, *24*, 2157–2169. [CrossRef]
105. Georgii, J.L.; Amadeu, T.P.; Seabra, A.B.; de Oliveira, M.G.; Monte-Alto-Costa, A. Topical S-nitrosoglutathione-releasing hydrogel improves healing of rat ischaemic wounds. *J. Tissue Eng. Regen. Med.* **2011**, *5*, 612–619. [CrossRef]
106. Amadeu, T.P.; Seabra, A.B.; de Oliveira, M.G.; Costa, A.M.A. S-nitrosoglutathione-containing hydrogel accelerates rat cutaneous wound repair. *J. Eur. Acad. Dermatol. Venereol.* **2007**, *21*, 629–637. [CrossRef]
107. Amadeu, T.P.; Seabra, A.B.; de Oliveira, M.G.; Monte-Alto-Costa, A. Nitric oxide donor improves healing if applied on inflammatory and proliferative phase. *J. Surg. Res.* **2008**, *149*, 84–93. [CrossRef]
108. Seabra, A.B.; Fitzpatrick, A.; Paul, J.; De Oliveira, M.G.; Weller, R. Topically applied S-nitrosothiol-containing hydrogels as experimental and pharmacological nitric oxide donors in human skin. *Br. J. Dermatol.* **2004**, *151*, 977–983. [CrossRef]
109. Seabra, A.B.; Pankotai, E.; Feher, M.; Somlai, A.; Kiss, L.; Biro, L.; Szabo, C.; Kollai, M.; de Oliveira, M.G.; Lacza, Z. S-nitrosoglutathione-containing hydrogel increases dermal blood flow in streptozotocin-induced diabetic rats. *Br. J. Dermatol.* **2007**, *156*, 814–818. [CrossRef]
110. Cao, J.F.; Su, M.Z.; Hasan, N.; Lee, J.; Kwak, D.; Kim, D.Y.; Kim, K.; Lee, E.H.; Jung, J.H.; Yoo, J.W. Nitric Oxide-Releasing Thermoresponsive Pluronic F127/Alginate Hydrogel for Enhanced Antibacterial Activity and Accelerated Healing of Infected Wounds. *Pharmaceutics* **2020**, *12*, 926. [CrossRef]
111. Parisi, C.; Seggio, M.; Fraix, A.; Sortino, S. A High-Performing Metal-Free Photoactivatable Nitric Oxide Donor with a Green Fluorescent Reporter. *ChemPhotoChem* **2020**, *4*, 742–748. [CrossRef]
112. Urzedo, A.L.; Goncalves, M.C.; Nascimento, M.H.M.; Lombello, C.B.; Nakazato, G.; Seabra, A.B. Cytotoxicity and Antibacterial Activity of Alginate Hydrogel Containing Nitric Oxide Donor and Silver Nanoparticles for Topical Applications. *ACS Biomater. Sci. Eng.* **2020**, *6*, 2117–2134. [CrossRef] [PubMed]
113. Hasan, S.; Thomas, N.; Thierry, B.; Prestidge, C.A. Controlled and Localized Nitric Oxide Precursor Delivery From Chitosan Gels to Staphylococcus aureus Biofilms. *J. Pharm. Sci.* **2017**, *106*, 3556–3563. [CrossRef]
114. Zahid, A.A.; Ahmed, R.; Rehman, S.R.U.; Augustine, R.; Tariq, M.; Hasan, A. Nitric oxide releasing chitosan-poly (vinyl alcohol) hydrogel promotes angiogenesis in chick embryo model. *Int. J. Biol. Macromol.* **2019**, *136*, 901–910. [CrossRef]
115. Najafi, H.; Abolmaali, S.S.; Heidari, R.; Valizadeh, H.; Jafari, M.; Tamaddon, A.M.; Azarpira, N. Nitric oxide releasing nanofibrous Fmoc-dipeptide hydrogels for amelioration of renal ischemia/reperfusion injury. *J. Control. Release* **2021**, *337*, 1–13. [CrossRef]
116. Fraix, A.; Gref, R.; Sortino, S. A multi-photoresponsive supramolecular hydrogel with dual-color fluorescence and dual-modal photodynamic action. *J. Mat. Chem. B* **2014**, *2*, 3443–3449. [CrossRef]
117. Fraix, A.; Kandoth, N.; Gref, R.; Sortino, S. A Multicomponent Gel for Nitric Oxide Photorelease with Fluorescence Reporting. *Asian J. Org. Chem.* **2015**, *4*, 256–261. [CrossRef]
118. Gutierrez Cisneros, C.; Bloemen, V.; Mignon, A. Synthetic, Natural, and Semisynthetic Polymer Carriers for Controlled Nitric Oxide Release in Dermal Applications: A Review. *Polymers* **2021**, *13*, 760. [CrossRef]
119. Chen, G.Q.; Li, J.L.; Song, M.C.; Wu, Z.Y.; Zhang, W.Z.; Wang, Z.Y.; Gao, J.; Yang, Z.M.; Ou, C.W. A Mixed Component Supramolecular Hydrogel to Improve Mice Cardiac Function and Alleviate Ventricular Remodeling after Acute Myocardial Infarction. *Adv. Funct. Mater.* **2017**, *27*, 1701798. [CrossRef]
120. Bruschi, M.L. Mathematical models of drug release. In *Strategies to Modify the Drug Release from Pharmaceutical Systems*; Bruschi, M.L., Ed.; Woodhead Publishing: Sawston, UK, 2015; pp. 63–86. [CrossRef]
121. Fu, K.; Wu, H.; Su, Z. Self-assembling peptide-based hydrogels: Fabrication, properties, and applications. *Biotechnol. Adv.* **2021**, *49*, 107752. [CrossRef] [PubMed]

122. Halpenny, G.M.; Olmstead, M.M.; Mascharak, P.K. Incorporation of a designed ruthenium nitrosyl in PolyHEMA hydrogel and light-activated delivery of NO to myoglobin. *Inorg. Chem.* **2007**, *46*, 6601–6606. [CrossRef] [PubMed]
123. Masters, K.S.B.; Leibovich, S.J.; Belem, P.; West, J.L.; Poole-Warren, L.A. Effects of nitric oxide releasing poly(vinyl alcohol) hydrogel dressings on dermal wound healing in diabetic mice. *Wound Repair Regen.* **2002**, *10*, 286–294. [CrossRef] [PubMed]
124. Picheth, G.F.; da Silva, L.C.E.; Giglio, L.P.; Plivelic, T.S.; de Oliveira, M.G. S-nitrosothiol-terminated Pluronic F127: Influence of microstructure on nitric oxide release. *J. Colloid Interface Sci.* **2020**, *576*, 457–467. [CrossRef]
125. Kang, Y.; Kim, J.; Lee, Y.M.; Im, S.; Park, H.; Kim, W.J. Nitric oxide-releasing polymer incorporated ointment for cutaneous wound healing. *J. Control. Release* **2015**, *220*, 624–630. [CrossRef]
126. Zhang, K.Y.; Chen, X.N.; Li, H.F.; Feng, G.W.; Nie, Y.; Wei, Y.Z.; Li, N.N.; Han, Z.B.; Han, Z.C.; Kong, D.L.; et al. A nitric oxide-releasing hydrogel for enhancing the therapeutic effects of mesenchymal stem cell therapy for hindlimb ischemia. *Acta Biomater.* **2020**, *113*, 289–304. [CrossRef]
127. Zhao, Q.; Zhang, J.M.; Song, L.J.; Ji, Q.; Yao, Y.; Cui, Y.; Shen, J.; Wang, P.G.; Kong, D.L. Polysaccharide-based biomaterials with on-demand nitric oxide releasing property regulated by enzyme catalysis. *Biomaterials* **2013**, *34*, 8450–8458. [CrossRef]
128. Durao, J.; Vale, N.; Gomes, S.; Gomes, P.; Barrias, C.C.; Gales, L. Nitric Oxide Release from Antimicrobial Peptide Hydrogels for Wound Healing. *Biomolecules* **2019**, *9*, 4. [CrossRef]
129. Park, K.; Dawson, J.I.; Oreffo, R.O.C.; Kim, Y.H.; Hong, J. Nanoclay-Polyamine Composite Hydrogel for Topical Delivery of Nitric Oxide Gas via Innate Gelation Characteristics of Laponite. *Biomacromolecules* **2020**, *21*, 2096–2103. [CrossRef]
130. Masters, K.S.B.; Lipke, E.A.; Rice, E.E.H.; Liel, M.S.; Myler, H.A.; Zygourakis, C.; Tulis, D.A.; West, J.L. Nitric oxide-generating hydrogels inhibit neointima formation. *J. Biomater. Sci.-Polym. Ed.* **2005**, *16*, 659–672. [CrossRef]
131. Deng, Y.; Chen, G.Q.; Ye, M.; He, Y.Y.; Li, Z.H.; Wang, X.B.; Ou, C.W.; Yang, Z.M.; Chen, M.S. Bifunctional Supramolecular Hydrogel Alleviates Myocardial Ischemia/Reperfusion Injury by Inhibiting Autophagy and Apoptosis. *J. Biomed. Nanotechnol.* **2018**, *14*, 1458–1470. [CrossRef]
132. Nacharaju, P.; Tuckman-Vernon, C.; Maier, K.E.; Chouake, J.; Friedman, A.; Cabrales, P.; Friedman, J.M. A nanoparticle delivery vehicle for S-nitroso-N-acetyl cysteine: Sustained vascular response. *Nitric Oxide-Biol. Chem.* **2012**, *27*, 150–160. [CrossRef]
133. Schanuel, F.S.; Santos, K.S.R.; Monte-Alto-Costa, A.; de Oliveira, M.G. Combined nitric oxide-releasing poly(vinyl alcohol) film/F127 hydrogel for accelerating wound healing. *Colloid Surf. B-Biointerfaces* **2015**, *130*, 182–191. [CrossRef]
134. Breijyeh, Z.; Jubeh, B.; Karaman, R. Resistance of Gram-Negative Bacteria to Current Antibacterial Agents and Approaches to Resolve It. *Molecules* **2020**, *25*, 1340. [CrossRef]

MDPI
St. Alban-Anlage 66
4052 Basel
Switzerland
Tel. +41 61 683 77 34
Fax +41 61 302 89 18
www.mdpi.com

Pharmaceutics Editorial Office
E-mail: pharmaceutics@mdpi.com
www.mdpi.com/journal/pharmaceutics

www.ingramcontent.com/pod-product-compliance
Lightning Source LLC
LaVergne TN
LVHW070454100526
838202LV00014B/1719